MASS MURDERING DOCTORS: THE TRUTH ABOUT ONCOLOGISTS, CHEMOTHERAPY AND CANCER

How Corrupt, Greedy "Doctors" The MHRA/FDA And Big Pharma Tried To Murder Me With The Lie That Is Chemotherapy And Obstruct My Cure.

By Teri Davis Newman

MASS MURDERING DOCTORS: THE TRUTH ABOUT ONCOLOGISTS, CHEMOTHERAPY AND CANCER

ACKNOWLEDGMENTS

First, I want to thank Dr. Yamamoto, First Immune and David Noakes. Without them, I would be dead from the cancer that killed my sister and tried to kill me. I owe Dr. Yamamoto and David Noakes (who owns First Immune) my life and we have made medical history as I am the ONLY known survivor of Peritoneal Carcinomatosis of the Pelvis originating as High-Grade Serous-cell Carcinoma of the Ovary & Uterus. I owe them my life and my cure which enabled the book you're about to read.

Second, I want to give my heartfelt thanks to my doctor of 11 years, Janet Alvarado, MD who is the best doctor in America. While she wasn't a believer in the beginning, she trusted my judgment and made sure that I had the correct medications requested by First Immune to make sure the GcMAF/Goleic worked and saved my life. She was there for me at every turn and made sure I had everything I needed to keep my pain managed and to fight for my life rather than writing me off as a dead woman walking. She was my doctor for 10 years before the cancer struck and will be my doctor until she retires. I owe her my life as well; as I could not have done this without her help.

Third, I am grateful to all of the authors of the technical papers I've included for reference purposes. They were invaluable to me in sharing the correct cancer information with my readers and are what enabled me to find GcMAF/Goleic, but it was Dr. Dan O'Connell, DDS a dentist friend of mine in Illinois who sent me the first article that mentioned the miracle of GcMAF/Goleic which saved my life.

To my friends and family who encouraged and prayed for me and listened to my frantic phone calls and terrified moments when I was afraid I would be joining my sister because my cancer was deemed incurable and there were NO known survivors. Kim, Dad, Mom, Elke, Gerilyn, Tammy, Keith, Justin, Kristen, Cody, Carliegh, Lindsay, JoAnn, Dave W, Guido, Charlie, Betty, Joan, Liz, Jane, Ginny, Brandy, Karen, Lanette, John C, and my beloved super-brave sister Sarah—thank you! I love you all and your love and support meant more to me than I can ever say.

Saving the best for last, my beloved and **AMAZING** husband, John. He risked his job, his career, his Top Secret security clearance, large fines and prison to help save my life. When the corrupt scumbags at the FDA grabbed my GcMAF/Goleic because it was "unapproved" my husband smuggled the medicine into the country for me at huge personal risk. I would not have survived if it hadn't been for him; I owe him my life because of it. Thank you for everything you did for me babe. You have ice-water in your veins and the nerves of a steely-eyed assassin; I love you more than anything!

INTRODUCTION: OVARIAN CANCER: A DEADLY ADVERSARY

"You are BRCA1 positive."

Those words spoken by my doctor sent a cold chill through me. In 3 seconds I went from being a career oriented political and management consultant with a great business, wonderful husband and living the American dream to a very frightened 56-year old woman facing the very real probability that I could die from cancer—and soon. I can develop ovarian or breast cancer at any time. This genetic defect means that I carry a genetic time bomb and I am going to defuse it with surgical intervention. I have an 87% chance of cancer if I do nothing, so I'm going to fight back proactively and have surgery that will save my life and give me a much better chance of living out to my projected life span.

This is the story of my fight against a killer that has silently lived inside my body since birth stealthily waiting to strike at any moment. However, by hearing those words, I also knew I had been given the chance to fight back BEFORE the cancer appeared; assuming it hadn't already started. The chance to fight back surgically with a radical hysterectomy taking out every single piece of my reproductive system and double mastectomy with reconstruction was mine but it had come at a terrible price:

My younger sister Lori paid for it—with her life.

This is a story of how cancer devastated my family, took my younger sister at 55 and orphaned my niece and nephews. It is also a story of survival and fighting back against a killer that spares no one young or old. It is a story of loss, of hope and of the rage that runs through me when I think of how she died at the hands of doctors who slashed her open, poisoned her with chemicals and radiated her until she practically glowed in the dark and worst of all, they sold her false hope as she lay dying after $750,000 worth of useless surgeries, chemotherapy and radiation. Even worse, I believe it was an infertility doctor that killed her by prescribing the fertility

MASS MURDERING DOCTORS: THE TRUTH ABOUT ONCOLOGISTS, CHEMOTHERAPY AND CANCER

drug Clomid for nearly 4 years in order to give her the 3rd child and to try for a 4th child. With the very strong connection between the drug and ovarian cancer in NON-BRCA1+ women, I am not sure that the Clomid wasn't the catalyst, exacerbated by the stress of a 4 year fight to get a divorce from her abusive former husband that started the disease. Cancer is an immunodeficiency disease and it is NOT beatable by chemotherapy. **If you have chemo, you'll either die from the cancer, the chemo or the cancer you will get from the chemo!**

Along with the rest of my family and her friends we watched her fight like a tiger, none of us knowing she never had a chance because of the BRCA1 genetic defect and it was too late when we started AND because the chemo killed her plain and simple. She didn't have to die from chemotherapy, she would be alive today if she had refused the chemotherapy that killed her—not the cancer. She believed the lies the scumbag oncologists told her about "the next chemo should do the trick" when they KNEW she had no chance of survival and they cheerfully reassured her as they happily poisoned her for profit until they killed her. She had been widowed 15 years earlier when her beloved husband Carl lost his fight to brain cancer, an astrocytoma that mutated into a glioblastoma multiforme, and she was determined that my 17 year old niece, Carliegh, would not lose her other parent to cancer. No one in the family but me believed she'd really die—they ALL bought into the lies and bullcrap shoveled by the "doctors" that murdered her. She was tough, beautiful, hard-working and extremely successful in her business and determined not to let cancer beat her. She wanted to live to see her 2 grandchildren grow up and marry and was anxious for more grandchildren from her second son who married in April 2015 at the height of her brave battle, and her 17 year old daughter who was graduating high school with honors in June of 2016. She was brave beyond words, a fierce competitor and a woman of strong faith in God, and she was very determined not to lose this fight. I begged her to listen to me and to stop the chemo, but she believed the outright lies of her scumbag doctors, not knowing or refusing to believe that they were murdering her for money, and she paid for it with her life.

I am telling our story though many tears because it is one that must be told. There are too many of us out there that carry this genetic time bomb, unaware of our risk

MASS MURDERING DOCTORS: THE TRUTH ABOUT ONCOLOGISTS, CHEMOTHERAPY AND CANCER

and not knowing the danger. There are too many of us that believe that chemo is the "only hope" which is a bullcrap LIE perpetuated by scumbag oncologists who profit hugely by pushing their poison as a cure. As painful as this is to tell, if just ONE BRCA1+ positive woman is saved by reading this and getting tested and surgically preventing her own cancer or getting the CORRECT treatment instead of being poisoned to death by profiteering lying scumbags masquerading as doctors, then it will be worth the agony of telling it to strangers and, in doing so, reliving all of it again. We are all from the same family tree and human race. This is the story of my family's fight against BRCA1, a silent killer waiting to strike at the most opportune time and starting a life-and-death battle with cancer. This gene has decimated my family but at least I know that they will not die from cancer even though ALL of my sister's 3 children carry the killer gene that endangers them. I prayed it would die with me and that my dad and I would be the last carriers of this horrible and deadliest of genetic defects, but it wasn't to be.

Epithelial ovarian cancer is a much more complex disease than anyone envisioned, when it was believed that extensive debulking (tumor reducing/removal) surgery and the newest cytotoxic (cell killing) chemotherapy would radically reduce the death rate from ovarian cancer in the United States. Chemotherapy with platinum and taxanes is the first line of treatment for all epithelial ovarian cancer (Epithelian Ovarian Cancer) patients after debulking surgery. Even though the treatment is initially effective in 80% of patients, recurrent cancer is inevitable in the vast majority of cases. Emerging evidence suggests that some tumor cells can survive chemotherapy by activating the self-renewal pathways resulting in tumor progression and clinical recurrence. These defined population of cells commonly termed as "cancer stem cells" (Cancer Stem Cells) may generate the bulk of the tumor by using differentiating pathways. These cells have been shown to be resistant to chemotherapy and, to have enhanced tumor initiating abilities, suggesting Cancer Stem Cells as potential targets for treatment. Recent studies have introduced a new paradigm in ovarian carcinogenesis (starting the cancer) which proposes in situ carcinoma at the fimbrial end of the fallopian tube to generate high-grade serous ovarian carcinomas, in contrast to ovarian cortical inclusion cysts (CIC) which produce borderline and low grade serous, mucinous, endometrioid, and clear cell carcinomas. Primary surgery followed by systemic

MASS MURDERING DOCTORS: THE TRUTH ABOUT ONCOLOGISTS, CHEMOTHERAPY AND CANCER

platinum-based chemotherapy is the cornerstone of management for ovarian cancer. However, the majority of patients have an advanced disease (stage III/IV) at the time of diagnosis rendering the optimal primary cytoreduction feasible in only a small percentage of cases. A large tumor bulk limits the success of subsequent antiblastic therapy. There are two alternatives to overcome this unfavorable situation: (1) employment of ultra-radical interventions such as peritonectomy (removal of peritoneum) procedures, to increase the optimal cytoreduction rate; or (2) neoadjuvant chemotherapy. For second-line therapies no consensus regarding treatment has emerged. **When previous effective drug combinations fail, there is <u>virtually no chance of inducing a significant response</u> with second-line treatment.** Salvage chemotherapy is often utilized in patients with advanced ovarian cancer, due to the high frequency of recurrent disease even after a clinical or pathological complete response after primary chemotherapy. Main objectives of salvage chemotherapy include: 1. improvement in quality of life and symptoms; 2. tumor load reduction and survival advantage; 3. evaluation of potentially active new drugs to be included in first-line. Since the goal is palliation in most cases, monotherapy is generally indicated. Extension of the platinum-free interval before re-treatment with platinum or taxanes may allow partial reversal of resistance to these agents which can therefore still show significant activity in relapsing patients. Unfortunately, durable response to salvage chemotherapy is rare and cure is impossible. Currently, standard primary therapy for advanced disease involves a combination of maximal cytoreductive surgery and chemotherapy with carboplatin plus paclitaxel or with carboplatin alone. Despite initial high response rates, a large proportion of patients relapse, resulting in a therapeutic challenge. Because these patients are not curable, the goal of therapy becomes improvement in both quality and length of life. The search has therefore been to find active agents for women with recurrent disease following platinum-based chemotherapy. Now, **40 years** after the first patient was treated with cisplatin and carboplaxin along with taxanes for epithelial ovarian cancer, (the standard treatment for ALL tumor cancers) the annual death rate from ovarian cancer continues to increase. Currently, standard primary therapy for advanced disease involves a combination of maximal cytoreductive surgery and chemotherapy with carboplatin plus paclitaxel or with carboplatin alone. As a general

MASS MURDERING DOCTORS: THE TRUTH ABOUT ONCOLOGISTS, CHEMOTHERAPY AND CANCER

categorization within what is actually a continuum, "platinum sensitivity" refers to disease recurrence 6 months or more after prior platinum-containing chemotherapy, and "platinum resistance" refers to a response to platinum-based chemotherapy followed by relapse less than 6 months after chemotherapy is stopped. "Platinum-refractory disease" refers to a lack of response or to progression while on platinum-based chemotherapy. For patients with platinum-refractory or platinum-resistant disease, the goals of treatment should be to improve quality of life by extending the symptom-free interval, by reducing symptom intensity, and by increasing progression-free interval, and, if possible, to prolong life.

Where's that **TRILLION DOLLARS** raised by the allegedly fraudulent charity the American Cancer Society? Why is a **FORTY-YEAR OLD** treatment STILL the front-line treatment for cancer? Just **in the past decade, the number of women in the United States dying from ovarian cancer has increased 18% with no cure or reduction in sight.** There won't be a cure until there a test to reliably detect this cancer in the early stages has been developed, and until Big Pharma decides to stop paying off the FDA to keep the cure off the market to protect their **200-300 BILLION** per year **EVERY YEAR** in cancer treatment profits. They do NOT care how many people die of cancer as long as they are making money from it—all Cancer, Inc. understands is PROFIT. They do not care how much human suffering and loss of life goes into their blood money profits every year. Failed chemotherapies are 80% of EVERY oncologist's annual income since "modern" cancer treatment has a "cure" rate of 2.1% which is pretty pathetic and wouldn't be even be considered as an "effective" treatment if the FDA wasn't totally bought and paid for with Big Pharma bribes to Congress through their vast lobbyist network. Because of that network, the FDA has been bribed and pressured by bribed lawmakers (yes—our Senators and Congressional Representatives who don't give a crap about America or us either as long as the money keeps rolling in) to consider a cancer treatment effective if it shrinks a tumor by 50% for 28 DAYS. Big fat hairy deal. Do you know what shrinking a tumor 50% does for curing your cancer? Jack shit. A big steaming hot cup of NOTHING. Also, oncologists buy the chemotherapy medicine for your treatment "Cocktail" from Big Pharma and mark them up enormously (they buy the "cocktail" drugs for about $5,000 then mark it up to $75,000-$100,000) and them resell them to

MASS MURDERING DOCTORS: THE TRUTH ABOUT ONCOLOGISTS, CHEMOTHERAPY AND CANCER

the patients to "save their lives". It's poisoning people for profit, unconscionable and no one does anything about it in the government because they are all bought and paid for scumbags as well. Chemo kills 50% of the people who use it—NOT the cancer they are desperate to cure. I hope President Trump cleans HOUSE when he gets to DC. However, here are the major risk factors for the deadliest cancer of all the female cancers, High-grade serous-cell carcinoma of the ovary. It's what we BRCA1+ gals get and it's what kills us. It struck my sister; she didn't have to die, the chemo killed her.

SIDEBAR: RISK FACTORS FOR OVARIAN CANCER OTHER THAN BRCA1/2

Age: Two-thirds of women diagnosed with ovarian cancer are age 55 or older.
Childbearing status: Women who have delivered at least one child, especially before age 30, are at a lower risk for developing the disease. The more children a woman has, the more her ovarian cancer risk declines. Women who breastfeed further reduce their risk.

Obesity: Women with a body mass index (BMI) of 30 or greater may have a higher risk of developing ovarian cancer.

GENETICS

Family history: Women with a mother, sister, grandmother or aunt who has had ovarian cancer have a higher risk of developing it.

Genetic mutations: Some women who develop ovarian cancer have an inherited mutation on one of two genes called breast cancer gene 1 (BRCA1) and breast cancer gene 2 (BRCA2). Women with the BRCA1 mutation, have a 35 to 71 percent higher risk of ovarian cancer. Women with the BRCA2 mutation have a 10 to 30 percent higher risk. However, the vast majority of women who are diagnosed with ovarian cancer don't have either mutation, BUT of the women who get High-grade Serous-cell Carcinoma, 38% of them are BRCA1+ or BRCA2+. If you are concerned about this risk factor for ovarian cancer, you can discuss getting tested for both of the BRCA mutations with your OB-GYN. If you have a family history of ovarian or breast cancer, and if you are of European or Ashkenazi Jewish heritage, your insurance company WILL pay for your genetic testing and DO NOT WAIT! Your risk of developing ovarian

MASS MURDERING DOCTORS: THE TRUTH ABOUT ONCOLOGISTS, CHEMOTHERAPY AND CANCER

cancer is close to 78% by age 70 and it WILL kill you. Don't make any mistake about that—and it is far easier to PREVENT cancer than it is to TREAT it. Also, your chances of surviving high-grade serous carcinoma are very small, even with the poison of chemotherapy, only 2.1% survive and those are all stage 1 cancers that do NOT recur. When it recurs after the chemo as peritoneal carcinomatosis, you WILL die if you had chemo; as I am the ONLY known survivor of this deadly cancer and I did it with NO chemotherapy. Chemo makes cancer immortal by destroying your immune system and cancer is an immunodeficiency disease. About 1.3 percent of women in the general population will develop ovarian cancer sometime during their lives. By contrast, according to the most recent estimates, 39 percent of women who inherit a harmful BRCA1 mutation and 11 to 17 percent of women who inherit a harmful BRCA2 mutation will develop ovarian cancer by age 70 years. Your risk of breast cancer is even higher. About 12 percent of women in the general population will develop breast cancer sometime during their lives. By contrast, according to the most recent estimates, 55 to 65 percent of women who inherit a harmful BRCA1 mutation and around 45 percent of women who inherit a harmful BRCA2 mutation will develop breast cancer by age 70 years. Harmful mutations in BRCA1 and BRCA2 increase the risk of several cancers in addition to breast and ovarian cancer. BRCA1 mutations may increase a woman's risk of developing Fallopian tube cancer and peritoneal cancer.

Although ovarian cancer is estimated to account for 26,700 cases and 14,800 deaths in 1996, it is a low-prevalence disease in comparison with breast cancer, which annually is estimated to account for 185,700 cases and 44,560 deaths. Inexplicably, similar to breast cancer, the lifetime risk for ovarian cancer in the United States continues to increase. The most recent Surveillance, Epidemiology and End Results (SEER) calculations of lifetime risk for ovarian cancer are that 1 in 55 women will develop ovarian cancer over their lifetime, or 1.8%, up from the 1970 figures of 1 in 70, or 1.4%. The 1.8% baseline lifetime risk for the general population is used to estimate the lifetime risk of known ovarian cancer risk factors. Given these sobering statistics, the public health issue is whether prophylactic oophorectomy for two select groups of women may be one measure in reducing the mortality from ovarian cancer in the United States. The two groups of women are: A) women age 40 or older who undergo hysterectomy for non-cancerous uterine conditions and B) those with a family history of ovarian cancer.

MASS MURDERING DOCTORS: THE TRUTH ABOUT ONCOLOGISTS, CHEMOTHERAPY AND CANCER

Men with BRCA2 mutations, and to a lesser extent BRCA1 mutations, are also at increased risk of breast cancer. Men with harmful BRCA1 or BRCA2 mutations have a higher risk of prostate cancer. Men and women with BRCA1 or BRCA2 mutations may be at increased risk of pancreatic cancer. Mutations in BRCA2 (also known as FANCD1), if they are inherited from both parents, can cause a Fanconi anemia sub-type (FA-D1), a syndrome that is associated with childhood solid tumors and development of acute myeloid leukemia. Likewise, mutations in BRCA1 (also known as FANCS), if they are inherited from both parents, can cause another Fanconi anemia sub-type. Most mutations in these other genes are associated with smaller increases in breast cancer risk than are seen with mutations in BRCA1 and BRCA2. However, researchers recently reported that inherited mutations in the PALB2 gene are associated with a risk of breast cancer nearly as high as that associated with inherited BRCA1 and BRCA2 mutations. They estimated that 33 percent of women who inherit a harmful mutation in PALB2 will develop breast cancer by age 70 years. The estimated risk of breast cancer associated with a harmful PALB2 mutation is even higher for women who have a family history of breast cancer: 58 percent of those women will develop breast cancer by age 70 years. Ovarian cancer is the most lethal gynecological malignancy. It is usually diagnosed at a late stage, with a 5-yr survival rate of <30%. The majority of ovarian cancer cases are diagnosed after tumors have widely spread within the peritoneal cavity, limiting the effectiveness of debulking surgery and chemotherapy. Owing to a substantially lower survival rate at late stages of disease than at earlier stages, the major cause of ovarian cancer deaths is believed to be therapy-resistant metastasis. Although metastasis plays a crucial role in promoting ovarian tumor progression and decreasing patient survival rates, the underlying mechanisms of ovarian cancer spread have yet to be thoroughly explored.

PREVIOUS CONDITIONS

Breast, colorectal or endometrial cancer: Women who've been diagnosed with one of these cancers have a higher risk of developing ovarian cancer

SIDEBAR: THE RISK OF BRCA1 and BRCA2

MASS MURDERING DOCTORS: THE TRUTH ABOUT ONCOLOGISTS, CHEMOTHERAPY AND CANCER

Women from families with multiple cases of breast and ovarian cancer, specifically those who carry cancer-associated mutations of BRCA1 or BRCA2 are at increased life-time risk for peritoneal carcinoma, (YO!! right here—that's me!) even after previous surgery to remove the ovaries, Fallopian tubes and uterus. Hereditary breast-ovarian cancer (HBOC) syndrome and the associated BRCA1 and BRCA2 mutations are particularly prevalent in women of Jewish lineage, and specific BRCA1 and BRCA2 germline mutations have been linked with peritoneal carcinoma and HBOC (Hereditary Breast and Ovarian Cancer) syndrome in Jewish populations, especially those of Ashkenazi descent. This review presents the currently available data and looks forward toward further and better understanding of peritoneal carcinoma in women with inherited susceptibility. Over 90% of peritoneal cancer in patients from HBOC syndrome families and associated with BRCA1 and BRCA2 mutations are serous carcinomas, which is equivalent with the proportion of ovarian cancers that are serous carcinomas in similar patients. The best indications are that while many peritoneal carcinomas in genetically susceptible women may arise directly from malignant transformation of the peritoneum, others might represent metastases from primary ovarian or Fallopian tube carcinomas. Although the incidence of borderline ovarian tumors may not be increased in HBOC syndrome and those who carry cancer-associated BRCA1 and BRCA2 mutations, these individuals could be susceptible to malignant transformation of borderline lesions of the ovaries and peritoneum. Moreover, recent reports raise the question of possibly increased risk in Jewish carriers of germline BRCA1 mutations for **uterine papillary serous carcinoma**, which could be the source of metastasis to the peritoneum in some cases. I believe that this is how my cancer spread as Dr. DallaRiva missed it in the original hysterectomy.   The penetrance of cancer-associated BRCA1 mutations for ovarian cancer is estimated to be 11%-54%, and for BRCA2 mutations the penetrance for ovarian cancer is 11%-23%. So far, available screening methods appear to be insufficient for early detection of many ovarian cancers. Prophylactic oophorectomy has been found to reduce the risk for ovarian cancer in women from HBOC kindreds and those who carry cancer-associated BRCA1 and BRCA2 mutations, leaving a residual risk for peritoneal carcinomatosis of less than 5% AFTER the preventative surgery, **ASSUMING** that the ovaries and Fallopian tubes are removed prior to developing cancer. Therefore, surgical removal of the ovaries, Fallopian tubes and uterus, after child-bearing has been completed and by early in the fifth decade of life, are appropriate prophylactic procedures in women whose genetic susceptibility puts them at increased risk for cancers of mullerian tract origin, including ovarian and Fallopian tube carcinomas and possibly papillary serous carcinoma of the uterus. Hysterectomy, as well as having the preventative salpingo/oophorectomy, removes the gynecologic organs targeted for malignant transformation in genetically susceptible women and simplifies decisions regarding hormone replacement therapy and chemical prophylaxis and treatment of breast cancer. Unless a transabdominal operative approach is otherwise indicated, laparoscopic-assisted transvaginal techniques are well suited for intra-abdominal exploration, cytology, biopsies and prophylactic salpingo-oophorectomy and hysterectomy in women with hereditary susceptibility to gynecologic cancer.

Women who carry BRCA1 or BRCA2 mutations have an estimated lifetime risk of between 60% and 85% of developing breast cancer, and a lifetime risk of between 26% and 54% of developing ovarian cancer for BRCA1, and between 10% and 23% for BRCA2. The factors associated with a decreased risk of ovarian cancer are the use of oral contraceptives, breastfeeding, bilateral tubal ligation or hysterectomy, prophylactic salpingo-oophorectomy (surgical removal of ovaries and Fallopian tubes where it is now beginning to be the accepted and settled belief that ALL ovarian cancers begins in the Fallopian tubes). Here's a nice new research paper quote about it, courtesy of PubMed and online here: https://www.ncbi.nlm.nih.gov/pmc/articles/PMC2745605/ that has the following statement: Recently, attention has been drawn to a lesion in the fallopian tube that has the cytologic appearance of high-grade serous carcinoma of the ovary and has been designated tubal intraepithelial carcinoma (TIC) These lesions are almost always detected in the fimbriated end of the fallopian tube. The fimbriated end is in close proximity to the ovarian surface, and it has been suggested that the tube is the origin of a subset of "ovarian" high-grade serous carcinomas. This is supported by the following: (1) early serous carcinomas in prophylactic bilateral salpingo-oophorectomy specimens from women with BRCA mutations (i.e., women who are at an increased risk for "ovarian" carcinoma) can be detected in the tube, especially the fimbriated end, in the absence of an ovarian tumor, (2) identical TP53 mutations have been reported in TIC and synchronous ovarian high-grade serous carcinomas, and (3) identical TP53 mutations have been reported in TICs and in small foci of histologically normal tubal epithelium that diffusely expresses p53, which has been termed "p53 signature". It has been suggested that p53 signatures are precursors of TICs which in turn precede the development of high grade serous carcinoma. Moreover, it has been proposed that when there is a synchronous TIC and ovarian high-grade serous carcinoma that the fallopian tube is the primary site of origin for the "ovarian" tumor. In one study, all fallopian tube tissue from consecutively accessioned pelvic serous carcinomas was submitted for histologic examination, and 48% of tumors initially interpreted as ovarian in origin contained a TIC. In an analysis of ovarian high-grade serous carcinomas at The Johns Hopkins Hospital in which all tubal tissue was submitted for histologic examination, 45% of cases contained TIC (unpublished data). It has, therefore, been hypothesized that neoplastic cells of TIC, or a small invasive high-grade serous carcinoma in the fallopian tube which developed from TIC, implant on the ovary, developing into a high-grade serous carcinoma that clinically and grossly appears to be an ovarian primary tumor. Thus, the morphologic and molecular observations detailed above suggest that possibly half of "ovarian" high-grade serous carcinomas may be of tubal origin. In the other half of tumors, primary origin may have been ovarian or peritoneal. It should be noted that the criteria for distinction of primary ovarian vs. peritoneal origin are quite arbitrary. Bona fide well-defined precursor lesions in the ovary are rare and have not been identified in the peritoneum. In summary, the pathogenesis of high-grade serous carcinoma (Type II pathway) is characterized by: (1) rapid development from what are now believed to be intraepithelial carcinomas very likely of tubal origin, (2) TP53 mutations, (3) a high level of chromosomal instability, (4) in hereditary tumors, BRCA germline mutations, and (5) absence of mutations of KRAS, BRAF, or ERBB2."   ----Adv Anat Pathol. 2009 Sep; 16(5): 267–282. doi: 10.1097/PAP.0b013e3181b4fffa

PMCID: PMC2745605
NIHMSID: NIHMS139803OVARIAN LOW-GRADE AND HIGH-GRADE SEROUS CARCINOMA: Pathogenesis, Clinicopathologic and Molecular Biologic Features, and Diagnostic Problems Russell Vang, M.D., Ie-Ming Shih, M.D., Ph.D., and Robert J. Kurman, M.D.

MASS MURDERING DOCTORS: THE TRUTH ABOUT ONCOLOGISTS, CHEMOTHERAPY AND CANCER

Here's some more technical stuff about genetics that explains how something most people never heard of kills you.

The major genetic risk factor for ovarian cancer is a mutation in BRCA1 or BRCA2 DNA mismatch repair genes, which is present in 48% of ovarian cancer cases. Only one allele need be mutated to place a person at high risk, because the risky mutations are autosomal dominant. The gene can be inherited through either the maternal or paternal line, but has variable penetrance. Though mutations in these genes are usually associated with increased risk of breast cancer, they also carry a substantial lifetime risk of ovarian cancer, a risk that peaks in a person's 40s and 50s. The lowest risk cited is 30% and the highest 80%. Mutations in BRCA1 have a lifetime risk of developing ovarian cancer of 15-45%. Mutations in BRCA2 are less risky than those with BRCA1, with a lifetime risk of 10% (lowest risk cited) to 40% (highest risk cited). On average, BRCA1 associated cancers develop 15 years before their sporadic counterparts, because people who inherit the mutations on one copy of their gene only need one mutation to start the process of carcinogenesis, whereas people with two normal genes would need to acquire two mutations. A study examining mutations in DNA repair genes in women with advanced ovarian cancer found that the disease remained at bay longer in women with the mutations than without, and that women having cancers with these mutations lived longer. The rate of relapse in ovarian cancers is highly dependent upon the initial stage at diagnosis, the histologic type, and the presence of residual disease at the time of primary or interval debulking. Women with Type II ovarian cancers, e.g. HGSC, are also likely to have higher rates of recurrence of the cancer and it is the Genghis Khan of cancers.

The original study, a phase III clinical trial (Gynecologic Oncology Group 218), was intended to examine the impact of adding the drug bevacizumab to standard chemotherapy for advanced ovarian cancer. In this new study researchers sought to determine whether having mutations in some DNA repair genes (called homologous recombination or HR genes) affected the response to the combined treatment and found that they did not. More importantly, however, the researchers found that the mutation status affected how long a woman may live overall survival (OS) and remain free from disease progression-free survival (PFS). Although many women with recurrent ovarian cancer will be symptomatic or have detectable signs of recurrence upon physical examination, an increasing number of women are being (or could be)

MASS MURDERING DOCTORS: THE TRUTH ABOUT ONCOLOGISTS, CHEMOTHERAPY AND CANCER

diagnosed with recurrent ovarian cancer through the detection of incremental rises in CA-125 and through the use of more sophisticated imaging technology. Two new agents have recently been approved by the FDA for patients with recurrent ovarian cancer. Bevacizumab, a humanized antibody that blocks vascular endothelial growth factor (VEGF), in combination with one of three chemotherapy regimens (i. e. dose-dense paclitaxel, liposomal doxorubicin, and topotecan), is now approved for the treatment of patients with platinum-resistant ovarian cancers. Olaparib, an orally given chemotherapy medication. is a PARP inhibitor, has been approved as a monotherapy for BRCA mutation–positive, recurrent ovarian cancer patients who have had three prior chemotherapy treatments. IP chemo (Intraperitoneal Chemotherapy which is only given to about half of women with ovarian cancer) has shown better effectiveness than IV chemotherapy alone but is difficult to tolerate. (They pump your pelvic cavity full of the same poison they run through your veins—only the poison is 400 times STRONGER. Does that sound like a sensible thing to do?) Studies have indeed shown that PARP inhibitors, alone or in combination with chemotherapy, are effective in women with recurrent ovarian cancer, particularly those with a BRCA1 or BRCA2 mutation. However, there are STILL NO KNOWN SURVIVORS of High-grade serous-cell carcinoma after it recurs as peritoneal carcinomatosis. NONE. It's universally fatal. Yet I am still alive.

Chemotherapy with platinum and taxanes is the first line of treatment for all epithelial ovarian cancer (EOC) patients after debulking surgery. Even though the treatment is initially effective in 80% of patients, recurrent cancer is inevitable in the vast majority of cases. Emerging evidence suggests that some tumor cells can survive chemotherapy by activating the self-renewal pathways resulting in tumor progression and clinical recurrence. These defined population of cells commonly termed as "cancer stem cells" (CSC) may generate the bulk of the tumor by using differentiating pathways. These cells have been shown to be resistant to chemotherapy and, to have enhanced tumor initiating abilities, suggesting CSCs as potential targets for treatment. Recent studies have introduced a new paradigm in ovarian carcinogenesis which proposes in situ carcinoma at the fimbrial end of the fallopian tube to generate high-grade serous ovarian carcinomas, in contrast to ovarian cortical inclusion cysts (CIC) which produce borderline and low grade serous, mucinous, endometrioid, and clear cell carcinomas. In particular, olaparib improves Progression Free Survival when used

MASS MURDERING DOCTORS: THE TRUTH ABOUT ONCOLOGISTS, CHEMOTHERAPY AND CANCER

as a maintenance therapy in the context of BRCA1 or BRCA2 mutations, platinum sensitivity, and recurrent disease. In December 2014, the FDA approved olaparib as a therapy for women with recurrent ovarian cancer who have a BRCA1 or BRCA2 mutation and who have had three prior chemotherapy treatments. Two months before that, in October 2014, the European Medicines Agency had approved olaparib as first-line maintenance therapy for women with platinum-sensitive, recurrent HGSC who are in complete or partial response to platinum-based chemotherapy. Additional evidence suggests that the addition of olaparib to chemotherapy improves PFS in platinum-sensitive recurrent ovarian cancer, but they all die anyway. Current trials are exploring the use of PARP inhibitors, including in combination with other molecularly targeted agents. Preliminary evidence suggests that the combination of the anti-angiogenic cedirinab and the PARP inhibitor olaparib may be as effective as cytotoxic chemotherapy regimens. (Not NEARLY as profitable though) Tests for alterations in BRCA1 and BRCA2 genes are currently of interest as possible predictive tests that could identify those patients most like to benefit from PARP inhibitors. The OVA1 test is approved by the FDA for use in guiding referral to a gynecologic oncologist. It is "a qualitative serum test that combines the results of five immunoassays into a single numerical score for women with an ovarian adnexal mass for which surgery is planned as an aid to further assess the likelihood that malignancy is present when the physician's independent clinical and radiological evaluation does not indicate malignancy" making it a diagnostic tool that is far better than the CA-125 test currently used by most doctors. The CA-125 test is only accurate about 50% of the time although a false negative is far worse than a false positive.

Median Progression Free Survival and optimum survival (OS) for women with no BRCA 1 or 2 mutations is 12.6 and 42.1 months, respectively until/unless it recurs as peritoneal carcinomatosis which is unsurvivable. For women with BRCA1 mutations, Progression-Free Survival (PFS) and OS were longer at 15. 7 and 55. 3 months. For BRCA2, median Progression Free Survival and OS were even longer at 21. 6 and 75. 2 months. For mutations in non-BRCA genes, median Progression Free Survival and OS were 16 and 56 months, similar to that seen for BRCA1 mutations. All three mutation-carrier groups had significantly better progression-free and overall survival when compared to those with no mutations. Researchers also found that these mutations were present in all histologic types of ovarian cancer (what the cells look like under the microscope). This underscores the message that women with any type of ovarian cancer should have genetic testing, and they should be included in clinical trials of drugs that work best in the setting of HR defects. If a clinician feels their patient is a candidate for bevacizumab, mutation status does not have a large impact on that decision."

Ovarian cancer usually has a relatively poor prognosis. It is disproportionately deadly because it lacks any clear early detection or screening test, meaning most cases are not diagnosed until they have reached advanced stages. However, in some cases, ovarian cancer recurrences are chronically treatable, but not high-grade serous carcinoma and not peritoneal carcinomatosis, these are 100% fatal.

Ovarian cancer metastasizes early in its development, often before it has been diagnosed. High-grade tumors, which are the most common in BRCA1+ genetic mutation carriers, (like my sister's cancer) metastasize more readily than low-grade tumors. Typically, tumor cells begin to metastasize by growing in the peritoneal cavity. More than 60% of women presenting with ovarian cancer have stage-III or stage-IV cancer, when it has already spread beyond the ovaries. Ovarian cancers shed cells into the naturally occurring fluid within the abdominal cavity. These cells then implant on other abdominal (peritoneal) structures, included the uterus, urinary, bladder, bowel, lining of the bowel wall, and omentum, forming new tumor growths before cancer is even suspected, making it a deadly and silent killer with a huge mortality rate. **It's also a very profitable cancer since it is virulent and recurs with alarming frequency requiring more expensive and ineffective treatment so it is the darling of Big Pharma as it is so very profitable to treat and recurs several times before the patient typically dies since chemo has only a 2.1% success rate. It's also PROOF that chemo makes cancer IMMORTAL.**

The five-year survival rate for all stages and kinds of ovarian cancer is 46%; the one-year survival rate is 72% and the ten-year survival rate is 35%, but this is for ALL kinds of ovarian cancer. The survival rate for HGSC ovarian cancer when it recurs as peritoneal carcinomatosis is ZERO percent. No known survivors. Period. The other 3 kinds of ovarian cancer are survivable, HGSC is not—unless you happen to have it discovered accidentally in a very early stage and don't die from the chemo, and it

MASS MURDERING DOCTORS: THE TRUTH ABOUT ONCOLOGISTS, CHEMOTHERAPY AND CANCER

never recurs because when it does, it's stage four peritoneal carcinomatosis from the get-go which is always fatal—just a matter of time.

For cases where a diagnosis is made early in the disease, when the cancer is still confined to the primary site, the five-year survival rate is 92. 7%. About 71% of women with advanced disease respond to initial treatment, most of whom attain complete remission, but half of these women experience a recurrence 1–4 years after treatment. Brain metastasis is more common in stage III/IV cancer but can still occur in cancers staged at I/II. People with brain metastases survive a median of 8. 2 months, though surgery, chemotherapy, and whole brain radiation therapy can improve survival. This is for all 4 kinds of ovarian cancers, of which Clear Cell Carcinoma, stromal-cell carcinoma, low-grade serous carcinoma are survivable, but High-grade serous-cell carcinoma is 100% fatal when it recurs as peritoneal carcinomatosis. IV chemo has NO effect on it, so the ONLY reason for chemo is to enrich your oncologist (who tells you he has to "shrink the tumors") while he poisons you until you're happy to die. Ovarian cancer survival varies significantly with subtype. Dysgerminomas have a very favorable prognosis. In early stages, they have a five-year survival rate of 96.9%. Around two-thirds of dysgerminomas are diagnosed at stage 1. Stage-3 dysgerminomas have a five-year survival of 61%; when treated with BEP chemotherapy after incomplete surgical removal, dysgerminomas have a 95% two-year survival rate. Sex-cord-stromal malignancies also have a favorable prognosis; because they are slow-growing, even those with metastatic disease can survive a decade or more. Low malignant potential tumors usually only have a bad prognosis when there are invasive tumor implants found in the peritoneal cavity.

Complications of ovarian cancer can include spread of the cancer to other organs, progressive function loss of various organs, ascites, and intestinal obstructions, which can be fatal. Intestinal obstructions in multiple sites are the most common proximate cause of death. Intestinal obstruction in ovarian cancer can either be a true obstruction, where tumor blocks the intestinal lumen, or a pseudo-obstruction, when tumor prevents normal peristalsis. Continuous accumulation of ascites can be treated by placing a drain that can be self-drained.

The 5-year survival rate for patients with HGSC (High-Grade Serous Carcinoma) is between 35% and 40%, and it is strongly influenced by the extent of disease at

MASS MURDERING DOCTORS: THE TRUTH ABOUT ONCOLOGISTS, CHEMOTHERAPY AND CANCER

presentation (stage) and the amount of residual tumor following primary debulking surgery. However, considerable variation in outcome is observed among HGSC patients matched for stage and debulking status, suggesting that other determinants of survival are at play. Although no molecular predictors of clinical outcome are currently in use, several factors are becoming increasingly apparent. **Women with a germline mutation in either BRCA1 or BRCA2 show higher response rates to chemotherapy, a longer progression-free survival, and improved overall survival compared with non-carriers. Improved survival is also seen in women with somatic mutations in BRCA1/2but not in those with methylation of the BRCA1 promoter. However, longer survival times does NOT mean there was, or is, a cure.** It seems that the defects in HRR associated with loss of BRCA function that create an initial susceptibility to ovarian cancer also render the tumors sensitive to platinum-based DNA cross linking agents. Intragenic BRCA1/2mutations that result in the partial restoration of defective germline alleles were observed in a significant fraction of tumors following platinum-based chemotherapy and the emergence of resistance. The apparently strong selective pressure for such germline BRCA reversion underscores the importance of BRCA dysfunction in influencing platinum sensitivity.

Case-control studies suggest that *BRCA1* and *BRCA2* mutation carriers have improved responses to chemotherapy when compared with patients with sporadic epithelial ovarian cancer. This may be the result of a deficient homologous DNA repair mechanism in these tumors, which leads to increased sensitivity to chemotherapy agents.

 Although most women with HGSC have excellent responses to initial chemotherapy (50% DIE from the chemo though) following primary surgery, 30% to 60% of patients relapse within 6 months of treatment.

Ovarian cancer frequently recurs after treatment. Overall, in a 5-year period, 30% of stage I and II cancers recur. Most recurrences are in the abdomen. If a recurrence occurs in advanced disease, it typically occurs within 18 months of initial treatment. **Recurrences can be treated, but the disease-free interval tends to shorten and chemo-resistance increases with each recurrence and are universally fatal.** When a dysgerminoma* (*rare malignant ovarian neoplasm composed of undifferentiated gonadal germinal cells) recurs, it is most likely to recur within a year of diagnosis, and other malignant germ cell tumors recur within 2 years 90% of the time. **Germ cell tumors other than dysgerminomas have a poor prognosis when they relapse, with a 10% long-term survival rate.** Low malignant potential tumors rarely relapse, even when fertility-sparing surgery is the treatment of choice. 15% of Low Malignant Potential (LMP) tumors relapse after unilateral surgery in the previously unaffected ovary, and they are typically easily treated with surgery. More advanced tumors may take up to 20 years to relapse, if they relapse at all, and are only treated with surgery unless the tumor has changed its histological characteristics or grown very quickly. In these cases, and when there is significant ascites, chemotherapy may also be used. **Relapse is usually indicated by rising CA-125 levels and then progresses to symptomatic relapse within 2–6 months.** Recurrent sex cord-stromal tumors are typically unresponsive to treatment but not aggressive.

In the United States, five of 100 women with a first degree relative (mother, sister) with ovarian cancer will eventually get ovarian cancer themselves, placing those with affected family members at triple the risk of women with unaffected family members. Seven of 100 women with two or more relatives with ovarian cancer will eventually get ovarian cancer. **In general, 5-10% of ovarian cancer cases have a genetic cause. BRCA mutations are associated with high-grade serous non-mucinous epithelial ovarian cancer.**

Dr. Brad Nelson, OVCARE researcher and Director of the BC Cancer Agency's Deeley Research Centre, has just published in the Journal of Pathology the results of a collaborative study that provides new insight into **high-grade serous carcinoma (HGSC), the most common and fatal form of ovarian cancer. While most tumors respond well to surgery and chemotherapy, the majority of HGSC patients experience recurrence of treatment-resistant tumors, and the mutations associated with recurrence are poorly understood.**

Women from families with multiple cases of breast and ovarian cancer, specifically those who carry cancer-associated mutations of BRCA1 or BRCA2 are at increased life-time risk for peritoneal carcinoma, even after previous surgery to remove the ovaries, fallopian tubes and uterus. Hereditary breast-ovarian cancer (HBOC) syndrome and

MASS MURDERING DOCTORS: THE TRUTH ABOUT ONCOLOGISTS, CHEMOTHERAPY AND CANCER

the associated BRCA1 and BRCA2 mutations are particularly prevalent in women of Jewish lineage, and specific BRCA1 and BRCA2 germline mutations have been linked with peritoneal carcinoma and HBOC syndrome in Jewish populations, especially those of Ashkenazi descent. Over 90% of peritoneal cancer in patients from HBOC syndrome kindreds and associated with BRCA1 and BRCA2 mutations are serous carcinomas, which is equivalent with the proportion of ovarian cancers that are serous carcinomas in similar patients. The best indications are that while many peritoneal carcinomas in genetically susceptible women may arise directly from malignant transformation of the peritoneum, others might represent metastases from primary ovarian or fallopian tube carcinomas. Although the incidence of borderline ovarian tumors may not be increased in HBOC syndrome kindreds and those who carry cancer-associated BRCA1 and BRCA2 mutations, these individuals could be susceptible to malignant transformation of borderline lesions of the ovaries and peritoneum. Moreover, recent reports raise the question of possibly increased risk in Jewish carriers of germline BRCA1 mutations for uterine papillary serous carcinoma, which could be the source of metastasis to the peritoneum in some cases. The penetrance of cancer-associated BRCA1 mutations for ovarian cancer is estimated to be 11%-54%, and for BRCA2 mutations the penetrance for ovarian cancer is 11%-23%. So far, available screening methods appear to be insufficient for early detection of many ovarian cancers. Prophylactic oophorectomy has been found to reduce the risk for ovarian cancer in women from HBOC kindreds and those who carry cancer-associated BRCA1 and BRCA2 mutations, leaving a residual risk for peritoneal carcinomatosis of well less than 5%. Therefore, surgical removal of the ovaries, Fallopian tubes and uterus, after child-bearing has been completed and by early in the fifth decade of life, are appropriate prophylactic procedures in women whose genetic susceptibility puts them at increased risk for cancers of mullerian tract origin, including ovarian and Fallopian tube carcinomas and possibly serous carcinoma of the uterus. Hysterectomy, as well as salpingo-oophorectomy, removes the gynecologic organs targeted for malignant transformation in genetically susceptible women and simplifies decisions regarding hormone replacement therapy and chemical prophylaxis and treatment of breast cancer. Unless a transabdominal operative approach is otherwise indicated, laparoscopic-assisted transvaginal techniques are well suited for intra-abdominal exploration, cytology, biopsies and prophylactic salpingo-oophorectomy and hysterectomy in women with hereditary susceptibility to gynecologic cancer.

A research team, led by Dr. Brad Nelson and Dr. Rob Holt, performed genomic sequencing on tumor cells of three patients at primary, first and second recurrence in order to compare mutations to healthy DNA over time. Their results proved—for the very first time—that recurrent HGSC arises from multiple clones present in the primary tumor, with very few new mutations in recurrent tumors, even after two rounds of treatment. The stability of the disease over time offers hope of identifying new therapeutic targets and ultimately preventing the tumors from recurring. Additionally, the researchers discovered commonalities among mutations that may point the way to more effective, targeted treatments. In particular, Dr. Nelson's team intends to use genomic sequencing information to develop customized vaccines for each patient. These vaccines will educate the patient's immune system to recognize and destroy mutation-containing cancer cells.

Stages of Ovarian Cancer (NOTE: This info is in several places in the book as a convenience to the reader. Readers won't have to thumb through to refer to this when it is mentioned in later chapters)

Once diagnosed with ovarian cancer, the stage of a tumor can be determined during surgery, when the doctor can tell if the cancer has spread outside the ovaries. There are four stages of ovarian cancer:

Stage I (early disease) to Stage IV (advanced disease). Your treatment plan and prognosis (the probable course and outcome of your disease) will be determined by the stage of cancer you have.

Following is a description of the various stages of ovarian cancer:

Stage I- Growth of the cancer is limited to the ovary or ovaries.

Stage IA- Growth is limited to one ovary and the tumor is confined to the inside of the ovary. There is no cancer on the outer surface of the ovary. There are no ascites present containing malignant cells. The capsule is intact.

Stage IB- Growth is limited to both ovaries without any tumor on their outer surfaces. There are no ascites present containing malignant cells. The capsule is intact.

Stage IC- The tumor is classified as either Stage IA or IB and one or more of the following are present: (1) tumor is present on the outer surface of one or both ovaries; (2) the capsule has ruptured; and (3) there are ascites containing malignant cells or with positive peritoneal washings.

Stage II- Growth of the cancer involves one or both ovaries with pelvic extension.

Stage IIA- The cancer has extended to and/or involves the uterus or the Fallopian tubes, or both.

Stage IIB- The cancer has extended to other pelvic organs.

Stage IIC- The tumor is classified as either Stage IIA or IIB and one or more of the following are present: (1) tumor is present on the outer surface of one or both ovaries; (2) the capsule has ruptured; and (3) there are ascites containing malignant cells or with positive peritoneal washings.

Stage III- Growth of the cancer involves one or both ovaries, and one or both of the following are present: (1) the cancer has spread beyond the pelvis to the lining of the abdomen; and (2) the cancer has spread to lymph nodes. The tumor is limited to the true pelvis but with histologically proven malignant extension to the small bowel or omentum.

Stage IIIA- During the staging operation, the practitioner can see cancer involving one or both of the ovaries, but no cancer is grossly visible in the abdomen and it has not spread to lymph nodes. However, when biopsies are checked under a microscope, very small deposits of cancer are found in the abdominal peritoneal surfaces.

Stage IIIB- The tumor is in one or both ovaries, and deposits of cancer are present in the abdomen that are large enough for the surgeon to see but not exceeding 2 cm in diameter. The cancer has not spread to the lymph nodes.

MASS MURDERING DOCTORS: THE TRUTH ABOUT ONCOLOGISTS, CHEMOTHERAPY AND CANCER

Stage IIIC- The tumor is in one or both ovaries, and one or both of the following is present: (1) the cancer has spread to lymph nodes; and/or (2) the deposits of cancer exceed 2 cm in diameter and are found in the abdomen.

Stage IV- This is the most advanced stage of ovarian cancer. Growth of the cancer involves one or both ovaries and distant metastases (spread of the cancer to organs located outside of the peritoneal cavity) have occurred. Finding ovarian cancer cells in pleural fluid (from the cavity which surrounds the lungs) is also evidence of stage IV disease.

This is what I am dealing with. I am prepared to fight tooth and nail. If I could change that I used to smoke cigarettes many years ago, I would. Believe me I would never have touched them if I had known—even though smoking isn't really a risk factor for this, it can't have been a good thing for me. Coulda-shoulda-woulda—didn't. I think my cancer is a stage II-A but the oncologist-gynecologist says it's II-C which I don't believe but he's the doctor so I'll leave it at that and let my reader decide what to believe. The doctors miss it because there is NO definitive test to say "Yes, it's cancer" when it is in early stages and you don't pop the CA-125 until you get into stage III (or not at all since it's a false negative 50% of the time) and the cancer cells are clogging your pelvic lymph nodes and your CA-125 skyrockets—and by then you might as well put your affairs in order if you are going to stick with conventional medicine as chemo has a 2.1% success rate with all ovarian cancers and with High-Grade Serous Carcinoma, a recurrence of ovarian cancer is the "always fatal" peritoneal carcinomatosis and there are no known survivors. With stage 2-C ovarian that had metastasized into both ovaries and my uterus my CA-125 was a 16—which is in the normal range with 0-35 being the range. The only reason my insurance decided to pay for my hysterectomy without symptoms or diagnosis of cancer was my family history—I am BRCA1+ and my paternal grandmother died of breast cancer and my younger sister died of ovarian cancer and she never had a chance. They found her ovarian cancer at stage 3-C which means she was riddled with it, she had cancerous tumors bigger than 2 cm all over her pelvis and abdominal cavity. Her CA-125 was 4400 and when they finished the surgery they told her she was terminal. They had already done 6 rounds of heavy duty chemo when they did the surgery and she wouldn't stop the chemo and try something else. She was BRCA1+ as well and told me to get tested and in doing so possibly saved my life. Had I not gotten tested and decided to have a PREVENTATIVE hysterectomy in early Feb 2016 which revealed the ovarian cancer, right about now, the cancer would have progressed to shedding cells which would be attaching to my pelvic walls and by Christmas I'd be swelling up with ascites and on Valentine's day they'd tell me I was terminal and July 4th 2017 I'd probably have died. It messes with your head when you realize the consequences of events to an action you take or DON'T take. Anyway, TIME IS OF THE ESSENCE as serous-cell carcinoma is the most malignant and most aggressive and most COMMON of the pelvic cancers. Because there's no way to detect it early means it's a killer and almost impossible to survive; and if it recurs as peritoneal carcinomatosis it is 100% fatal. There are 4 kinds of ovarian cancer, three of them are survivable but the statistics lump all of them together and are misleading. 89% survival at stage 1, 40% survival by stage 2, 20% survival by stage 3, 3% survival at stage 4. The survivors are the ones who do NOT have a recurrence of HGSC as peritoneal carcinomatosis, as that is 100% fatal. Given the chemo-sensitive nature of this disease, as well as the fact that it remains largely incurable in advanced stages, efforts continue to be made to improve initial therapy. Your ONLY chance with chemo is to get it ALL and hope it never comes back. Don't play around with this bad boy! I've always thought I was pretty tough but I am really scared, more scared than I have ever been in my life. I do not want to die, I want to enjoy my golden years with my husband and drop dead of a heart attack when I get to be too infirm to live alone. I don't know if I will manage to achieve that goal but I am absolutely going to try! I've been eating beef, butter and cheese my whole life and I do not want to die at 58 from an inherited cancer I never saw coming! I want to die of the massive heart attack I've been training for my whole life—as God intended when He invented steak. If this cancer comes back after chemotherapy which happens in 85% OR MORE of the time, you are going to die. End of story.

CHAPTER ONE: FAMILY CANCER HISTORY: GRANDMA BOBBIE

My paternal grandmother died of breast cancer in February of 1960 when I was 14 months old. My sister Lori was on her way but Grandma Bobbie died two months before my sister was born and never met or held her second grandchild. Ironically, my grandmother carried the gene that eventually killed Lori in 2015 but none of us knew

MASS MURDERING DOCTORS: THE TRUTH ABOUT ONCOLOGISTS, CHEMOTHERAPY AND CANCER

it at the time; as genetics and the massive research about it was 50 years in the future. There's no doubt that Grandma Bobbie was the possessor of the killer gene, but life's a crap shoot and you get what you get. God has a sense of humor and he drinks. My father was an only child and as luck would have it; has never had any kind of cancer and, as I write, is still with us at the age of 87. My mother's side of the family had no cancer whatsoever other than my uncle, a Vietnam veteran whose cancer is from Agent Orange, like so many others. My father, not having ever contracted cancer lends itself to the myth that BRCA1 "skips a generation". It does NOT and the genetic defect DOES NOT DILUTE. It was just good luck that my dad never had cancer as he is also BRCA1 positive. I never had the chance to know my grandmother as BRCA1+ took her from me before I was old enough to know her as a person. I do know she was of European and Ashkenazi Jewish descent both of which, which we now know, are huge risk factors for the BRCA1+ genetic defect she MUST have carried. I never met her but the genetic gift that she gave us all keeps on giving. I hoped and prayed that it didn't get passed on to Lori's children or grandchildren!

When you have a parent that is BRCA1 positive, you have a 50% chance of also being BRCA1+ and it doesn't dilute to future generations. I had a 50% chance of passing it on to my children and Lori had a 50% chance of passing it on to her children as well. If her children are BRCA1+ they each have a 50% chance of passing it on. My younger brother Keith is NOT BRCA1+ so his children are safe and have no chance of passing it on to the next generation and I am grateful for that, and happy for them that they will never have to make the choice I made.

I have urged my sister's children to be tested, and I am hoping that they will be. Being tested for the genetic defect; no matter what the outcome, gives them the chance to fight back proactively with surgical intervention. Not knowing is rolling the dice and when I received my BRCA1 test results, I chose surgeries to reduce my risk. I did it for two reasons. The first reason was my husband was adamant that we had to try anything to avoid cancer developing and BRCA1 means an 87% chance of cancer by age 70 which is why my health insurance was fine with paying for surgeries to remove tissue that had not already been determined to be cancerous. The other was more personal. My sister made it possible for me to be able to have the chance to intervene and prevent cancer before it happened but the price of knowing I am BRCA1+ was very high, my sister paid for it with her life.

If you have a 1st degree relative: Mother or Sister, with breast, uterine or ovarian cancer you may be at risk. If you have two or more second degree relatives: maternal or paternal Grandmother, Aunt or Cousin, again you should consider testing and if you have one or more of each, in any combination, you also should be tested for the defect. I had NO idea I was BRCA1. NONE. It's a silent and potentially deadly condition and you should be tested. Most insurance will pay for the test if you have relatives with the aforementioned cancers. Your doctor, by sticking a needle in your arm may give you the opportunity to intervene and save your own life by doing so. Where's the down side? It's almost painless although it may take up to a month to get the results. If you are at risk I implore you to take the test, you've nothing to lose and it may save your life. At the very least, it gives you the knowledge you will need to proactively fight the cancer before it rears it's ugly head.

My sister wasn't tested until her idiot doctors told her they couldn't figure out why she wasn't beating the cancer with the "best and most expensive care" available. When they tested her, they knew why she got it, they already knew they couldn't stop it after the biopsy came back. Then they sold her more false hope with this statement: "Your cancer is incurable but treatable and you could live for years with treatment". Do you know what that REALLY means? It's doctor-speak for "We can't help you and you're going to die soon but we'd like to keep billing your insurance fifty to a hundred grand a pop for your chemotherapy that is poisoning you and never had any chance of curing you. Is that OK with you? Great—sign here." They told her this knowing she had cancerous tumors all over the peritoneum larger that 2 cm in diameter, a belly FULL of cancerous growths. I will never forgive her doctors for selling her false hope and filling her with poison. They knew they couldn't help her and didn't care—it was all about being able to keep billing her insurance over and over again for chemotherapy treatments that had no chance of helping her. Cancer doctors are the scum of the earth as are most doctors, with the exception of plastic surgeons. Doctors take money from sick people, plastic surgeons take money from the vain. Huge difference. Huge. I have gotten extremely good at telling which doctors are there for

MASS MURDERING DOCTORS: THE TRUTH ABOUT ONCOLOGISTS, CHEMOTHERAPY AND CANCER

the money and which are there because they like healing the sick. I find my doctors for technical excellence in surgeons and I toss in some bedside manner in my internist.

I have no love for or patience with money-grubbing doctors and don't think for ONE second that medicine isn't a business—it is. Cancer treatment is insanely expensive as well. Lori's medical bills were nearly three quarters of a million dollars. Chemotherapy is fifty to a hundred grand PER TREATMENT in the cycle of six so $600K is what ONE cycle of chemo costs. Think about that—and you'll know why cancer policies are sold. **EIGHTY PERCENT OF EVERY ONCOLOGIST'S INCOME IS FAILED CHEMOTHERAPY TREATMENTS and oncologists BUY the DRUGS for the Patient's chemo MARK THEM UP ABOUT 10,000% AND RE-SELL THEM TO THE PATIENT.** Think about that one too. Luckily for my sister, she (although it didn't matter because she was BRCA1+) had great health insurance and ironically as her late husband was in insurance sales and died of cancer, she also had a cancer policy. I have always found that to be eerily prescient of her. Carl was a great insurance salesman and he had a unique motto:"Buy life insurance—it doesn't have to be a sad day for everybody!" It did take her 6 months for disability payments from Social Security to start up, but of course if she went back to work they stopped immediately. Just one more way the government screws us out of our own money. While the BRCA1 genetic defect along with late discovery of the cancer at stage 3-C prevented her from beating the cancer I strongly believed that the root cause was the fertility drug Clomid or possibly the fact that we both used baby powder our whole lives which is now supposed to cause ovarian cancer. There's now a 6 month lifetime limit of Clomid administration now, but 20 years ago it was not in place and she took it for over THREE YEARS. There's a strong link between Clomid and ovarian cancer. Lori had THREE PRIMARY CANCERS including triple negative breast cancer, ovarian and uterine cancer and the BRCA1 genetic defect may have prevented her medical treatment from working on the cellular level. There is a lot of anecdotal evidence as well as some research showing that when one carries the BRCA1 genetic defect that your immune system will NOT gear up as effectively to fight the cancer cells which is what helps let it get started, but the major killer of cancer patients is chemotherapy,

MASS MURDERING DOCTORS: THE TRUTH ABOUT ONCOLOGISTS, CHEMOTHERAPY AND CANCER

not the cancer. 50% of cancer patients die from the chemotherapy long before the cancer would have killed them—FIFTY PERCENT!

Three primary cancers is a medical condition that does NOT appear in nature. It is exposure to SOMETHING. In my sister's case I believe it's Clomid or talc that we both used our whole lives. There is a lot of research into this at the moment as the huge numbers of ovarian cancer among former users of Clomid is a huge red flag. Clomid is an old drug, commonly prescribed for fertility issues and is still on the market. I believe it should be taken off the market but it's profitable and effective. Clomid does what it's supposed to do—help women get pregnant. Sadly, far too many women are greeted with ovarian cancer as their college freshman leaves for school and they don't make the connection between the two as it was 20 years ago when they took the drug and the BRCA1+ and BRCA2+ carriers die from it for previously stated reasons. I think that there should be a genetic test given to women seeking fertility drugs because of the cancer risk. It's too high for BRCA1/2 women and I believe future research will bear this out. I beg you all to use my family's loss to prevent a similar loss in your family, it is why I am writing this!

Prophylactic surgical removal of the ovaries has been offered for many years as a potential preventative of ovarian cancer in women deemed to be at increased hereditary risk for this disease. Now, it is possible to test for specific mutations of the BRCA1 and BRCA2 genes that render members of hereditary breast ovarian cancer (HBOC) syndrome families susceptible to cancer. Widespread intra-abdominal or peritoneal carcinomatosis, which mimics metastatic ovarian serous carcinoma, has been reported following oophorectomy in individuals at increased hereditary risk. This study was undertaken to examine and report particularly the occurrence of intra-abdominal carcinomatosis, as well as other cancers, following prophylactic oophorectomy in patients who carry cancer susceptibility mutations of BRCA1 and BRCA2 and to assess the cumulative risks for this disease in order to assist in developing appropriate surgical interventions, based on currently available information, and to counsel patients who choose prophylactic surgery, concerning the potential prognosis, thereafter. The calculated cumulative risks of developing intra-abdominal carcinomatosis after prophylactic oophorectomy in members of HBOC syndrome families, specifically those who carry deleterious mutations, are well below the estimated risks of ovarian cancer published in the literature for similar patients. Breast cancers, which tended to be small and localized, were the most common malignancy in BRCA1 and BRCA2 mutation carriers after prophylactic oophorectomy. Prophylactic oophorectomy has been recommended in patients with a strongly positive family history for ovarian carcinoma. A prophylactic oophorectomy does not afford complete protection in women with familial ovarian cancer syndrome. Any tissue derived from the coelomic epithelium may potentially undergo malignant transformation. Prophylactic oophorectomy remains a controversial issue among gynecological surgeons. A woman's history of hereditary ovarian cancer syndrome is currently considered the most important indication for prophylactic oophorectomy. This is because of the high risk of ovarian cancer developing in these women and the poor prognosis that is generally associated with ovarian cancer. The purpose of prophylactic oophorectomy in women with no family history of hereditary ovarian cancer syndrome who present for hysterectomy because of other gynecological indications is, however, less clear. The attitude of the patients toward removal of normal ovaries deserves special consideration when counseling for prophylactic oophorectomy in this group of women. Knowledge about the risk of ovarian cancer in the conserved ovaries, cancer phobia, possible psychological effects of prophylactic oophorectomy, and the need for long-term hormone replacement therapy if prophylactic oophorectomy is carried out, are all important considerations in the counseling process but with documentation as a BRCA1/2+ the risk is so high that insurance companies leap to pay for the surgery in hope of avoiding having to pay for million-dollar chemotherapy in the future. Prophylactic oophorectomy in pre-menopausal women has been recommended to prevent ovarian cancer. Ovarian cancer is the fourth leading cause of cancer deaths in American women. About 10% of cases are thought to have a hereditary basis, and family history is the strongest known risk factor. In the past, prophylactic oophorectomy has been advocated for women with two or more affected first-degree relatives. More recently, with the identification of the genes responsible for most hereditary ovarian cancers (BRCA1, BRCA2), oophorectomy can now be offered specifically to women who are mutation carriers. Conversely, non-carriers in these families can be reassured that their risk of ovarian cancer is not increased. The value of oophorectomy in mutation carriers has not yet been proven, however, and concern exists that the benefit may be less than intuitively expected.   However, serous carcinoma of the peritoneum, which is indistinguishable from ovarian carcinoma, can and does occur after oophorectomy in BRCA+ women. In view of the uncertainty regarding the efficacy of prophylactic oophorectomy, chemo-preventive and early detection approaches also deserve consideration as strategies for decreasing ovarian cancer mortality in women who carry mutations in ovarian cancer susceptibility genes. It's also now believed that ovarian cancer begins at the fimbriated ends of the Fallopian tubes rather than in the ovaries so they should always be removed as well. Hereditary ovarian cancers exhibit distinct clinical pathologic features compared with sporadic cancers. The cumulative lifetime risk of ovarian cancer is 40% to 50% for BRCA1 mutation carriers and 20% to 30% for BRCA2 mutation carriers. Both BRCA proteins participate in transcriptional regulation of gene expression as well as the recognition or repair of certain forms of DNA damage, particularly double-strand breaks.

Most ovarian cancers associated with germ line BRCA mutations are diagnosed at a younger age and are high-grade and advanced-stage serous carcinomas. BRCA mutations do not seem to play a significant role in the development of mucinous or borderline ovarian tumors. Hereditary ovarian cancers have a distinctly better clinical outcome with longer overall survival and recurrence-free interval after chemotherapy than sporadic cancers. Women with a family history including 2 or more first- or second-degree relatives with either ovarian cancer alone or both breast and ovarian cancers should undertake prophylactic oophorectomy immediately after childbearing has been completed to reduce the risk of ovarian cancer. Unfortunately, despite an initial response to chemotherapy in the majority of patients, relapse is a frequent problem and is often detected by a rise in the serum tumor marker CA-125 in the absence of symptoms or signs of disease by physical examination or radiographic studies. In such cases, a hormonal maneuver is oftentimes considered in order to avoid the toxic effects of chemotherapy when the patient is asymptomatic and the goal of treatment is largely palliation, although eventually the development of clinical progression mandates the institution of second-line chemotherapy. If the treatment-free interval is > 6 months from the completion of first-line treatment, treatment with the same 40 YEAR OLD platinum-based chemotherapy is STILL considered a reasonable first step, even though there are no survivors. For those patients who develop resistance to second-line platinum or who have difficulty tolerating this agent, multiple other options are available for relapse management, including liposomal doxorubicin, topotecan, gemcitabine and etoposide. Eventually the disease becomes resistant to multiple chemotherapy agents, and reorienting management toward supportive care and pain control is necessary until they kill you. Ongoing efforts to identify more effective multi-agent first-line regimens, to develop more effective strategies for early detection and to incorporate agents with novel mechanisms of action, such as anti-angiogenesis compounds (which should be a front-line treatment and would be if it were as profitable as poisoning patients with chemo) that have no chance of success. The only way that High-grade serous-cell carcinoma is survivable is IF the first surgery gets it all AND THERE IS NO RECURRENCE. Chemo makes this cancer immortal and when it relapses, put your affairs in order because there are NO survivors when HGSC recurs as peritoneal carcinomatosis. Low-grade serous-cell, clear-cell and stromal-cell have some known survivors but not high-grade serous-cell. Epithelial (HGSC) ovarian cancer is always fatal, and is the number one cause of death of all the gynecological cancers. It's the only known "Weed-and-Seed" cancer.

CHAPTER TWO: THE SEARCH FOR MY SURGEON

One would think it would be easy to handle this. Find a surgeon and make an appointment, schedule the surgery, have it done and recover. This is not the case in the age of the horrific insurance "reforms" commonly called Obamacare. It has totally destroyed medical care and placed the government in the doctor's office with us. This is not an opinion about what a mess Obamacare is, just a sidebar on to how much more difficult it is to find and get competent care with health insurance in such disarray with tons of ridiculous paperwork that exponentially LOWERS our quality of care by forcing doctors to demonstrate compliance with the outrageous and expensive boondoggle that is Obamacare rather than focus on patient care.

I searched the website of my insurance provider to find the best surgeon I could find. I went to every medical ratings website and cross-checked them against each other and against court records for medical malpractice cases my choices were involved in.

MASS MURDERING DOCTORS: THE TRUTH ABOUT ONCOLOGISTS, CHEMOTHERAPY AND CANCER

Then I checked the lists against disciplinary records with the State Medical Boards in Missouri and Illinois. Your care and outcome are directly related to the competence of your doctor and due diligence is a very important part of the search for the right doctor. While a medical malpractice suit or two is common in these litigious times, a large number of them should be a huge red flag. For a hysterectomy you will need an OB-GYN specialist and they are commonly sued for malpractice even when it's not their fault something went wrong. Most of the OB-GYN suits are for damaged babies in these days of plaintiff mining and advertising for large numbers of plaintiffs. Take this into account during your search and expect to find five to ten cases even with the BEST of surgeons. I finally settled on Dr. James DallaRiva who was rated the best surgeon in town and his partner was rated the second best surgeon in town. Their office staff had horrific ratings (which were justified in my experience with them, the front window wench who is in charge of the sign-in clipboard is a first rate c**t) although I thought Cindy and Teri, (his surgical scheduler) were wonderful. I didn't factor the office staff into my doctor choice decision, in since I was never going to have to see him again after the initial consultation and surgical follow-up visit. If I had been pregnant and/or seeking regular care, I might have made a different decision rather than dealing with the window wench regularly for 9 months. However, since I make my internist do my gynecological work, I don't see a separate doctor and she gets to make a few extra bucks.

After you settle on a surgeon, you will need to make an appointment (and probably get a referral depending on the terms of your insurance coverage) to see the surgeon of your choice. Make a list of questions to ask. Pay attention to the demeanor of your surgeon and also his office staff. Many doctors have TERRIBLE office staff and if his office staff is terrible you won't be happy with him or her. Most of the doctor rating websites have a section to rate the staff—pay attention to what they say as it WILL make a difference. I have seen great doctors with office staff so horrid that I went elsewhere just because the office staff was comprised of miserable bitches that were impossible to deal with. I can't understand why Dr. DallaRiva keeps this woman employed, but his management standards aren't my problem. I've found the window wenches in most doctor's offices at least try to be civil, with the ones at Dr. Janet's office being so very sweet. Most of the miserable ones are behind a 1/16th inch of

MASS MURDERING DOCTORS: THE TRUTH ABOUT ONCOLOGISTS, CHEMOTHERAPY AND CANCER

glass that they think will protect them from an enraged, hormonal, pregnant and crazed woman when they treat her like crap. I would pay a $20 cover charge to be there on the day one of these window wenches goes too far and one of these hormonal-crazed women snatches the window wench by the hair and drags her through the window. The way this woman treats Dr. DallaRiva's patients means it's just a matter of time before this happens. I just want to watch—and laugh my ass off.

Doctors as a rule are usually lousy businessmen and don't realize that since we are now customers rather than patients we're not going to put up with abuse from his office staff when there are so many doctors out there to choose from. However, I was looking for a technically excellent surgeon and his bedside manner and office staff were not my primary concern. However, to my delight, Dr. DallaRiva turned out to be wonderful all the way around, (other than leaving the cancer that recurred behind which I thought wasn't his fault until he told my husband about a "tacky patch" he left behind) and I was glad I went to him. He's a right guy and he gets me. I also believed at the time that he saved my life but I don't any more since it took me 9 weeks and 18 calls, 12 messages and a nasty Facebook post to shame him on social media to get his staff to give me my surgery report—like he was hiding something.

Excellent surgeons tend to be rather abrupt as they feel bedside manner and hand-holding are for Primary Care doctors. This is an observation rather than a slam. After more than 30 surgeries in my lifetime, I don't look for bedside manner as much as I look for surgical talent combined with technical competence. Dr. DallaRiva is one of the few surgeons that successfully combine both, so it was a plus for him.

I made my appointment and was happy that his office staff (other than the wretched window wench) didn't live up to their online reputation. Luckily, Dr. DallaRiva was everything I could have hoped for so I scheduled my surgery for 4 days later, February 12, 2016. Women who carry inherited mutations in the genes BRCA1 or BRCA2 have a lifetime risk of breast cancer of more than 80 percent, as well as a high risk of ovarian cancer, according to the most comprehensive study to date of these women and their families. The study, published by The New York Breast Cancer Study Group in the Oct. 24 edition of Science, also found that many women with these inherited mutations come from families with few if any reports of breast or ovarian cancer. The good news from the study is that even among women at very high risk, exercise and healthy weight as an adolescent delayed the onset of breast cancer.

"It was a surprise, but a source of hope, to learn that factors over which we have some control made a difference in the age at which these highest-risk women developed breast cancer," said the lead author, Mary-Claire King, Ph.D. King is American Cancer Society Professor of Genome Sciences and Medicine in the University of Washington School of Medicine in Seattle and a pioneer in the study of the link between inherited genetic alterations and disease. "Women with inherited mutations were at extremely high risk, but exercise and appropriate weight during their adolescent years clearly delayed the onset of breast cancer." (I fail to see how they can prove this considering that you can't count what doesn't happen, so it's essentially research bullcrap on a par with the hoax that is global warming.)

"The possibility that lifestyle changes such as increased exercise and weight control could modify the impact of genetic risk has very intriguing implications, not only for BRCA-related cancers but for other breast cancers as well," said Dr. Larry Norton, head of the Division of Solid Tumor Oncology and Norna S. Serafim Chair in Clinical Oncology at Memorial Sloan-Kettering Cancer Center. The research was conducted with financial support from The Breast Cancer Research Foundation of New York.

Courtesy of: https://www.sciencedaily.com/releases/2003/10/031024063314.htm?trendmd-shared=0

CHAPTER THREE: THE FIRST STEP: MY HYSTERECTOMY

I arrived at Anderson Hospital for my pre-surgery blood work and EKG two days before my surgery. Defensive medicine is the name of the game these days, so you will have to run around and do a lot of pre-surgery testing to make sure you don't die on the table. The better your general state of health means the less testing you will have to endure. Luckily for me, Monica at Anderson was terrific. She got me in and we went over the paperwork for consent and such, and she was very good at her job.

I also STRONGLY recommend you read and strike out and initial any changes you want to make in the boilerplate agreement they will give you to sign. Hospitals are FAMOUS for getting patients to accept financial liability for all your bills but you do

MASS MURDERING DOCTORS: THE TRUTH ABOUT ONCOLOGISTS, CHEMOTHERAPY AND CANCER

NOT have to accept it. They also don't care about making sure that the other doctors ("Providers") they use for your anesthesia are on your insurance as they will just stick you with the bill and then sue you if you don't, won't or can't pay for it when your insurance denies the claim. Most people do not realize you can make changes to the agreement. **Two you should definitely add to the agreement are:**

1. <u>**Do NOT accept financial responsibility for bills not covered by your health insurance.**</u> If you are on an HMO you are NOT required to pay for anything other than your contracted co-pays UNLESS YOU AGREE TO IT BY ACCEPTING FINANCIAL RESPONSIBILITY. You do not have to accept it and they cannot refuse treatment if you don't accept it. They have a CONTRACT with your insurance company and they are required to live up to it. Draw a line through the sentence that reads something like: "I accept responsibility for all charges not paid by my insurance company, etc." and initial it. At the bottom also write these words: **"I do not accept financial responsibility for any charges not paid by my insurance company."** This prevents huge bills being sent directly to you in order for you to fight it out with your insurance provider. Most people accept it without realizing they do NOT have to do so and are sent huge bills where NO attempt by the hospital has been made to collect the bill from your insurance company AND you are billed for payments higher than what the rate is that the hospital is contracted to provide services to you. For example if you have a hysterectomy, your insurance has a "Fee Schedule" that pays $3500 to the hospital for your surgery. Now of course the hospital would like to have more money for your services and IF YOU ACCEPT RESPONSIBILITY they will bill you for another $2500 OR MORE than the contracted fee for your service and YOU WILL BE OBLIGATED TO PAY IT. "Why?" you ask. **Because you AGREED TO PAY IT by accepting financial responsibility** and they WILL come after you for the money, **read the agreement, it tells you they will and also bill you for the collection and legal fees to sue you.**

2. <u>**Write the words: "I do NOT authorize and WILL NOT PAY FOR treatment by ANY PROVIDER not listed as an authorized provider on my insurance plan."**</u> If you don't do this, the hospital will call in anyone they want to call in and

send you the bill for it. They tell you it's not their job to make sure the provider is on your plan, and doctors are famous for calling in their buddies for "assistance" and billing YOU for their services when your insurance refuses to pay for an "out of network" provider. Without writing the above statement on your admittance forms, you WILL get the bill and they will do their best to collect it along with interest, penalties and legal fees for THEIR attorneys. Why go through this along with all the other stress when you are NOT legally required to accept responsibility as part of the conditions of being admitted and treated by the hospital? Hospitals like to brush off your concerns with a line like "Oh—that's just standard boilerplate language, just sign it." Believe me when I tell you that **NO BOILERPLATE AGREEMENT IS EVER WRITTEN TO YOUR ADVANTAGE. EVER.** They are ALWAYS written to benefit the party who wants you to sign it.

After you decline financial responsibility and refuse treatment by any provider not on your plan, you can be pretty sure you won't be getting a huge surprise bill in the mail while you are recovering from your surgery. Believe me when I tell you that writing these few word on EVERY SINGLE FORM you are ever asked to sign will save you money and stress—even in the doctor's office write these words on the consent forms. READ EVERY WORD on the forms because they wouldn't be there if they weren't important—and the smaller the print the more important the information.

There are many places on these forms that are asking for your consent to test you for all kinds of things AND SHARE THE INFORMATION with those you may not wish to be informed—the government comes immediately to mind. Read the entire agreement AND **DO NOT BE HURRIED OR PRESSURED** (if you are bleeding to death/life-threatening condition have your spouse/whomever read it and make the changes while you go get your life saved) into signing something you haven't read. I know that the agreement is long and boring but it is a **LEGAL DOCUMENT** and it is also a BINDING contract. The smaller the print, the more important the information it contains. **Don't screw yourself by not looking over the agreement because believe me when I tell you the hospital's lawyers sweated over every word to make SURE it was to their advantage and so did the doctor's office.** Protect yourself because no one else will—and that's some solid truth.

MASS MURDERING DOCTORS: THE TRUTH ABOUT ONCOLOGISTS, CHEMOTHERAPY AND CANCER

After the EKG and the blood draw, there was just the wait for surgery. Being BRCA1+ means you don't wait months for surgery. I saw Dr. DallaRiva for the first time on Monday February 8th 2016. I had my surgery four days later on February 12, 2016. Time is of the essence when you are in your 50s and BRCA1+ because your risk of cancer is 87% by the time you turn 71 years old. Think about that number for a few minutes. It means that of every hundred women who are BRCA1+ EIGHTY-SEVEN of them will have cancer by age seventy. Almost NINE OUT OF TEN will have cancer by age seventy. That's a huge risk. It's why my insurance company was willing to pay for a full hysterectomy, and is ALSO willing to pay for a double mastectomy and reconstruction for what they know AT THIS MOMENT are healthy ovaries, uterus, Fallopian tubes and breasts with no CURRENT diagnosis of cancer. They do NOT expect to find cancer in my reproductive system yet they are STILL willing to pay tens of thousands of dollars to remove my CURRENTLY HEALTHY reproductive system, my CURRENTLY HEALTHY breasts and additionally pay to have them reconstructed.

What do you think that says about what my risk of contracting very expensive to treat cancer? It says that they think my risk of cancer is SO HIGH that they are willing to pay a lot of money to keep from having to pay even more for exponentially more expensive cancer treatment. If you have family history of ovarian and breast cancer and fit the other pieces as well, you NEED TO BE TESTED. Being DOCUMENTED as a BRCA1+ or BRCA2+ and having it on your records means doctors will look harder at symptoms that could be cancer rather than just blowing you off. I would NEVER have gotten a covered and paid-for hysterectomy with ZERO symptoms and a normal value CA-125 test (0-35 is normal, I was 16, my sister was over 1100 when she went for her last surgery) if I hadn't been a documented BRCA1+, there's NO WAY they would have paid for it. GET THE TEST! It made the difference (hopefully) between life and death, because if I hadn't been BRCA1+ and documented as such, I would have to have been showing symptoms of something LIKE MY BABY SISTER and by then it would be too late, I would be terminal—just like her, so GET TESTED!! If you want to save your life, you have to be proactive. She wasn't a documented BRCA1+ so the idiot gastroenterologist gave her antacids for 8 MONTHS and until her routine mammogram revealed sub-clinical breast cancer NOTHING WAS DONE TO CHECK FOR CANCER UNTIL SHE WENT IN FOR A DOUBLE MASTECTOMY. Finally they did a

MASS MURDERING DOCTORS: THE TRUTH ABOUT ONCOLOGISTS, CHEMOTHERAPY AND CANCER

CT which revealed—you guessed it—HGSC. Had she been a documented BRCA1 she would have been scanned for cancer with the first visit to the gastroenterologist and might have had a chance to survive it. They drained nearly a GALLON of MALIGNANT ascites out of her belly in the hospital and she never had a chance, she bought some time but because she bought into the lie that is chemotherapy, she was doomed from the get-go. Chemo will not help you survive ovarian cancer, but it WILL ensure that you die miserable, bald, scrawny and vomiting.

We all know how insurance companies hate to part with money. That they are willing and eager to pay for all this surgery for me with no cancer diagnosis speaks volumes about just how dangerous it is to have this genetic defect and how huge my risk must be or they would roll the dice. The knowledge of this is what made me decide to have the surgery, because the price of knowing about my genetic defect was my little sister's LIFE because she was BRCA1+ as well but no one KNEW so she went to a gastroenterologist who spent 8 months telling her she had "Irritable Bowel Syndrome" which virtually NEVER presents for the first time after age 50 (she was 54) when she had a belly swollen SO FULL of ascites and cancer that she looked 6 months pregnant and it wasn't until her MAMMOGRAM showed breast cancer and she went into the hospital for a mastectomy that her ovarian high-grade serous-cell carcinoma was diagnosed. The takeaway from this is that my orphaned niece is suing the living crap out of him for medical malpractice and a chaser of wrongful death and he has it coming without a doubt. However, had she been DOCUMENTED as a BRCA1+ there's a possibility the incompetent doctor MIGHT have figured out she didn't have IBS!

CHAPTER 4: SURGERY DAY

Four days later I was being prepped for a total hysterectomy. Ovaries, uterus, Fallopian tubes, cervix; like a fire sale: Everything must go! I have a double mastectomy planned in April or May when I recover from the hysterectomy and a mammogram as soon as possible. Hubby and I arrive at the hospital and I change into my spiffy hospital gown complete with stupid crunchy, papery booties and the weird hairnet hat. Dr. DallaRiva shows up and talks to me briefly. I can't wait to get this over with so that I don't have to worry about cancer any more. When I have the mastectomy and reconstruction, I will be happy to have it done with. The

MASS MURDERING DOCTORS: THE TRUTH ABOUT ONCOLOGISTS, CHEMOTHERAPY AND CANCER

hysterectomy is the first step on the road to preventing the cancer that killed my baby sister. The anesthesiologist comes by and we chat briefly and he orders up my favorite happy juice combo: Versed and Demerol and the very sweet nurses start pushing them into my IV line. I am comfortable and woozy and on my way to the operating room. I apparently put up a little struggle with the mask after they numbed my throat for the intubation tube and the last thing I remember is trying to push the mask away as I am a little tiny bit claustrophobic and the local anesthetic made my throat feel like it was thick and closing and I panicked with the mask over my mouth and nose and the last thing I remember was fighting to push the mask off my face and I apologize to the sweet anesthesiologist for that. I'm sorry, I was on drugs!!

The next thing I remember is pain like the worst combination of severe menstrual cramps along with abdominal cramps that feel like I spent a week in Mexico and drank ALL the water I could swallow. I feel like I have been gang-raped by the Jolly Green Giant and his coven of giant friends. My throat is raw from the intubation tubes and as luck would have it, I vomited several times—that wonderful green acid-filled bile that burns like fire—the kind you dry-heave when you've been food poisoned on a Carnival Cruise to and from HELL—but that's another story. Don't cruise Carnival by the way, feel free to ask me why—nothing I love more than telling the story of how Carnival food poisoned me and the swell kitchen tour that showed me why it happened. I had told Dr. DallaRiva to give me Phenergan for nausea but he ordered up the brand new anti-nausea drug Zofran—which causes me to projectile vomit. At least I got my Demerol, Dilaudid is like speed for me.

I was beyond miserable when my angel nurse Irene gave me an IV push of Demerol. There's nothing better than feeling pain stop hurting along with the rush of an intravenous push of a scheduled narcotic—I can sure see how people get addicted to it. My doctor has also popped in a Foley catheter so I don't even have to get out of bed to urinate. Irene brings me more Demerol every 3 hours with an IV push and the vomiting stops after 3 or 4 episodes. I suck ice cubes for my sore throat and try to sip water. I also have a HUGE maternity sanitary pad strapped between my legs that's about the size of an ironing board but WAY less comfortable. I know I'm going to be compelled to get up and sit in the chair at some point this evening and I am not

MASS MURDERING DOCTORS: THE TRUTH ABOUT ONCOLOGISTS, CHEMOTHERAPY AND CANCER

looking forward to it. Dr. DallaRiva stops by and tells me everything went well and he didn't see anything to worry about and that he will call me ONLY if there is a problem with the pathology as my organs were sent to a lab to be checked for cancer.

Later that evening my wonderful husband stops by and offers me food or anything else and I am sore, miserable and totally not in the mood to eat or have visitors. My night nurse, Kathi comes in with Irene and she's just the best nurse as well. They have different personalities but both of them are the best nurses I've had in a hospital in a long time. I'm in the maternity ward at Anderson Hospital where they have the sweetest nurses (at every hospital the nicest nurses work in L&D). Kathi tells me she's had the same surgery done by my doctor and that he's wonderful and I don't need to worry about a thing. She tells me that the first 8-10 hours are the very worst and I will start feeling better in a few hours. I got up for a few minutes and sat in the chair while my husband and mother in law were visiting but I still felt pretty bad so I went back to bed and they went home. Kathi dropped by with some more Demerol and pushed it into my IV and about 10 pm I started feeling much better just as she had predicted. She disconnected my IV drip but left the saline lock for medication administration and we talked a bit. She brought me a little smorgasbord of red jello, chocolate pudding and some graham crackers (that were really FRESH and crispy too) and I was hungry and ate them all and a second round as well. Graham crackers dipped in chocolate pudding are very good by the way, and I was feeling better and the next morning as planned, I was released from the hospital and sent home with orders to take it easy for the next two weeks. He told me that he would not call me unless there was a problem with the biopsy and that everything looked normal. I dressed and left the hospital and went home to recover under the watchful eyes of my husband and my mother in law. I was sore but not suffering terribly although I still felt like I had been gang-raped by the Jolly Green Giant & Co.

The next few days I hung out around the house, making plans for work and deciding I should write all this down as it would be cathartic. It would also be a tale that would help other women who have a background similar to mine. If after reading my story they got tested and prevented cancer by proactive surgery like I have done and even one life was saved from the terrible death of cancer then the effort would be more than worth it. I was planning getting on with my life and thinking of having the double mastectomy in the summer—perhaps in June or July. Then the other shoe dropped and suddenly my journey through BRCA1+ took another twist.

CHAPTER 5: "SURPRISE, SURPRISE, SURPRISE!" (AS GOMER PYLE USED TO LIKE TO SAY).

On February 18th I was working on writing the story you are reading. The phone rang. When I answered it, the woman on the other end told me that she worked for Dr. DallaRiva and he wanted to see me. TODAY. At that moment I knew that this story was about to end much differently than I had originally believed. I bullied her over the phone until she told me what I already knew from the second she identified herself. I have cancer. High-grade Serous Carcinoma that was at least Stage 2-A in my ovaries and not sure of the stage of the cancer in my uterus. Both my ovaries had cancer and so did my uterus. I did what every normal, successful well-adjusted career woman would do at this moment: I started to cry uncontrollably.

I called my husband at work and told him he needed to come home. He demanded to know what was going on and I didn't want to tell him because I didn't want him to be upset on the 35 minute drive home but he made me tell him. He came home and we talked and Dr. DallaRiva called and told me that he wanted me to see an oncologist immediately and that I probably should have the double mastectomy immediately. I thought I had escaped the BRCA1+ cancer fate but my journey was now longer and much more complicated that I thought it would be, but I wasn't too worried. It was early and they said they got it all and I'd see the oncologist as a precaution and go on living life. This was before started researching my cancer. I had NO idea what I was up against and I wasn't expecting to have to battle the Genghis Khan of cancer. I just figured that I might have to have a second surgery (which after 30+ surgeries is—to ME—about on a par with having my TEETH CLEANED since I've been through it so many times for assorted injuries). So, I was pretty chill about it since I didn't think it was a big deal because I didn't know much about ovarian cancer other than it was a bad one but "early detection is the key to the cure" and all that BS lulled me into a false sense of security. Also, I did not know there were several different kinds of ovarian cancer and not knowing what kind of ovarian cancer my sister had because

MASS MURDERING DOCTORS: THE TRUTH ABOUT ONCOLOGISTS, CHEMOTHERAPY AND CANCER

my asshole ex-brother in law wouldn't tell any of us anything, I had not been able to research her cancer or find out anything other than "ovarian cancer" which I DID look up and there were several different kinds and most of them very survivable—other than high-grade serous carcinoma—and at the time we did NOT know we were both BRCA1 genetic defect carriers that almost exclusively get HGSC. It's how we die, apparently.

I still get the cold chills when I think about how I wanted to put off the hysterectomy until summer of 2017 and my husband John was adamantly against it and nagged me to get my butt in to the surgeon so that I wouldn't GET ovarian cancer. It was all for nothing because we are too late. While I sat with my parents and my sister putting on a brave front for her, and pretending that we believed her when she said she was going to be OK, the same cancer that killed her came to kill me as well. I had ZERO clue that I had cancer. NONE. I was totally asymptomatic and assumed that Dr. DallaRiva was taking out healthy ovaries, uterus, cervix and Fallopian tubes. I felt fine, healthy and happy with no pains of any sort or ANY KIND OF WARNING that the most deadly of all reproductive cancers was taking up residence in my reproductive system to kill me.

I never dreamed I could have cancer. NEVER. Not in a million years did I think that fate would be so cruel to my parents or my beloved husband. I was now faced with the reality that a mere 12 weeks—90 DAYS to the DAY—after my parents watched their other daughter die from a ruptured esophagus brought on by chemo-induced vomiting; that there was now a very real probability that they would bury me as well. I didn't think I could tell them and that they would be better off NOT knowing anything until or unless I was declared terminal. My sister's cancer was extremely aggressive. In October of 2014 she was diagnosed as stage zero breast cancer and on November 18th 2015 she died of the stage 4 ovarian cancer (later I found out she died from the chemo, NOT cancer) that her belly was full of—discovered accidentally during her hospital stay for her mastectomy. Now all I can think of is whether or not the same fate awaits me. Am I going to die from this?

Dr. DallaRiva appeared to be extremely concerned and told me his office was setting up an appointment with "the best gynecological oncologist" in St. Louis. I couldn't

MASS MURDERING DOCTORS: THE TRUTH ABOUT ONCOLOGISTS, CHEMOTHERAPY AND CANCER

think about anything but that I needed to get the double mastectomy done as soon as possible and start the most aggressive chemotherapy that was available to me. No matter how bad I felt or how much I puked or if my hair all fell out, I HAD planned to pursue aggressive treatment. I believe with all my heart that if I die from this cancer that it will kill both my elderly parents. They stressed out and suffered horribly through my sister's battle with cancer, culminating in watching her die in front of them as she bled to death from the ruptured esophagus brought on by chemo-induced vomiting. I just didn't see how I could put them through the hellish deja vu of another adult child having to battle cancer with the outcome possibly being the same. I am writing this as I go through this so as I write, I do not know if I will die or not by the end of this story—that's ONE way to keep you turning the pages! Most writers know how their story will end, but I do not have that luxury. My story is literally happening as I write. It's now a first-person account of the nightmare of cancer in the age of the worse nightmare that is Obamacare in 2016. Instead of a loving tribute to my sister I was writing so that other women with family cancer history would get the BRCA1 test and possibly be saved Lori's fate, I am now swept up in my sister's story. It has become OUR story not just her brave battle. Every day when I have to deal with the horrible program that is Obamacare; I swear to myself that when I get better I am going to lobby non-stop to repeal this horrific assault on our health insurance and health care because it is horrible beyond words. I already had health insurance and it was excellent and Obamacare ruined my plan and cost me my doctor of 10 years so I am NOT a fan. It doubled the cost of my health insurance and halved my coverage. Obamacare is the worst law in the long sad story of bad politics and history will excoriate Obama for it.

They say there are seven stages of loss. I've experienced several in a very short time. First, there was disbelief which lasted about 3 minutes. Then grief which I cried my way out of in about 5 minutes. Then there was anger which is where I am right now. I'm PISSED OFF. Really really really pissed off. How DARE this cancer return to further torment my family? Hasn't it taken ENOUGH?? My grandmother. My sister. My sister's children and grandchildren who are all potentially BRCA1+ and maybe me as well. With it comes the stress and worry that if I tell my parents that they will not hold up for a second round of a child with cancer—and the very real possibility that if my

MASS MURDERING DOCTORS: THE TRUTH ABOUT ONCOLOGISTS, CHEMOTHERAPY AND CANCER

cancer is as virulent and aggressive as Lori's—and I have since discovered I have the exact same kind of cancer that killed her—that in their late 70s (Mom) and mid-80s (Dad) they will bury a second child in a short time. My brother was not gifted with the BRCA1 gene so he is safe and so are his children. It won't follow them through their lives with a constant threat. How can this be happening to my family AGAIN—wasn't losing Lori enough? It's not fair—but instead of whining and self-pity which I've always found totally counter-productive, I'm so mad I could spit!

I went to dinner with my husband and we talked about what to do. He told me my parents have a right to know and that I need to tell them. I disagree. They can't do anything but worry and stress out. Why do they need to know? There's plenty of time to tell them if it turns out I am not going to make it. However, they will be upset if I don't tell them. I decided to talk to my dad's wife, Elke. She's my stepmother and we are close. She's also not an ethnic American, she is a German national who is a naturalized citizen. She is smart, kindhearted, but also stoic and pragmatic, which is something I could use a good dose of right about now. She and my dad have been married for 20+ years. If I knew NOTHING else about her, that my father loves her and seeing how happy he is every time I see him would be all I would ever need to know. She's a lovely person and I love her like a second mom. At 75, she is still working full time and owns her own business and another one with my dad. She looks about 65 and she is a terrific wife to my dad. I call Elke and we talk and she tells me that I must tell my father, but that I should wait until Monday. Dad is studying and is taking the re-licensing continuing education courses the state of Florida requires to renew his professional license. Dad is an eye doctor and one of the best there is in the state of Florida and probably the South. At 87, he still sees patients and has no plans to retire. He told me that if he stopped working that he would have nothing to do but sit on the couch, watch TV and wait to die. He wants to keep working because he says it is good for him. He must be right as he also looks about 65 and is sharp as a tack. If you didn't KNOW he was 87, you would NEVER know and most people are stunned to find out he's 87. I dig my dad—he's a great guy and even though he is the source of my BRCA1 genetic defect, I don't care. He's been the best dad anyone could ever ask for and I wouldn't trade him for anything. Raising a textbook Meyers-Briggs INTP personality with a 167 IQ couldn't have been easy but my dad is a laid back guy and

MASS MURDERING DOCTORS: THE TRUTH ABOUT ONCOLOGISTS, CHEMOTHERAPY AND CANCER

he gets me MOST of the time. My beloved husband John gets me about 99% of the time, and I can see how worried and upset he is as well. I've always been buddies with my dad—he's a lot of fun and has always supported my decisions even when he didn't agree with them. I'm a daddy's girl all the way. My mother and I have a much more complicated relationship. She's way different than my dad, and has a much more volatile personality and we crack heads more than we should at our age but she's mellowing and losing the golden child rocked her—HARD. Mom and my sister Lori never cut the umbilical cord after it was reattached when Lori was first born. She was a very sick infant and my parents were afraid she was going to die as an infant and something my dad and I never understood happened that two weeks. I could never get between Lori and Mom there was no room; no one could—but that's just how it was and since it started when I was only 16 months old, it was never a shock, it was just how things were all my life so I really didn't know that wasn't how it was supposed to be until I got older and by then it was something I was used to—and it didn't matter to me because my dad has always been my hero and there wasn't much room for her in my life either.

Mom and I still have a complicated relationship which was exacerbated during Lori's battle with her cancer. Mom thought I should spend lots of time with Lori but I didn't. Lori and I had 54 years to have a relationship with each other and we never did. We loved each other but we had NOTHING in common. I never had any hostility toward her and as far as I know she never had any toward me. We just weren't close and each of us had very very different lives. She was about home and family and I have gypsy feet—I went off to see the world while she built a hugely successful business in Jupiter, Florida with her salon and day spa. Our contact was family events and she was my hairdresser for 35 years so we talked regularly but that was it. No one got it or understood our relationship but we were both fine with it. If she had wanted me to come spend time with her, she would have said so, and she didn't. So I came to Florida several times to see her while she was sick but I didn't go to the funeral as I just couldn't get away. I was in Chicago on a business trip when Lori died and since it was just before Thanksgiving I couldn't get a flight and they had the funeral the Saturday after Thanksgiving when there were no flights under $1500 even if you could get a seat which I could not. I had to eat a great deal of crap for skipping the funeral,

MASS MURDERING DOCTORS: THE TRUTH ABOUT ONCOLOGISTS, CHEMOTHERAPY AND CANCER

but there were literally hundreds of people there—my dad said he never saw such a funeral crowd even for cops that get killed in the line of duty. Truthfully, I'm stunned they even noticed I wasn't in attendance.

Meanwhile, back to the phone call with my stepmother: Elke and I talk for a while and she is upset. I feel bad having to tell her, but she is my youngest parent at 75 and she's tough. She grew up starving in post-WW II Germany and has been married to my dad for more than 20 years. She tells me to call her anytime and is so wonderfully supportive that I start to cry all over again. I must beat this cancer at all costs because I don't want my dad to die of grief from losing both his daughters; one right after another. I also realized at this point, and for the first time, that the entire time my sister was battling her cancer that mine was silently growing and waiting to strike and now it's trying to kill ME. I had decided to be proactive and have the surgery even though I was sure I didn't have cancer and wasn't going to GET cancer either. God has a sense of humor and a drinking problem. Elke tells me that my dad is studying and asks me to wait until the test is over on Monday February 22, 2016 and I am fine with that. My dad could probably write the book he's studying from, but he doesn't need to be distracted right now. I can't tell my mother yet because she can't keep a secret to save her life and telling her means my dad will know about my cancer about 12 seconds after I hang up the phone.

I am going to have to call my dad in 3 days and tell him some terrible news. I can't put into words how much I do NOT want to do this. My husband (John) tells me he will do it if I can't, but it needs to come from me. I'm really mad now. I'm going to fight this evil disease with everything I have. My family needs me. I can't let them down and I can't lose this fight. Still, telling my dad is going to be equal to having to tell my husband which was the hardest thing I've ever done in my life.

We went out to dinner with some friends, a retired colleague that John used to work with until he retired and his wife. John has known Dr. Knickmeyer for longer than I have but he and Patrice came to our wedding and we've kept in touch after he retired. They are concerned and I asked Dr. Knickmeyer as a parent if he would want to know if his daughter had cancer—in THIS SITUATION—having just lost his other daughter to the SAME cancer just 12 weeks earlier and being 86 years old when she died on top of it. Would he want to know? I told him to think about it and email me and he said he'd get back to me in 24 hours. He's a college professor these days, and he's a smart guy and thoughtful and introspective but he has such a way with words and is a joy to converse with. He sent me such a wonderful contemplative answer that I thought it should be shared with my readers:

SIDEBAR: EMAIL REPLY FROM DR. KNICK

Hey, Teri.

Standing on the deck and watching the clouds stream past the moon, I reflected on your question, and came to this conclusion: Were I your father, I would prefer to be informed. A way of seeing why this seems correct to me is to ask yourself this question: If you were your father, what would you prefer? If worse came to worst, how would your father feel if you had not seen fit to let him know about your illness? The announcement, so close on the heels of his other daughter's death, will certainly be a shock—and it will also be an extraordinarily difficult conversation for you. But will that shock be greater or less if the facts are concealed until some possible point in the future? The great likelihood, as far as I can tell, is that you will pass safely through these shoals, and your father could remain forever in the dark on the matter. But that deprives him both of the opportunity to be afraid for you (and that is indeed a gift), and the chance to rejoice at a favorable outcome. All that said, you know your father, and I do not. Perhaps his physical and emotional state are too fragile to cope with your situation. Nonetheless, I think the considerations above are robust. So there is some more of that common commodity: advice. Free, and as you said earlier today, likely worth its cost. Love, Knick

Thank you Dr. Knick. I'm so blessed to know you and Patrice!

CHAPTER SIX: THE OFFICIAL DIAGNOSIS (WITH LOTS OF TECHNICAL STUFF!!)

The next day I call Dr. DallaRiva and talk to Teri his wonderful surgery scheduler and ask her what is the name of my cancer. She is sweet and helpful and tells me what I need to know, the name of my oncologist and that they are putting all my records and pathology reports in a package and that the oncologist's office will be calling me to set up an appointment. I look up my cancer on the internet so I don't go nuts worrying.

MASS MURDERING DOCTORS: THE TRUTH ABOUT ONCOLOGISTS, CHEMOTHERAPY AND CANCER

I'm looking for some hope and some reassurance that I am going to survive this and that I will not force my parents to attend my funeral while they are still grieving for their other daughter that was killed by this horrific genetic defect that has struck my family for the THIRD time. Will I be third time lucky? Or will I die from this cancer as well? Right now it's CANCER 2, FAMILY 0.

Actually it will be the hospice nurse that kills me if it comes to that. You don't die from the cancer. You die when the amount of medication it takes to control the pain is also enough to stop your heart. Will I leave my husband to fend for himself if I die? I have no idea. I am living this as I write and I don't know how it's going to end. I feel so bad for my husband—who nagged me relentlessly until I had the surgery that I thought was totally unnecessary. If I beat this cancer it will be due solely to John's continuous insistence that I stop screwing around and schedule the surgery as I am a terrible procrastinator—there's always time, right? Except one day the phone rings and a strange voice tells you there isn't any more time. I owe him my life for not relenting and letting me procrastinate to the point where a cure is no longer possible or likely. In the interim, let's talk about it. Meet my cancer:

SIDEBAR: HIGH-GRADE SEROUS CARCINOMA (HGSC)

HGSCs account for approximately 71% of malignant ovarian surface epithelial carcinomas in North America and in Europe, although this subtype is less common in other parts of the world. Almost 90% of HGSCs present with advanced-stage (stage III or IV) disease. Most HGSCs have spread beyond the pelvis at the time of diagnosis, accounting for low median survival times. It is now believed that most HGSCs arise from the distal, fimbriated end of the Fallopian tube, a finding supported by the observation that both familial or sporadic cases of HGSCs have synchronous tubal intraepithelial carcinoma in most cases and that these lesions share *TP53* mutations and immunoreactivity for PAX8, a transcription factor expressed in secretory tubal epithelium; examination of telomere length in tubal intraepithelial carcinomas also supports the tubal lesions being precursors rather than metastases. (The cancer STARTS there, it hasn't SPREAD THERE) The propensity of HGSCs to spread transcelomically, with bulky intraperitoneal disease, makes it challenging to determine the primary site of the serous carcinoma (ovarian, peritoneal, Fallopian tube, among

MASS MURDERING DOCTORS: THE TRUTH ABOUT ONCOLOGISTS, CHEMOTHERAPY AND CANCER

others) in an individual case. The designation 'pelvic HGSC' has been suggested for such cases, to avoid speculation about the primary site. While the primary site (Fallopian tube vs. ovary) has profound implications for screening or prevention strategies, it does not have any implications on the management for advanced-stage HGSCs cancer since everyone dies from it. The biology of ovarian carcinoma differs from that of hematogenously metastasizing tumors (spread through bloodstream with normal circulation carrying the cancer) because ovarian cancer cells primarily disseminate within the peritoneal cavity and are only superficially invasive. However, since the rapidly proliferating tumors compress visceral organs and are only temporarily chemo-sensitive, (responsive to chemotherapy) my kind of high grade serous ovarian adenocarcinoma is a universally deadly disease.

SIDEBAR: MORPHOLOGY OF HGSC (HIGH-GRADE SEROUS CARCINOMA)

Macroscopically, HGSCs of the ovary are usually large, bilateral and demonstrate a mix of solid, cystic and papillary growth. The solid regions are tan-white, and typically contain regions of necrosis and hemorrhage. The carcinoma often invades through the capsule and grows on the surface of the ovary. The Fallopian tube may be overgrown and obliterated; however, sometimes a polypoid tumor growth is seen at the fimbriated end. The omentum often shows diffuse involvement with multiple discreet and coalescing tumor nodules (referred to as 'omental cake'), and the peritoneal surface may be studded with metastatic carcinoma (also called miliary tumors) as this cancer is a weed and seed—it doesn't invade the organs but instead crowds out visceral organ function since the explosive growth and non-responsiveness or immediate chemo-resistance to all known forms of chemo make it virtually impossible to kill. The ONLY chance for survival is an early stage one discovery, no chemo and no recurrence. IV chemo is totally ineffective against HGSC once it recurs as peritoneal carcinomatosis but this doesn't stop oncologists worldwide from poisoning you for profit. Platinum-based chemotherapy for high-risk stage I ovarian cancer does not appear to improve survival over non-platinum regimens. I think that is what pisses me off the most: EVERY SINGLE ONCOLOGIST TRIED TO CHEMO ME WHEN THEY KNEW—HAD TO KNOW—THAT IT IS TOTALLY INEFFECTIVE. This tells you everything you will ever need to know about what kind of scumbag oncologists are—the do not care about your quality of life or that they are killing you for money

MASS MURDERING DOCTORS: THE TRUTH ABOUT ONCOLOGISTS, CHEMOTHERAPY AND CANCER

long before the cancer would kill you—when you are so miserable that death is welcome after the nightmare that is chemotherapy.

This is what I am up against and if Lori's ex-husband, (that jag-off!!) had ever told ANY OF US she had the deadly serious high-grade serous-cell carcinoma and peritoneal carcinomatosis, I would have researched it but he wouldn't tell any of us anything—and she didn't have to die. I begged her to let me help her and she just wouldn't—she was just too scared to do anything and let him make her decisions which were the slash, poison and burn of conventional treatment that has a 2.1% survival rate (ONLY in stage one, so after that, Sayonara baby) which is abysmal and ineffective but SO loved by oncologists and Big Pharma that makes 200 billion in cancer profits a year—every year—and should they ALLOW a cure all; that profit goes up in a puff of smoke. There is never going to be a cure for ANY long-term chronic disease that can be managed with ever-more-expensive medications which are paid for by the now government-required boondoggle that is "Obamacare" that is creating more government intervention in you life. Here's the scam: Insurance; that you are required to buy, is required to pay for prescription medication. The rates will go up for everyone, but the subsidies that are handed out by the federal government will go up as well (and the taxes that pay for them) but Big Pharma KNOWS that they can charge anything because health insurance policies are required to pay them so it's an unending spiral UPWARD with NO end in sight. Hopefully President Trump will get Obamacare repealed and undo all the other crap that Obama and Pelosi crammed down our throats and will clean up the slime that is Washington D.C. and that the voter will send these corrupt House and Senate members home—regardless of party affiliation. But I digress...so back to our regularly scheduled medical information! Reading and learning about what a killer cancer I am up against is TERRIFYING and for the first time I realize than not only am I in trouble, I am very probably going to DIE from this killer cancer. I am seriously scared!

SIDEBAR: THIS CANCER CAME TO KILL ME AND IT JUST MIGHT SUCCEED

The statistics on ovarian cancer is grim. 69% of all patients with ovarian cancer will succumb to their disease when it recurs as the 100% fatal peritoneal carcinomatosis, as compared with 19% of those with breast cancer. The vast majority of the 31% that survive did not have HGSC and the other types of ovarian cancer are treatable and

MASS MURDERING DOCTORS: THE TRUTH ABOUT ONCOLOGISTS, CHEMOTHERAPY AND CANCER

MUCH more survivable. The high mortality of this tumor is largely explained by the fact that the majority (75%) of patients present at an advanced stage, with widely metastatic disease within the peritoneal cavity. I presented with a very early case because of the preventative nature of my surgery, albeit about a year too late. Ovarian high-grade serous-cell carcinoma metastasizes either by direct extension from the ovarian/Fallopian tumor to neighboring organs (bladder/colon) or when cancer cells detach from the primary tumor. Exfoliated tumor cells are transported throughout the peritoneum by the physiological movement of the naturally occurring peritoneal fluid and spread within the abdominal cavity. Extensive seeding of the peritoneal cavity by tumor cells is often associated with ascites, particularly in advanced, high-grade serous cell carcinomas. **These cancers grow rapidly, metastasize early, and have a very aggressive disease course.** Current treatment strategies for advanced ovarian carcinoma consist of aggressive surgery ("cytoreduction" or "tumor debulking"). To clear the cancer in the pelvis, surgery often involves an *en bloc* resection of the ovarian tumors, reproductive organs, and the sigmoid colon, with a primary bowel reanastomosis ("posterior exenteration"). This is technically possible because ovarian tumors stay within the peritoneal cavity, only invade the mesothelium-lined surface, and grow above the peritoneal reflection in the pelvis. Even large omental tumors only invade the superficial bowel serosa and never the deeper layers, which is why removal of the transverse colon is rarely necessary. The omentum, normally a soft $20 \times 15 \times 2$-cm fat pad covering the bowel and the abdominal cavity, is almost always transformed by tumor into what is called "omental cake". This generally causes the patient significant pain because the omental tumor tends to obstruct the stomach and the small and large bowel. The surgical treatment goal is to remove as much tumor as possible, because several studies have convincingly shown that cytoreduction results in improved patient survival (which to me is just common sense). **This effect of cytoreduction is indicative of a dramatic difference in the biological behavior of ovarian cancer as compared with other malignancies, because in most other cancers the removal of metastatic tumors has not been found to improve survival.** Post-operatively, all women, except those with very well-differentiated early-stage cancer, receive chemotherapy with platinum (carboplatin, rarely cisplatin) and a taxane (Taxol, rarely taxotere) a nearly 50 year old treatment that started as mustard

MASS MURDERING DOCTORS: THE TRUTH ABOUT ONCOLOGISTS, CHEMOTHERAPY AND CANCER

gas and KILLS 50% of cancer patients. You read that right, FIFTY PERCENT of cancer patients DIE FROM THE CHEMO, NOT THEIR CANCER. The optimal route of administration is still a matter of significant debate, but there is some evidence that in patients who have undergone optimal debulking (no residual tumor >1 cm), intraperitoneal (IP) delivery of these drugs increases progression-free survival by 5 months and overall survival by 15 months when compared with IV administration, however, they STILL DIE from the cancer or the chemo, so there are still NO known survivors. The rationale for this treatment modality is based on the observation that ovarian carcinomas are generally restricted to the abdominal cavity and on pharmacodynamic studies that show that i.p. chemo can achieve very high peritoneal drug concentrations. However, because pathologists were generally unable to find an *in situ* ovarian lesion, doubt remains that ovarian carcinoma originates in the ovarian surface epithelium. Indeed, high-grade ovarian serous carcinoma is the only epithelial cancer currently **without** an established precancerous component. Fallopian tube origin is also supported by a detailed understanding of pelvic organ embryology. **Type II cancers, which are most prevalent in postmenopausal women, are initially very chemo-sensitive to platinum containing chemotherapy, but patients have a median survival of only 30 months.** (WHOA!! Definitely NOT GOOD!) The task of metastasis appears to be easy for ovarian carcinoma. **Once the cancer cells have detached as single cells or clusters from the primary ovarian tumor, it is thought that they metastasize through a passive mechanism, carried by the physiological movement of peritoneal fluid to the peritoneum and omentum.** Clinical observation and retrospective clinical studies suggest that **high-grade serous ovarian carcinomas grow very efficiently within the peritoneal cavity, but rarely metastasize outside of it.** This was confirmed in patients who had peritoneovenous shunts implanted to palliate intractable ascites. The shunts, which were intended to relieve the discomfort of ascites without the risks associated with repeated paracentesis (draining the ascites from the pelvic cavity which fills with fluid because the lymph nodes become so filled with cancer cells that they block the drain function of the nodes), infused billions of cancer cells into the venous system through the jugular vein. After up to 2 years of continuous shunting, most patients did **not** develop disseminated hematogenous metastases (blood-borne cancer spread). This unusual result, a byproduct of a

MASS MURDERING DOCTORS: THE TRUTH ABOUT ONCOLOGISTS, CHEMOTHERAPY AND CANCER

palliative clinical intervention, confirms that Dr. Paget's "seed and soil" theory holds true for ovarian carcinoma. **The "soil" for ovarian carcinoma is the mesothelium that covers all organs within the peritoneal cavity, including the omentum and the diaphragm. It is an interesting, but poorly understood, feature of ovarian carcinoma that the tumor implants invade the mesothelial cell layers but rarely invade deeper into the peritoneum.** TP53 (Tumor Protein 53, previously known as p53) is probably the best known of all tumor suppressor genes, and is mutated in nearly all (96%) high-grade serous ovarian cancer (HGS-OvCa), which is the most common histopathological type of epithelial ovarian cancer Epithelial Ovarian Cancer. Recently, TP53 is found to involve in regulating cell metabolic pathways besides its classical tumor suppressive functions. In addition, emerging evidence suggests that mutant TP53 is associated with cancer metastasis. Through summarizing and comparing the roles of wild-type TP53 and mutant TP53 in the progression of various types of cancer, we hypothesize that mutant TP53 in HGS-OvCa cells interacts with sterol regulatory element-binding proteins (SREBPs) and guanidinoacetate N-methyltransferase (GAMT), leading to increased gene expression of key enzymes involved in fatty acids (FAs) and cholesterol biosynthesis and the inhibition of fatty acid oxidation (FAO), thus promotes lipid anabolism to accelerate tumor growth and progression. Elevated platelet number in patients' tumor microenvironment results in increased TGF-β production. Then, TGF-β acts in concert with mutant TP53 to promote HGS-OvCa metastasis by assembling a mutant-TP53/p63/Smads protein complex, in which p53's functions as metastasis suppressor are antagonized, and by enhancing the activities of the Slug/Snail and Twist families to drive induce EMT-like transition. Then adipocyte-derived IL-8 facilitates the metastasis of transformative cancer cells to abdominal adipose tissue (e.g., omentum). Once metastasis is established, mutant TP53 together with adipocyte-derived IL-8 upregulates Fatty acid-binding protein 4 (FABP4) expression and then promotes FAs absorption from adipocytes to support rapid tumor growth in adipocyte-rich metastatic environments. In summary, these indicate that mutant TP53 may play determinant roles in the progression of HGS-OvCa. Ovarian carcinoma is associated with the highest death rate of all gynecological tumors. On one hand, its aggressiveness is based on the rapid dissemination of ovarian cancer cells to the peritoneum, the omentum, and organs located in the peritoneal cavity,

MASS MURDERING DOCTORS: THE TRUTH ABOUT ONCOLOGISTS, CHEMOTHERAPY AND CANCER

and on the other hand, on the rapid development of resistance to chemotherapeutic agents. In this review, we focus on the metastatic process of ovarian cancer, which involves dissemination of, homing to and growth of tumor cells in distant organs, and describe promising molecular targets for possible therapeutic intervention. We provide an outline of the interaction of ovarian cancer cells with the microenvironment such as mesothelial cells, adipocytes, fibroblasts, endothelial cells, and other stromal components in the context of approaches for therapeutic interference with dissemination. The targets described in this review are discussed with respect to their validity as drivers of metastasis and to the availability of suitable efficient agents for their blockage, such as small molecules, monoclonal antibodies or antibody conjugates as emerging tools to manage this disease. Ovarian carcinoma is associated with the highest death rate of all gynecological tumors. On one hand, its aggressiveness is based on the rapid dissemination of ovarian cancer cells to the peritoneum, the omentum, and organs located in the peritoneal cavity, and on the other hand, on the rapid development of resistance to chemotherapeutic agents. One of the most interesting parts of GcMAF/Goleic is that you must take high doses of vitamin D3 along with it, which is interestingly supported by this research finding: Epithelial ovarian cancer is the leading cause of gynecological cancer death in women, mainly because it has spread to intraperitoneal tissues such as the omentum in the peritoneal cavity by the time of diagnosis. In the present study, we established in vitro assays, ex vivo omental organ culture system and syngeneic animal tumor models using wild type (WT) and vitamin D receptor (VDR) null mice to investigate the effects of $1\alpha,25$-dihydroxyvitamin D3 (1,25D3) and VDR on Epithelial Ovarian Cancer invasion. **Treatment of human Epithelial Ovarian Cancer cells with 1,25D3 suppressed their migration and invasion in monolayer scratch and transwell assays and ability to colonize the omentum in the ex vivo system, supporting a role for epithelial VDR in interfering with Epithelial Ovarian Cancer invasion.** Furthermore, VDR knockdown in OVCAR3 cells increased their ability to colonize the omentum in the ex vivo system in the absence of 1,25D3, showing a potential ligand-independent suppression of Epithelial Ovarian Cancer invasion by epithelial VDR. In syngeneic models, ID8 tumors exhibited an increased ability to colonize omenta of VDR null over that of WT mice; pre-treatment of WT, not VDR null, mice with EB1089 reduced ID8 colonization, revealing a role for stromal VDR in suppressing Epithelial

MASS MURDERING DOCTORS: THE TRUTH ABOUT ONCOLOGISTS, CHEMOTHERAPY AND CANCER

Ovarian Cancer invasion. These studies are the first to demonstrate a role for epithelial and stromal VDR in mediating the activity of 1,25D3 as well as a 1,25D3-independent action of the VDR in suppressing Epithelial Ovarian Cancer invasion. The data suggest that VDR-based drug discovery may lead to the development of new intervention strategies to improve the survival of patients with Epithelial Ovarian Cancer at advanced stages.

Epithelial ovarian cancer, primarily high-grade serous-type ovarian cancer (HGSOC), is **one of the most deadly threats to women's health worldwide**. Over 70% of HGSOC patients are diagnosed at advanced and metastatic stages, and their 10-year survival rate is below 30% and survival is limited to those who do NOT have a recurrence. Also, the current treatment of ovarian cancer is largely dependent on the limited success of chemotherapeutic agents, such as paclitaxel and carboplatin, thereby being strongly associated with rapid drug resistance and poor clinical outcomes. Hence, the improvement in treatment options, including the use of target-based therapies, is urgently needed to combat the malignancy of human ovarian cancer. Courtesy of: http://www. ncbi. nlm. nih.gov/pmc/articles/PMC2928939 and the **American Society for Investigative Pathology**

The peritoneal cavity is the primary site of ovarian cancer metastases. It is believed that the intraperitoneal invasiveness of the malignancy is determined by interactions between cancer cells and the normal peritoneal mesothelum. The nature of these interactions is, however unclear which is the reason for divergent opinions about the role of mesothelial cells in disease progression. According to some authors, the mesothelium acts as a barrier which prevents the expansion of the tumor cells. However other researchers claim that these cells actively promote various elements of cancer cell invasiveness, but the underlying mechanisms involved in ovarian cancer spread are not well understood. Intra-abdominal tumors, such as ovarian cancer, have a clear predilection for metastasis to the omentum, an organ primarily composed of adipocytes (fat cells). Currently, it is unclear why tumor cells preferentially home to and proliferate in the omentum, yet omental metastases typically represent the largest tumor in the abdominal cavities of women with ovarian cancer. Primary human omental adipocytes promote homing, migration and invasion of ovarian cancer cells, and that adipokines including interleukin-8 (IL-8) mediate these activities. Adipocyte ovarian cancer cell co-culture led to the direct transfer of lipids from adipocytes to ovarian cancer cells and promoted in vitro and in vivo tumor growth. Furthermore, co-culture induced lipolysis in adipocytes and β-oxidation in cancer cells, suggesting adipocytes act as an energy source for the cancer cells. A protein array identified upregulation of fatty acid-binding protein 4 (FABP4, also known as aP2) in omental metastases as compared to primary ovarian tumors, and FABP4 expression was detected in ovarian cancer cells at the adipocyte-tumor cell interface. FABP4 deficiency substantially impaired metastatic tumor growth in mice, indicating that FABP4 has a key role in ovarian cancer metastasis. These data indicate adipocytes provide fatty acids for rapid tumor growth, identifying lipid metabolism and transport as new targets for the treatment of cancers where adipocytes are a major component of the micro-environment. Here, we used a para-biosis model that demonstrates preferential hematogenous metastasis of ovarian cancer to the omentum. Our studies revealed that the ErbB3-neuregulin 1 (NRG1) axis is a dominant pathway responsible for hematogenous omental metastasis. Elevated levels of ErbB3 in ovarian cancer cells and NRG1 in the omentum allowed for tumor cell localization and growth in the omentum. **Depletion of ErbB3 in ovarian cancer impaired omental metastasis.** These findings have implications for designing alternative strategies aimed at preventing and treating ovarian cancer metastasis. Microscopically, HGSC is characterized by a wide variety of architectural patterns, which may coexist within the same tumor and in the same tissue section. The most common pattern is 'papillary', consisting not of well-formed fibrovascular cores in most cases, but instead of highly stratified epithelium with a fenestrated, tufted, or slit-like architecture. Less common patterns include solid, glandular and transitional like. All growth patterns share the same cytological features; the tumor cells are usually intermediate to large in size, with prominent nucleoli visible at low magnification. The nuclei are distinctly pleomorphic, showing more than a threefold variation in size; the primary diagnostic criterion in distinguishing HGSCs from LGSCs. Sometimes, bizarre mononuclear giant cells are seen. High mitotic rate and abundant apoptotic bodies are characteristic of HGSCs. In cases where the nuclear pleomorphism is equivocal in establishing a diagnosis of HGSC versus LGSC, a mitotic rate of greater than 12/10 high-power field supports a diagnosis of HGSC. Intra-abdominal tumors, such as ovarian cancer, have a clear predilection for metastasis to the omentum, an organ primarily composed of adipocytes. Currently, it is unclear why tumor cells preferentially home to and proliferate in the omentum, yet omental metastases typically represent the largest tumor in the abdominal cavities of women with ovarian cancer. FABP4 deficiency substantially impaired metastatic tumor growth in mice, indicating that FABP4 has a key role in ovarian cancer metastasis. These data indicate adipocytes provide fatty acids for rapid tumor growth, identifying lipid metabolism and transport as new targets for the treatment of cancers where adipocytes are a major component of the micro-environment. In English this means the cancer cells love the yummy fat cells in the omentum. No shock there—fat tastes good as we all know, and apparently even on the cellular level fat is still delicious. Good to know.

SIDEBAR: MOLECULAR FEATURES OF HGSC

Approximately half of all patients with ovarian HGSCs have either hereditary (germline) or somatic mutations in *BRCA1* or *BRCA2*, or loss of *BRCA1* expression in tumor cells as a result of methylation of its promoter (*BRCA2* is not inactivated by promoter methylation). The prevalence of germline mutations varies between populations studied (16–26%), **with mutations in *BRCA1* consistently being more common than *BRCA2* mutations.**
***BRCA1/2*mutations are almost exclusively seen in HGSC subtype of ovarian carcinoma.** Given the high frequency of *BRCA1/2*mutations in patients with HGSC, and the lack of sensitivity of family history in identifying these patients, it is believed that all such patients should be referred for genetic counseling and testing. For those patients with mutations, there can then be counseling regarding breast cancer screening and risk-reducing surgery.

Genetic counseling is, in my view, total BS by the way—it's just one more way the medical community has added another expensive layer of medical treatment. What kind of "counseling" do you think I need for God's sake? I'm either BRCA1 or I'm not. Why do I need a "specially trained genetic counselor" to tell me I have a genetic defect I was BORN WITH that predisposes me to this deadly, aggressive and virulent cancer. That's a black and white thing—you either ARE a BRCA1/2+ or you are not—there's no in-between. Why would ANYONE need some over-educated moron to bill your insurance for a few thousand bucks to "counsel" you over your genetic makeup? It's not like you can do jack about it, so it's another stupid Obamacare regulation and pushes insurance costs even higher adds another layer of cost and bureaucracy to your medical care. I had done all of this and my cancer was discovered as a result of a risk-reducing hysterectomy.

Loss of BRCA1/2 is lethal to normal cells; however, 95% of HGSCs have TP53 mutations early in oncogenesis, permitting cells to survive subsequent loss of BRCA1/2 These two changes result in loss of ability to repair DNA breaks, resulting in chromosomal instability. As a result, HGSCs are typically aneuploid with complex karyotypes. The landmark Cancer Genome Atlas study of HGSCs showed many somatic copy number alterations, which is a characteristic feature of this cancer subtype, but that recurrent mutations (apart from *BRCA1*, *BRCA2* and *TP53*) are uncommon. Among immuno-histo-chemical markers, immunoreactivity to WT-1 is particularly useful in the distinction of serous ovarian carcinomas from other subtypes. Approximately 71% of LGSCs and 80% of HGSCs are positive for WT-1, compared with less than 5% positivity of other ovarian subtypes. Estrogen receptor (ER) is positive in more than two-thirds of serous carcinomas, (this means that estrogen replacement feeds these tumors) and is also expressed in ECs, but is negative in almost all CCCs (clear-cell carcinoma) and MCs. With respect to the differential diagnosis between HGSCs and LGSCs, (Low-Grade Serous Carcinoma) abnormal p53 staining (i. e., either strong diffuse staining or complete absence of staining) and a high Ki-67 index are supportive of a diagnosis of HGSC. HGSC can be confused with LGSC, EC and CCC (Clear Cell Carcinoma). The differential diagnosis with LGSC has been discussed previously, which is based primarily on identification of at least threefold nuclear variation in HGSCs.

SIDEBAR: TREATING HIGH-GRADE SEROUS CARCINOMA

The initial therapeutic approach for HGSCs is usually surgical tumor removal (debulking) followed by chemotherapy. However, a recent randomized clinical trial has shown that for some patients with advanced-stage HGSC, equivalent outcomes (since they ALL die when it recurs—and it recurs MORE THAN 90% OF THE TIME) can be obtained if they first receive three to four cycles of chemotherapy, followed by interval debulking. With either strategy, optimal debulking, with no macroscopic residual disease, is the most important prognostic indicator. Most HGSCs (80%) respond well to platinum/taxane therapy initially, with drug resistance emerging during subsequent treatment cycles. Of course it destroys your immune system so you can easily die from a hospital staph infection. Chemo before surgery is ridiculous and nothing but a moneymaker for the scumbag oncologists. A minority of cases of HGSCs (20%) are refractory to platinum-based chemotherapy from the time of presentation, but the basis for this drug resistance is not known. Poly (ADP-ribose) polymerase (PARP) inhibitors represent a possible therapeutic intervention. PARP is a key enzyme involved in DNA repair, and its inhibition can be used to exploit the loss of DNA double-strand break repair in HGSCs. PARP inhibitors cause the death of cells also lacking double-strand break repair capability, while normal cells are unaffected. Initial studies have shown that the PARP inhibitor, olaparib, extends survival in a BRCA2-mutated ovarian cancer xenograft model, and the results of an initial clinical trial show activity against HGSC in patients with BRCA mutations and also in patients without such mutations. Unfortunately, routine use of PARP inhibitors remains some time in the future, with additional trial data needed (but not anticipated in the near future, based on currently active trials) **Olaparib has been approved as of December 2014.** As noted previously, targeting angiogenesis with bevacizumab has been used, but the improvements in outcome have been modest and there is a need for predictive bio-markers to identify those patients who stand to benefit from this therapy.Courtesy of Medscape. orghttp://www. medscape. org/viewarticle/776491_3

SIDEBAR: WHY WE ALL DIE FROM CANCER

Barriers To Prevention: Why Conventional Cancer Research Does Not Find 'The Cure'
http://preventdisease.com/home/tips93.shtml

For almost a century, cancer research has been devoted (so they say) to finding a cure. Isn't it amazing how this cure is so elusive, for such a long period of time, in the hands of thousands of skilled scientists with billions and billions of dollars in research grants? Have you ever wondered who the beneficiaries are of all the donations to cancer support groups and charities for the "war against cancer"?The 'cancer industry' is a generic term for the ever-expanding industry which has grown up around the disease of cancer. It is a vast industry incorporating all services, products, materials and technologies required for the orthodox management of the disease. As major fundraisers for research and major providers of public information and patient support services, cancer charities and societies work in close association with the cancer

MASS MURDERING DOCTORS: THE TRUTH ABOUT ONCOLOGISTS, CHEMOTHERAPY AND CANCER

industry. Primary prevention is not their objective; never has been and never will be. The reason is simple. **Prevention does not generate profits.**

Evidence for this situation is brazenly obvious in the long-prevailing silence from the industry on environmental, nutritional and occupational factors in cancer. This type of silence has a very basic goal. It deprives citizens of control over their health and their lives by depriving them of basic right to know information that keeps them healthy and prevents disease. Year after year, more and more money is spent on a virtual potpourri of money-seeking cancer foundations, and year after year cancer incidence grows higher and higher. What little progress is reported by the Pollyanna members of the cancer industry can primarily be attributable to early detection and prevention - activities which cannot begin to address, quantitatively, the large sums invested each year in cancer research and treatment. When informed, many will reject the reality of how the cancer industry really works. A typical response might be "I don't believe this...I don't want to hear it. It can't be true". Many refuse to be torn apart and angered by the human suffering caused by the horrendous activity of the cancer industry. Millions of people have suffered and died painful deaths. Millions more will die with this type of mentality, so how can it be true? Most will never question why cancer patients are restricted to the approved cancer therapies given by a medical community that has openly admitted they do not know the cause of cancer.

We have been conditioned over time to accept cancer as a fact of life (and death). Statistics tell us that cancer affects 1 in 3 of the population. These frequently reported figures influence the gradual acceptance of cancer as both a 'normal' disease and one that must inevitably affect some of us. Doctors insist that we must detect the cancer to prevent it. The slogan 'early detection is the best prevention' has attained the status of a 'truth' in the public mind. In fact, early detection, by whatever means, is only detection. For example, the conventional medical community persists on the promotion of regular mammograms as a 'preventive measure'. Mammography is a tool for detecting breast problems, not for preventing them. A new study by researchers from the Nordic Cochrane Centre in Denmark found that mammograms may harm ten times as many women as they help. The researchers examined the benefits and negative effects of seven breast cancer screening programs on 500,000 women in the United States, Canada, Scotland and Sweden. The study's authors found that for every

MASS MURDERING DOCTORS: THE TRUTH ABOUT ONCOLOGISTS, CHEMOTHERAPY AND CANCER

2,000 women who received mammograms over a 10-year period, only one would have her life prolonged, but 10 would endure unnecessary and potentially harmful treatments."

The main error of the biomedical approach is the confusion between disease processes and disease origins. Instead of asking why an illness occurs, and trying to remove the conditions that lead to it, medical researchers try to understand the biological mechanisms through which the disease operates, so that they can interfere with them. These mechanisms, rather than the true origins, are seen as the causes of disease in current medical thinking and this confusion lies at the very centre of the conceptual problems of contemporary medicine. This is why contemporary western medicine continues to fail every cancer patient it treats. For example, there is absolutely no reliable scientific evidence showing that chemotherapy has any positive effect whatsoever on cancer. Artificially reducing the size of a tumor does nothing to reverse the physiology of cancer in a patient's body. It doesn't initiate the healing that needs to take place to reverse cancer and stay cancer free. It will temporarily shrink a tumor, but it can never cure or improve the quality of a cancer patient's life.

At present, this establishment that continues to makes the rules (even if not by law) for dealing with cancer have their precepts practically frozen and unyielding. Surgery, radiation, and chemotherapy are the cardinal principles by which the medical profession and government funding dominate cancer therapy. So why do treatments of this sort persist over more cost-effect preventive strategies? MONEY!! The disease of cancer has spawned a major world industry and it is unlikely that such a massive and multi-faceted industry will welcome the prospect of its own demise in the shape of primary prevention. A firm alliance between the established cancer institutions and the chemical, pharmaceutical and nuclear industries has formed the medical-industrial complex. This complex will always, by it's own omission, fail to embrace any successful program for preventing cancer. What is stopping us [from getting serious about prevention] is the almost suffocating hold the medical industrial complex retains over cancer policy, and the hugely powerful chemical industry's interest in protecting its products.We generally trust advice when it comes to us from government, especially when it is reinforced by the media and cancer charities. That's why the public continues to financially support such conglomerates in the cancer industry

MASS MURDERING DOCTORS: THE TRUTH ABOUT ONCOLOGISTS, CHEMOTHERAPY AND CANCER

through specialized non-profit groups and societies. Most never question who the actual beneficiaries of such groups are. However, nearly 100% of the funds donated are used to recruit more cancer patients into highly-lucrative treatments that do more harm than good. The following is one such example of a grant list at the Komen for the Cure organization, which details grant recepients for breast cancer http://www.komenphoenix.org/site/c.nsKZ.... Note that not a single grant is provided for nutritional education or effective prevention strategies.

Most national governments establish cancer plans which target lifestyle factors (exercise, diet, alcohol consumption and smoking) as the key to cancer prevention. This narrow focus perpetuates ignorance that dietary and environmental contaminants are significant sources of human exposure to carcinogens which are impossible to avoid. The focus on lifestyle often obscures cancer's environmental roots. It presumes that the ongoing contamination of our air, food, and water is an immutable fact of the human condition to which we must accommodate ourselves. For example, the disinformation about sunlight has reached a level of absurdity that's virtually unmatched in the history of medicine. The cancer industry authorities know that vitamin D prevents almost 80% of all cancers. Since sunlight exposure causes the skin to generate vitamin D in the human body (for free, no less), the cancer industry has come to the realization that in order for it to continue surviving, it has to scare people away from anything that might actually prevent or cure cancer. This is the primary objective behind the sunlight scare campaigns. It's just a clever profit strategy to keep people sick and diseased by enforcing widespread vitamin D deficiency across the human population.

The cancer industry is well organized, unbelievably well funded, and also has total control over the news media due to the massive amounts of advertising dollars spent by Big Pharma. The media is the main source of public information in today's world. It is an all-pervasive global force in society and is becoming an integral part of the public debate about cancer. However, the information industry - print and broadcast - is largely controlled by market forces and these exert strong influences on society, especially through advertising. This can compromise editorial decision-making or it can obscure core issues. For example, the survival of a women's magazine or a TV channel in a very competitive marketplace will depend upon revenue from advertisers selling products—often directed at women—that should arguably be part of the debate on causes of breast cancer. Therefore, it is impossible to get issues like 'primary prevention' taken up by mainstream media. One result, for example, is the widespread misconception that breast cancer is a largely inherited disease.

Proscrastination has been one of the biggest barriers to primary prevention for cancer. There is a widespread tendency (among scientists, industrialists and politicians) to claim the need for more research when challenged by prevention measures based on existing scientific knowledge. In the case of cancer prevention this delaying tactic devalues a century of scientific endeavour, leaving policy makers forever in the grip of 'paralysis by analysis'. The illusion of science finalized and published in books and journals has led to a poor track record of prevention and often devaluing natural treatments and approaches that have been effective in practical applications for hundreds, even thousands of years. Ironically, technology has now empowered a growing internet savvy public to obtain the facts with just a few hours of research. Numerous cancer cures are a few clicks away. Vitamin D, cat's claw herbs, the Essiac formula, medicinal mushrooms, spirulina, cruciferous vegetables, green tea, graviola herbs, Chinese medicinal herbs, oxygen therapy, alkalizing water therapies and many more are all promising alternatives, and possibly far more effective than any existing conventional treatment.

Historically, easy solutions were found for a multitude of diseases because they came from traditional cultures without commercialized medicine (i.e. it came from an indigenous culture) and there were no established, highly funded, self-serving organizations around to suppress them. This is, admittedly, a simplification of the historical facts, but the fundamental principle is not easily debated. Money does not aid the search for cures; in fact, on balance it actually acts more as a deterrent. If the cancer industry wants to make themselves bigger (and they will) then they must make the problem bigger. Big budgets cannot be sustained in the presence of easy solutions. That means that their very survival demands that they use whatever means are at their disposal to suppress alternatives by rivals that would prove compellingly contrary. Advancing their cause requires a maximum, sustained effort to destroy those capable of providing an end to their grand 'raison d'etre' and the many growing, demanding, and expensive projects which it consequently spawns.

MASS MURDERING DOCTORS: THE TRUTH ABOUT ONCOLOGISTS, CHEMOTHERAPY AND CANCER

After a century of suppression by the cancer industry, and with the help of the internet, a very small percentage of the population is slowly and steadily being informed of the truth about cancer. Many are now realizing that these highly funded establishments set up to prevent or find a cancer cure will never effectively work to that aim. To ask the multitude of cancer organizations, societies and charities to find a cancer cure is to say, 'Now go. Be successful. And once you have achieved your aim, promptly commit suicide.' For once a real cancer cure or cures are announced, the need for these organizations, which collect hundreds of billions of dollars in the aggregate annually for treatment and research from governments, agencies, foundations, corporations, insurance companies, and private individuals—all of them, without exception, will have lost their reason for existence. That is why a prevention strategy or cancer cure will never come from their quarter: the very nature of their mandate is a violation of Natural Law. It is a grand act of political expediency and managerial stupidity that has made what should have been an easy-to-solve medical puzzle and turned it into the single greatest act of man-made carnage in history—a fraud of unspeakable magnitude that has spanned almost a century, and has needlessly caused the premature deaths of tens of millions of people. ----From the internet http://preventdisease.com/home/tips93.shtml

I hope everyone understands all the medical terms above. I am without evidence of neoplasm which is a good thing. I have cancer in both ovaries and my uterus. I'm going to beat it or die trying. Literally. Here's some less technical information:

The classification of a serous carcinoma as low grade or high grade has important clinical implications in that patients with high grade serous carcinoma are almost invariably treated by chemotherapy following surgical resection, even when stage 1. In contrast, patients with stage 1 low grade serous carcinoma do not usually receive adjuvant therapy as it is not considered effective. In addition, there is now a tendency among medical oncologists not to treat advanced stage low grade serous carcinomas with adjuvant chemotherapy if total surgical debulking (removal) has been achieved. It is also important to distinguish between low grade and high grade serous carcinoma on a core biopsy because chemotherapy is considered to be relatively ineffective in low grade serous carcinoma and so oncologists are less likely to treat these neoplasms with upfront chemotherapy.

MASS MURDERING DOCTORS: THE TRUTH ABOUT ONCOLOGISTS, CHEMOTHERAPY AND CANCER

High-grade serous carcinoma is the most malignant form of ovarian cancer and accounts for up to 71% of all ovarian cancer cases. The majority of high-grade serous ovarian cancers have recently been found to originate in the Fallopian tube, not the ovary with a survival rate of only 30% of which 80% will relapse WHICH IS UNSURVIVABLE. Approximately 35% of women with this form of ovarian cancer have an inherited abnormality in BRCA1/2genes. **Because of their origin in the Fallopian tube, serous carcinomas spread through the abdomen very early in the course of disease, and by the time they become symptomatic they are usually high stage tumors, with resulting poor outcomes.** High grade serous cancer of the ovary represents about 2/3rds of the cases of ovarian cancer. **These cancers are often diagnosed at an advanced stage as they have almost no symptoms until later stages.** Peritoneal cavity is the primary site of ovarian cancer metastases. It is believed that the intraperitoneal invasiveness of the malignancy is determined by interactions between cancer cells and the normal peritoneal mesothelium. The nature of these interactions is, however unclear which is the reason for divergent opinions about the role of mesothelial cells in disease progression. According to some authors, the mesothelium acts as a barrier which prevents the expansion of the tumor cells. However other researchers claim that these cells actively promote various elements of cancer cell invasiveness. The reciprocal interplay of cancer cells and host cells is an indispensable prerequisite for tumor growth and progression. Cells of both the innate and adaptive immune system, in particular tumor-associated macrophages (TAMs) and T cells, as well as cancer-associated fibroblasts enter into a malicious liaison with tumor cells to create a tumor-promoting and immuno-suppressive tumor micro-environment (TME). Ovarian cancer, the most lethal of all gynecological malignancies, is characterized by a unique TME that enables specific and efficient metastatic routes, impairs immune surveillance, and mediates therapy resistance. A characteristic feature of the ovarian cancer TME is the role of resident host cells, in particular activated mesothelial cells, which line the peritoneal cavity in huge numbers, as well as adipocytes of the omentum, the preferred site of metastatic lesions. Another crucial factor is the peritoneal fluid, which enables the transcoelomic spread of tumor cells to other pelvic and peritoneal organs, and occurs at more advanced stages as a malignancy-associated effusion. This ascites is rich in

MASS MURDERING DOCTORS: THE TRUTH ABOUT ONCOLOGISTS, CHEMOTHERAPY AND CANCER

tumor-promoting soluble factors, extracellular vesicles and detached cancer cells as well as large numbers of T cells, TAMs, and other host cells, which cooperate with resident host cells to support tumor progression and immune evasion. In this review, we summarize and discuss our current knowledge of the cellular and molecular interactions that govern this interplay with a focus on signaling networks formed by cytokines, lipids, and extracellular vesicles; the pathogenic physiological roles of TAMs and T cells; the mechanism of transcoelomic metastasis; and the cell type selective processing of signals from the TME.

This is what happened with my sister. She went to a gastroenterologist for SIX MONTHS who was treating her for Irritable Bowel Syndrome (which virtually NEVER presents for the first time after the age of 50, and she was 54) when she was quickly growing a belly full of cancer. My orphaned-at-age 17 niece is suing this doctor for medical malpractice and wrongful death AS SHE SHOULD. You don't just sue doctors to get money for damages, you also sue to prevent them from harming someone else. This went on for months with her bloating so badly she looked 6 months pregnant, yet the idiot doctor did nothing. She went in for her routine mammogram that revealed she had stage 0 breast cancer and scheduled a mastectomy so she wouldn't have to do chemo and they found her ovarian cancer at the hospital while she was under anesthesia for her mastectomy. She was at Stage 3-C when they discovered it, so she never had a chance with conventional medicine but with immunotherapy, she could have had a chance. Because her ex-husband wouldn't tell me or anyone else ANYTHING about what kind of cancer she had it was impossible for me to find out what she needed since NO ONE knew what kind of ovarian cancer she had but her. It was all through her pelvis when they discovered it with deposits of cancer over an inch in diameter, and it very quickly became resistant to chemotherapy. When she went for surgery after 6 rounds of chemo they told her she was terminal at that time. The scumbag oncologists at Moffit Cancer Center in Tampa Florida KNEW she was terminal from the get-go, but this didn't stop them from giving her $750 THOUSAND dollars worth of useless chemo while lying to her and selling her a bunch of false hope to go with it. **While this cancer usually responds to initial treatment, it frequently recurs and is not curable when it recurs**. There are NO known survivors of HGSC when it recurs as peritoneal carcinomatosis. A growing body of knowledge reveals that the majority of cases of high grade serous "ovarian" cancer actually are Fallopian tube cancers. The precursor lesions begin in the fimbriated end of the Fallopian tube and the cancer spreads from there. **The prognosis for cure is poor at later stages and the recurrence rate is very high.** None of this is good news for me, but I do have a slight advantage over Lori. Because it was too late when they found her cancer, and she wouldn't consider any other treatment but the chemotherapy that killed her, she really never had a chance but she fought like a tiger nonetheless. Her kids and the family were everything to her and she was determined that she would beat this. The rest of her friends and the family all thought she could because she was such a fighter and tough as nails but they found her cancer when it was already too late to do anything other than put her affairs in order and hope for as much time as possible, but I am also certain that she would be alive today if it wasn't for her ex-husband who just knew better than anyone else. I begged her to listen to me and not do the chemo but she just would not listen to anyone but her ex-husband. She was told during her original debulking surgery that she was terminal. I am trying to avoid hearing those words for as long as possible. That is why I am treating my cancer with an alternative medication regime because I don't trust big Pharma as they have a cure rate of 2.1% with their 200 TO 300 billion A YEAR in chemotherapy cancer treatment PROFITS. This is NOT an acceptable cure rate in my view and I am NOT going to do it. I will roll the dice with my treatment since I believe that if I go for chemotherapy, that it will kill me sooner rather than later. I have to decide if I am willing to take the risk of not going for the chemotherapies that the oncologist assures me that I will die if I do not have. I find it very odd that when I did refuse the chemotherapy protocols that Dr. Xynos NEVER CALLED ME. Wouldn't you think that if he was so concerned that I would die, that he would call me himself to try and persuade me to do the chemo? He never did. This is one more reason that I am confident in the protocols that I am going to use.

CHAPTER 7: TELLING FRIENDS & FAMILY I HAVE THE SAME CANCER THAT KILLED MY SISTER 90 DAYS AGO

I am now officially scared to death. I now have the disease that killed my sister a VERY short 90 days ago and it has come to kill me and it is the most aggressive, most malignant and most deadly of all the gynecologic cancers. Lori started chemo treatment at a later stage of the cancer and it was too late for her to have a chance with conventional treatment. I am praying it won't kill me as well. I am also faced with the horrific task of telling my parents that I have cancer—the same cancer that killed my sister, their other daughter—just twelve short weeks ago. I can't imagine how they are going to take it. I can't imagine how I am going to find the words to tell them that the 14 months of watching their younger daughter die are about to be repeated and they may have to watch their oldest daughter die as well. If there's ever been a worse kind of nightmare than this, I haven't lived through it yet, and if this isn't the worst thing I've ever had to do, it will do until the worst thing comes along. I don't have the words to tell them and I don't have the time NOT to tell them either. I'm out of time to do ANYTHING other than fight for my life and I do NOT want them stressed to death. Literally. I told my oldest nephew Justin, but swore him to secrecy other than his wife Kristin and his recently married brother Cody and his wife Lindsay. Their kids, Lori's grandchildren are too young to be told anything. Justin is a rock. A total rock. He's a great kid (well he's 36 now) but he's a fine family man with a good career and he's married to his soul mate and they have two great kids who are the closest thing to grandchildren I will ever get, and of course they are perfect! I'm so blessed to have them in my life.

I also had to tell three of my dearest friends, Kimberly, she's my oldest and dearest friend and we have been best friends for almost my entire life. I've known her since I was 11 or 12 and we went through school and then life together. Her daughters are my nieces and her oldest is my goddaughter. I was honored beyond words when she told me she was pregnant and asked me to be Jennifer's godmother. I don't want to tell the kids right now, but Kim and I had a long talk and she wanted to get on a plane immediately but she has a brand new grandson and he's her first and only grandchild and he's about a month old. The other thing is that she is terribly allergic to cats and I have SEVEN of them, so I told her not to come now. I couldn't enjoy her visit knowing that she was suffering because of my cats. I also called my friend Betty who is a nurse. We used to work together about 20 years ago and we've been friends a long time. I am going to call JoAnn and tell her as well. I hate to do it but I know they will be ticked if I don't tell them. I think I'm practicing to tell my dad later today.

MASS MURDERING DOCTORS: THE TRUTH ABOUT ONCOLOGISTS, CHEMOTHERAPY AND CANCER

If telling my parents I have the same cancer that killed my sister wasn't the hardest phone call I've ever had to make, it will do until the hardest thing comes along. My dad is a pretty stoic guy in front of me. The only time I've ever seen my dad cry was when Uncle Lester died (I could write a BOOK about him. He was a WWI vet and about the grandest old gentleman you could ever meet. Family, God and Country were his entire reason for being and I loved him to pieces—we all did) and he cried for sure at Lori's funeral but I wasn't there and we cried a couple of times talking on the phone while she was dying and we were helpless to do anything about it.

I inherited my BRCA1 gene from my dad as, obviously, did my sister. He feels guilty about it. When I was down visiting my sister in the hospice during her last few days of this life, I had dinner with my nephews and their wives and the kids who were fantastically well-behaved. I hate screaming out of control brats in restaurants. Anyway. They told me that my dad had lunch with them and started crying and telling them he was sorry he killed their mom and they were just so torn up. They told dad that there was NO possibility he could ever have done this on purpose and that there's no way of knowing what in your genes. When my dad and I were talking about this he said he wished he could go back in time and punch out the relative who passed this down the line. We talked a little about politics and then I told him that if I could get a different dad that wouldn't have given me the BRCA1, I wouldn't even consider it. We exchanged "love yous" and I told him I'd keep him in the loop. Telling Mom was not as hard as I thought it would be. She and I have had a lot of ups and downs over the years and our relationship is exceptionally complicated. She and Lori were inseparable from the time Lori was born. No one could get between them. She raised Lori's kids while Lori built a million-dollar business in the beauty for sale game. Lori always thought she was a great mom because her kids turned out well, but her kids turned out well because MY MOTHER raised them, not my sister. This is not to say Lori wasn't a good mom—she was—But when it came down to enforcing the rules, it was my mother who did it—took them to and from school, activities, fed and bathed and in general did the child-care thing for 30 years for Lori and the kids adored and still adore her.

MASS MURDERING DOCTORS: THE TRUTH ABOUT ONCOLOGISTS, CHEMOTHERAPY AND CANCER

Justin named his daughter Leilani after my mother, and Cody and Carliegh (who was just 17 when her mom died in November of 2015) are very close to her as well. I didn't have any kids for her to raise but Lori bought Mom an annuity before she died so that mom would keep getting her paycheck every week for the rest of her life. I'm grateful that she did that. Mom told me some things about Lori's cancer that will be helpful to my oncologist and we exchanged loves and I also promised to keep her in the loop. It KILLED ME to tell mom and dad but everyone I talked to told me they needed to know. Luckily, that didn't make it one bit easier to tell them.

I see the gynecological oncologist tomorrow and I will know a LOT more after talking to him, so tomorrow's update will have a bit more information. I'm having a mammogram on Weds (or Friday as I had to schedule a backup due to a pending godawful snowstorm Tuesday night) because my last mammogram was at least 18 months ago but it was clean as a whistle. If I have a clean mammogram, that will go a long way toward calming down family and friends and would also be a huge plus for my treatment plan.

HOWEVER, even with a clean mammogram, I am still having a double mastectomy and reconstruction as I had already decided to do that. I've given both my girls a thorough feel (I made Dr. DallaRiva and Dr. Xynos do a PROFESSIONAL feel-up and both of them said they didn't feel anything) and they seem to be the same as always when I do my monthly self-exams so I'm thinking that's a good sign. I'm not concerned about getting rid of them-they're old. I'll get new and better ones! I am going to have the bilateral mastectomies BEFORE starting any kind of chemotherapy because chemo destroys the immune system and I do NOT want to go in for major surgery with a compromised immune system. I feel that would be stupid and open me up to potentially more serious problems than a 2-3 week delay in starting chemotherapy. I don't care as much about reconstruction but I'd like to do that too before chemo if there's going to BE chemo; if there's going to be a NEED for chemo.

I am not inclined to start chemo unless absolutely necessary because it does a tremendous amount of damage to the body PLUS my particular cancer becomes chemo-resistant EXTREMELY QUICKLY and I'd rather save my kill shot for a recurrence than to use it on a cancer than has been removed surgically and is GONE.

MASS MURDERING DOCTORS: THE TRUTH ABOUT ONCOLOGISTS, CHEMOTHERAPY AND CANCER

That's just stupid but since the going rate for chemo is 50-100K a pop, they love to do it because medicine is all about MONEY. They don't give a crap about me. You know how you can tell doctors only care about money? Whenever you call for an appointment to see a new doctor they never ask what's wrong with you. The FIRST question is always "Who's your insurance company?" and I am not about to let them chemo me for a cancer that is already gone just because they have kids in college or want a new BMW. Homey don't play that!! I see my surgeon Thursday. I am going to talk to him and see if he wants to go back in and look around to make sure he got it all. He says feels very confident that the cancer was confined to my ovaries and that he DID get it all, but he was wrong. The "tacky patch" he expressed his concern about to my husband is the cancer he left behind. The tumors were inside each ovary, and on the uterine surface and the pelvic fluid washings weren't done, a violation of the standard of care. However, the gynecologist-oncologist would be the one to do any additional surgery which will suck since they're in St. Louis which is a 50 mile hike each way and will probably not do surgery at Anderson which was just about the nicest hospital I've ever been in—although I WAS in the maternity section which is where the sweetest nurses and nicest rooms are located in ANY hospital!

I'm cautiously optimistic that it's going to be OK. The cancer hasn't spread as far as I know and I am confident that, unless I have breast cancer to go along with my other cancers, I'll be OK and should have a good outcome. I have my Alzheimer's stricken mother in law and my husband with me, so I'm in good hands with him and I don't know what we are going to do with her. I can't go back to Louisiana with her as I can't get medical treatment in Louisiana (Thanks Obama, you lying sack of crap) and she is whining and complaining about not being in her cluttered home with her mangy vicious cat that would have a home with us as well if she didn't attack everyone that gets near her—other than mom. She's about to complain herself into a nursing home for a few months until this is over because we can't deal with her and with cancer and since she's being totally uncooperative we are running out of options. I've been living in Louisiana with her for the last 27 months while John was looking for a job in Louisiana and he's been looking for nearly 3 years. Hopefully she will get with the program because I would have addressed this quite some time ago when Lori first got sick if I hadn't been in Louisiana looking after my mother in law which has caused treatment to be delayed in trying keep her OUT of a nursing home.

CHAPTER 8: THE FIRST ONCOLOGIST VISIT

I am not looking forward to this. I'm thinking that I'm probably looking at some more exploratory surgery to take a look inside my pelvis but this one is gonna be a b*tch because they may have to make the belly-button to pubic bone incision that will leave me with a 3-4 day hospital stay and a ruined abdominal wall muscle so if they can tunnel in through my hoo-ha and take a look around that's the plan I am in favor of. The oncologist visit wasn't encouraging AT ALL. I am more scared now than I was before. My oncologist is Dr. Francisco Xynos, M. D. who is reputed to be the BEST gynecological oncologist in the Midwest.

Good News: Dr. Xynos, at first glance, turns out to be from Europe a delightful man with a massive God complex and Greek chauvinist to to core who doesn't listen to a word I say and just talks over me. His attitude is "I'm the doctor, I know everything" so shut up, sit down and be quiet while I do exactly as I please. Bad news: The first surgeon didn't take out the Omentum or the lymph nodes and the oncologist said that if they find I have cancer in the omentum and/or the lymph nodes that I'm at stage 3 not stage 2A where I think I am. They won't know until they do a pelvic wash, then pull out the omentum and the lymph nodes, and the pathologist examines it. If they are clean then I'm at 2A stage, but if they are not and the pelvic wash isn't clean they will move me to stage three. If that happens, I am in real trouble.

The cure rate for stage 3A is WAY lower than for Stage 2A. If the lymph nodes and omentum are clean, my mathematical or I guess statistical chances to skate out of this are close to 90%. If they aren't, then my chances drop to about 20% which isn't a cheery thought. John is a rock but he's freaking out inside and I'm worried about him. Not to mention the fact that I have been eating beef and butter and cheese most of my life because I planned to go out with a quick heart attack—and I am NOT going to be cheated out of my planned massive heart attack—I've earned it by GOD and I'm going to have it!! Also, my first gynecological surgeon Dr. DallaRiva didn't follow the standard of care by doing a pelvic wash to check the fluid for cells. He didn't think it was needed because he wasn't looking for cancer, however anytime you open the

MASS MURDERING DOCTORS: THE TRUTH ABOUT ONCOLOGISTS, CHEMOTHERAPY AND CANCER

pelvic cavity in this sort of surgery ESPECIALLY ON A BRCA1+ patient, a pelvic wash is the absolute standard of care. I am extremely unhappy about that, so I don't know that the pelvic wash was clean maybe it would have been, maybe not but after this I'm betting he never fails to do another wash. However they're scheduling me for more surgery ASAP to remove the omentum and the pelvic lymph nodes which are not normally removed in a standard hysterectomy even with one as extensive the surgery I had. Additionally, Dr. Xynos said that I would have to have chemotherapy because even if I was at stage one this is such an aggressive cancer that they want to do major chemotherapy. However, this guy works at when I can only classify as a medical factory that has GOT to be the worst place I have ever been. An assembly-line style check in that refers to me by NUMBER and window wenches that; while not as openly hostile as the DallaRiva window wenches, have all the warmth, charm and bedside manner of Dr. Josef Mengle but not **QUITE** as much compassion for their patients. Notwithstanding the delightful experience with the window wenches, I take a seat in a waiting room filled with crying and screaming babies and a screaming, running **BRAT STAMPEDE** causing a decibel level just slightly louder than your average rock concert. This continues until I am so shattered and stressed that I begin to seriously consider choking the living crap out of one of them as an example to the rest to shut the f**k UP!! I'm not interested in anything but QUIET while I try to wrap my head around the fact that I may not live another year if this goes sideways. Just as I am selecting my intended victim, the door opens and the backroom wench calls my name, she saved lives and doesn't know it—5 more minutes of that screaming and I would not have cared about prison or the electric chair—it would have been SO worth it.

This is the appointment that tells the future. If my omentum and lymph nodes are clean and the pelvic wash is clean then I am not inclined to do chemotherapy for a cancer I do not have. If the cancer was contained in the ovary and uterus, and the omentum, nodes and wash are all clean I don't see any reason to have chemo for a cancer that is no longer there. Chemo is way too damaging to the body to have it for a cancer that's not there at 50K-100K a pop for my insurance company to pay just because they want to bill for it—plus **EVERY oncologist in America makes 80% of their annual income from FAILED chemotherapies. EIGHTY PERCENT. Let**

MASS MURDERING DOCTORS: THE TRUTH ABOUT ONCOLOGISTS, CHEMOTHERAPY AND CANCER

that number sink in for a minute. They also MARK UP the drugs they BUY FOR YOUR CHEMOTHERAPY, the only doctors that sell medications directly to the patients at a **HUGE** profit. They pay 5 grand for your chemo "cocktail" and bill your insurance for a hundred thousand (and the patient for the REST of the bill IF you agree to it), and keep the difference so don't think for a second that they don't have a HUGE financial motive to sell you that worthless treatment with an abysmal 2.1% cure rate— if Lincoln sold cars and 97.9% of them killed the driver, would they still be in business? Not bloody likely! While I sort of trust Dr. DallaRiva (until I discovered later that he left cancer behind and did a sloppy surgery job) I am not sure about Dr. Xynos. He has an excellent reputation as the best in the Midwest but I have many reservations. First, he's 71 years old. It's unlikely, in my view, that he has kept up on the latest changes and improvements in chemotherapy since he will likely be retiring soon, and I need an oncologist who is at the top of his game. As it turns out, that doesn't matter since these dipcraps are still pushing 39 year-old chemotherapy with its negligible cure rate. **There is no lobby in Washington as large, as powerful or as well financed as the pharmaceutical lobby, and according to a report from Public Citizen, more than half of the drug industry's 625 registered lobbyists [that is more than the number of members of Congress!] are either former members of Congress or former Congressional staff members and government employees ... Other evidence suggesting possible FDA bias turned up in a study revealing that 37 of the 49 top FDA officials who left the agency moved into high corporate positions with the company they had regulated. Over 100 FDA officials owned stock in the drug companies they were assigned to manage.**

When morality comes up against profit, it is seldom that profit loses.
----Shirley Chisholm

Just for giggles, here's the mark-up of common drugs:

The Commerce Department came up with some interesting numbers:

- •Celebrex 100 mg
  Consumer price (100 tablets): $130.27
  Cost of general active ingredients: $0.60
  Percent markup: 21,712 percent

MASS MURDERING DOCTORS: THE TRUTH ABOUT ONCOLOGISTS, CHEMOTHERAPY AND CANCER

•Claritin 10 mg
Consumer Price (100 tablets): $215.17
Cost of general active ingredients: $0.71
Percent markup: 30,306 percent

•Norvasc 10 mg
Consumer price (100 tablets): $188.29
Cost of general active ingredients: $0.14
Percent markup: 134,493 percent

•Prevacid 30 mg
Consumer price (100 tablets): $44.77
Cost of general active ingredients: $1.01
Percent markup: 34,136 percent

•Prilosec 20 mg
Consumer price (100 tablets): $360.97
Cost of general active ingredients $0.52
Percent markup: 69,417 percent

•Prozac 20 mg
Consumer price (100 tablets) : $247.47
Cost of general active ingredients: $0.11
Percent markup: 224,973 percent

•Tenormin 50 mg
Consumer price (100 tablets): $104.47
Cost of general active ingredients: $0.13
Percent markup: 80,362 percent

•Vasotec 10 mg
Consumer price (100 tablets): $102.37

MASS MURDERING DOCTORS: THE TRUTH ABOUT ONCOLOGISTS, CHEMOTHERAPY AND CANCER

Cost of general active ingredients: $0.20
Percent markup: 51,185 percent

•Xanax 1 mg
Consumer price (100 tablets) : $136.79
Cost of general active ingredients: $0.024
Percent markup: 569,958 percent

Big Pharma claims that these prices are necessary for them to continue with their expensive research. Not so. Most of their mark-up is designed to cover other costs such as lobbyists and advertising. I'm definitely going to get a second opinion on the need for chemotherapy, I trust Dr. Xynos to do the surgery but his reputation is as an excellent surgeon which does not necessarily a clinician make. If I have stage 3 cancer, I want a top oncologist clinician after the surgery. I don't trust and am totally uncomfortable with the medical mill that is SLU-care. It's so obviously about money and volume of patients; that I would not even take my precious Siamese cats there. They are not about anything but money there and medicine is nothing but a profitable business to these people and the patients are nothing but faceless numbers with no one caring what happens to them as long as they have insurance to pay the hugely inflated bills to cover cost of care for illegals and other uninsured, pushing my rates through the roof, to the tune of $1800 a month at last count.

I have a mammogram scheduled tomorrow and if the mammogram is clean Dr. Xynos wants to wait and do the mastectomy somewhere down the road as a preventative measure because breast cancer is much less virulent then the ovarian cancer that I have. I'm hoping it's clean to buy some time to address the ovarian cancer. Hopefully the omentum will be clean along with the lymph nodes because if it's not, then I'm in REAL trouble. While this is a life-threatening cancer at any stage, my survival chances are increased exponentially by this cancer being caught at and staying at stage 2. I dislike Dr. Xynos, although he appears to know what he's doing but I'm still so scared. No more wise cracks and joking about this cancer, it came to kill me and I'm pissed OFF. Cancer took my grandmother before I had the chance to

MASS MURDERING DOCTORS: THE TRUTH ABOUT ONCOLOGISTS, CHEMOTHERAPY AND CANCER

know her. It let me have my father all my life but it killed my sister 90 days ago, and now it has come to kill me. Will it come for my nieces and nephews and their children as well? Are they also BRCA1+ as well? The thought of losing any of them to the horror of ovarian or some other horrid cancer is more than I can deal with right now. I don't have children of my own but Justin, Cody and Carliegh are as close as I will ever get! My other nieces and nephews are not BRCA1+ as my brother is not BRCA1+ so they are safe thank GOD but if Lori's children carry this deadliest of all cancer genes, they can get cancer at any time that will likely kill them—and their children and future children are also at risk. This cancer is extremely aggressive and virulent and the oncologist told me that they would be doing chemo even if I was stage 1 and they want to do it intravenously and also do intra-peritoneal chemo where they would fill my pelvic cavity with chemo drugs as well which are FOUR HUNDRED TIMES STRONGER THAN WHAT THEY CAN GIVE ME INTRAVENOUSLY. This cancer becomes chemo-resistant after the first treatment so if they got all the cancer the first surgery and my omentum, pelvic wash where they pump sterile fluid into my pelvic cavity (then shake me to mix well LOL) and suction it out and check it for cancer cells. If the wash is negative, meaning the cells are all clean this time then I'm really not inclined to have chemotherapy for a cancer that is gone because the recurrence rate is so high. I don't want to waste my potentially best kill shot on a cancer that has been sliced out—particularly when chemo is so HORRIFICALLY damaging to the body and if there's no cancer, they have NO reason to chemo me other than for profit. Chemo is 100 grand a pop so it's a big moneymaker for them but my husband is an engineer and he agrees no chemo if the omentum, wash and nodes are clean. Cancer Inc. has a 2.1% cure rate (because if they allowed a REAL cure THREE HUNDRED BILLION DOLLARS a year—EVERY YEAR would vanish in a puff of smoke). The chemo they want to use on my is what they have been using as a front-line gold standard since 1978!!?? Are you f**king kidding me?? THIRTY-NINE YEARS of the research of the American Cancer Society and those Komen women running for that cure and the American Cancer Society and other cancer charities begging for more money for research (only about 10% of what they collect goes to research BTW so ACS is a scam as well). Their cure rate is abysmally low but they think I'm just going to sign up like a blind sheep for an almost 40 year-old treatment, they are flipping NUTS. All this

MASS MURDERING DOCTORS: THE TRUTH ABOUT ONCOLOGISTS, CHEMOTHERAPY AND CANCER

research and money for a 2.1% cure rate is the best they've got after 40 years and a TRILLION dollars in research? WHERE'S THE MONEY GONE (to trash real cures??) WHERE'S MY CURE?? These people are crazy if they think I'm going to be voluntarily poisoned by a moron who has no clue if it will even work and from what I read about it (not to mention it killing my sister who died from her chemo, not her cancer) the "cure" rate of 2.1% is LOWER than medications that HAVE BEEN REMOVED BY THE FDA for lack of efficacy!

I am also having a preventative double mastectomy ASAP. I haven't had a mammogram for a couple of years but my last one was clean—every one has been clean—and if I don't have breast cancer (Lori had 3 primary cancers—breast, ovarian and uterine—not related to each other and ALL triple negative) that will go a long way to calming everyone down and give me some breathing room. I would hate to have to fight three cancers at once, but the mastectomies and immediate reconstruction are a given no matter what. The gynecological oncologist gave the girls a thorough going over feel-up exam yesterday and said he didn't feel anything out of the ordinary, and I'm was supposed to have a mammogram today at 10 am but we are having a snowstorm or blizzard if you listen to channel 4 which seem to be always in "STORM MODE" so I have a backup appointment on Friday since I am probably not going to be able to get in today due to weather issues. Florida natives and snow on the roads are not a good mix, and I am a poor snow driver due to total lack of experience with snow driving!

They want to do a 3-D imaging but they don't know if they will get my HMO to authorize that by Friday and tell me I might be billed for the difference. They also floated the line that if my HMO didn't authorize it, I'd have to pay for it. HMOs NEVER BUT NEVER post-authorize anything. EVER. I'm fine with just the ultrasound and the mammogram. I'm confident that will give me a good enough image to know if I have active cancer right now TODAY. I don't give a flip about anything else—the old girls are GONE regardless of what the mammogram shows. I just need to know if I'm going to be fighting two cancers or just one and if the omentum and lymph nodes are clean then I'm pretty much home free as far as Round 1 of cancer killing me off and we'll

MASS MURDERING DOCTORS: THE TRUTH ABOUT ONCOLOGISTS, CHEMOTHERAPY AND CANCER

make a determination on whether or not we want to do the chemotherapy. It's a game time decision as they say.

I have the hysterectomy surgical follow-up tomorrow with Dr. DallaRiva which I don't anticipate being anything other than routine. I'm going to grill him a little about the pelvic wash and see what he thinks about this. If he tells me he's confident about the cancer being confined that will help calm me down a lot. I am seriously EXTREMELY uncomfortable with the place Dr. Xynos works. It's a straight up medical mill that is running people through there as fast as they can. It was horrible, like the busiest ER I've ever seen with screaming kids and so noisy and it seems like they are trying to cram in as many patients as possible to bill the insurance for as much higher bill. I do NOT trust them. I am not sure I will ever want to go there ever again. It's so hectic and noisy that it just shatters my already tightly strung nerves to the point of pain.

Believe me, I am not a little snowflake. I'm a rough and tumble kinda gal, grew up in rural (at the time) Florida, grew up with horses and ended up having to battle stage 2 or possibly 3 ovarian cancer. Lori was way tougher than me. She raised 3 really good kids and built a million dollar business in her spare time. My oldest nephew, Justin is an accountant with a wonderful wife and they are so pathetically in love that watching them with each other is sweet enough to make you pop positive on a diabetes test. The have two cute kids, a boy Banyan who looks EXACTLY like Justin did when he was that age. They also have Leilani Grace who was named after my mother and she is the picture of Kristen but I can see some of her daddy as well. I love them all and they just lost their mother and grandmother who was my baby sister.

I expected to be telling you all about her fight for life and to beat this genetic killer of women and how brave she was. Then I wanted to tell you about how I found out I was BRCA1 and my decision to have my breasts and reproductive system removed as a preventative measures since I am BRCA1 and how important it is to be tested if you have a family history of cancer. Then all of a sudden in the blink of an eye, her fight became my fight as well, but I may have a better chance of survival because of her. With her death, she reached out and gave me a chance to save my own life and I foolishly procrastinated and I may pay for that with MY life. I really need to start doing everything my beloved, brilliant engineer husband tells me to do—he's never

MASS MURDERING DOCTORS: THE TRUTH ABOUT ONCOLOGISTS, CHEMOTHERAPY AND CANCER

wrong and I should listen to him more carefully but I foolishly always think I know better. I know when he reads that I will never live it down but I do not care. When John is right, he's REALLY right.

Stage 2 is survivable, hopefully and almost 40% of Stage 2 BRCA1 make 5 years but even at then the recurrence rate is very high, 88% of all stages have a recurrence within six to eighteen months and the diagnosis of ovarian cancer when you have no ovaries and it comes back is peritoneal carcinomatosis, which is unfailingly fatal because IV chemo won't reach it and it's inoperable, you cannot remove the peritoneum and you can't radiate the intestines—so you die. PERIOD. There are no known survivors of High-grade serous-cell carcinoma when it recurs as the "always fatal" peritoneal carcinomatosis. I fully expect that I will eventually die of some kind cancer because of my genetic defect but I hope it won't be THIS round that puts my lights out. I want to spend time with my husband and don't want him to be old and alone because I croaked. I like John as a person in addition to loving him and I like spending time with him. He retires in a few years and I am looking forward to that time with him when we don't have work stresses and money isn't a worry because we've worked and saved. This is why I am grateful we have an excellent HMO and I try to keep them from being ripped off by the medical profession.

SIDEBAR: HMOs vs. PPOs: THE VIEW FROM THE STIRRUPS

THANK GOD we have an HMO (Health Maintenance Organization) instead of a PPO (Preferred Provider) because this wouldn't be affordable if we didn't. A PPO means we pay 30% of our health costs, prescriptions, hospitals, doctors, etc. and the insurance companies pay the rest. The premiums are lower because you pay a bigger part of the cost of your care out of pocket. You save $200-$300 a month on the premiums but if you get sick, you are on the hook for a 1/3 of the cost. 30% doesn't SOUND like a lot, but on a 100K hospital bill it's 30 grand—and a hundred grand bill can take less than a week to ring up—so choose HMO! My one night stay at Anderson Hospital was over EIGHTEEN THOUSAND DOLLARS!!The lab work was ELEVEN HUNDRED DOLLARS!! The surgeon's fee was $3800. There were other charges too, but these are the big ones. On a PPO, our responsibility would be 30% or just under SEVEN THOUSAND DOLLARS. With our HMO the Hospital co-pay was $250, and the

MASS MURDERING DOCTORS: THE TRUTH ABOUT ONCOLOGISTS, CHEMOTHERAPY AND CANCER

Surgeon's co-pay was $40 for the surgical office visit co-pay and no co-pays on the labs so about $300 makes way less of a dent in the retirement than $7100!! The second hospital stay for 1 night was THIRTY-EIGHT THOUSAND DOLLARS—twenty thousand MORE than the first hospital for the same exact surgery and lab work. I've never seen such blatant thievery in my entire life and they weren't even embarrassed. It's called "cost-shifting" where the hospital bills my insurance company for 10-20 times what it SHOULD cost and try and bill the patient for the rest. **Never accept financial responsibility past what your insurance will pay and write it on the form—legally they cannot refuse to treat or admit you for this.** They are under contract with your insurance company to treat you for what the insurance company pays, NOT to take your insurance company's negotiated fee and try and sue YOU for the rest which they WILL do. More on that later.

I highly recommend HMOs by the way. I have always used HMOs and never had a problem with any kind of treatment I needed. If my primary care doctors said I had to have it, I got it. It might take a few days but I got it and for almost 30 years I've used HMOs for my health care needs. I'm a big fan of HMOs. The co-pays have gone up but it saves money in the long run. It used to be $5 to see the doctor and $5 for a generic prescription, but this was too cheap and caused people to go to the doctor when they had a splinter in their finger. At $40 to see the doctor, that's enough of a bite (after the monthly premiums) that you don't run to the doctor's office for every little sniffle resulting in a $500 or so bill for your HMO insurance company to pay and people going to the doctor when they aren't really sick enough to need medical attention but they figure it's only $5 so might as well go. $40 would at least make them THINK about it first.

This keeps the premiums down but those $40 a pop co-pays add up fast so try to combine visits or talk on the phone because it's free and bring a list of questions with you to the doctor—and don't go to the office to hear what they can tell you on the phone because THAT is also $40 just like an office visit. Still, I wouldn't trade my HMO for any other type of policy. They also have one more big advantage—NO lifetime limit on the amount they will pay. NONE. Many PPOs now have a ONE MILLION DOLLAR Lifetime Limit which seems like plenty of money—but it is not enough for cancer treatment. My sister's cancer was $750,000. 00 in 13 months. Mine is $67,000 for two days in the hospital and 2 robot surgeries. An HMO means you never run out of insurance money to fight for your life.

CHAPTER NINE: FOLLOW-UP VISIT AFTER 1ST HYSTERECTOMY

I am seeing Dr. DallaRiva at 8:45 for my follow-up after surgery. I've got a few questions to ask and of course I'll get to ride the iron pony again. I have the mammogram scheduled for 9 am Friday morning and hopefully by Tuesday I will have some answers I desperately need but am terrified to hear. We meet with Dr. DallaRiva and I rode the iron pony and he said I looked good and healing great and we talked about the cancer. I like what I heard and what Dr. DallaRiva had to say and so did John. He's not thinking about pushing chemo down my throat like the oncology people are scaring the crap out of me in doing so and they are pushing chemo hard. With this cancer you get 6 chemo treatments and that's it. No more. It recurs in 88% of the people who have it EVEN WITH CHEMO because chemo demolishes your immune system and makes cancer cells immortal because your body has nothing left to fight with. I'd like to monitor it closely and if it recurs THEN I will bang it with the chemo and hope for the best. Chemo is so damaging to the body that my quality of life would be crap even if the cancer didn't come back—and I wouldn't want to live like that—sick and suffering all the time from chemo side effects sitting on the couch dependent on a caregiver—and doing what? Miserably waiting to die? That's no life for me—and if you KNOW me, you KNOW that. The group I've been sent to is a very aggressive oncology group and I am certainly going to get a second opinion from a more conservative group. We are all going to die—it's just a question of your state of health up to the end. I don't see the point of beating this cancer at the price of being an invalid or semi-invalid for the rest of my life. I've got bigger and better things to do that spend a couple of decades going back and forth to doctor's appointments all the time. That's not life—that's an existence.

If you have cancer in your family and your mother and/or other 1st and 2nd degree relatives have died of either breast, ovarian or uterine cancer you NEED to be tested for the BRCA1+ genetic defect. Your health insurance will pay for it and your LIFE may depend on it. My sister fought her cancer not knowing until the end that she was

MASS MURDERING DOCTORS: THE TRUTH ABOUT ONCOLOGISTS, CHEMOTHERAPY AND CANCER

BRCA1+ and telling me to get tested. I had the test in October (takes 3 weeks to get the results) and I found out I was also BRCA1+ and that's why I arranged the surgery that may now NOT save my life. Now I'm waiting to see if I have a death sentence in my belly. I'm hoping and praying that I don't. The clean mammogram was a big psychological boost, but now I'm scared again. The wait until Thursday night is a long wait. I'm alone in the house and John and Mama G are on their way back to Louisiana to check on the house and do Mama G's income tax and drive back to Illinois for my surgery on Thursday. So, while I wait I want to tell you about my baby sister. We had a strange relationship but it worked for us.

CHAPTER 10: ME AND BABY SISTER

Lori and I had exactly 3 things in common. We are both allergic to morphine. We are both BRCA1+ and we have the same parents. That's about it. Now I can add a fourth thing: we may die of the same cancer. We are opposites in that we have literally NO shared interests. We never ever had a lunch when it was just the two of us and we only did hostage lunches—Mother's day, Mom's or Dad's birthday, Easter, Christmas, etc. We had only one mutual friend, Gerilyn Hughes who is an RN and Lori's REAL sister, they were best friends all of her life and I love Geri, she is an amazing person. I didn't hang out with her but she and Lori were always hanging out and when I saw them we'd all talk. It was so much easier to talk to Lori with Gerilyn around. Anyway, we loved each other and I love her kids, my niece and nephews and even though the only time we ever really talked was when she did my hair—and she was the BEST hairdresser in the world—no kidding. Over the years we never really argued but we knew we didn't agree on anything—so we never talked about anything but family stuff. She was a good mom and loved her kids and grandkids. She was a hell of a businesswoman too. She took a high school diploma and a cosmetology license and built it into a multi-million dollar salon and spa. She worked hard and spend a lot of time with her church but I'm not religious, I'm more spiritual. She was a lovely person but I don't regret that we never spent a lot of time together. I've lived all over the world so I just wasn't around much and we would catch up when we saw each other. Not seeing each other very often or for long periods of time worked perfectly for us and kept the family tiffs to an absolute minimum.

MASS MURDERING DOCTORS: THE TRUTH ABOUT ONCOLOGISTS, CHEMOTHERAPY AND CANCER

She called me and told me she was having a boob lift and a tummy tuck as a divorce present for finally getting rid of Dave, her ex-husband and one of life's more major asshole douche-bags. She had this surgery done the same day I did my face lift and we both had great results which we shared on my next visit to FL, and her surgeon did a spectacular job on her new boobs and tummy tuck. I went back to Illinois and 10 months later in August of 2014 she calls me and tells me she has a small breast cancer and she's going to have a mastectomy so that she doesn't have to do chemo. I tell her it's really early; give her the standard spiel about "early detection is the key to a cure" and told her that she will be fine. She says she's not worried, she just doesn't want to take two weeks off from work because she's really busy and she is seeing someone who turns out to be her piece of crap ex-husband. I tell her to call me when she feels better and that everything will be OK; at the time, I had no reason to think it wouldn't. Three days later she calls me to tell me that they found ovarian cancer when she was waking up from surgery and that they had drained 4 liters of ascites out of her belly and I knew she had to be in at least stage three and I called my Mom and she told me the fluid was FULL of cancer cells and this cancer is like the Red Tide: unstoppable. The ascites were happily doing what they do, they were seeding her peritoneal cavity with High-Grade Serous Carcinoma tumors that were already large and all over her pelvic cavity in golf ball size when they did her hysterectomy. When she woke up from the anesthesia they told her that she was terminal which she never told us, (but they NEVER DID THE INTRA-PERITONEAL CHEMOTHERAPY that they were so eager to do to me; they did IV chemo until they KILLED HER.) and my mother told me that they pulled 4 liters of malignant ascites out of her. It was at that moment I realized that she was going to die from this, and as it turns out, she sure did. She believed the lies that Cancer, Inc. told her and she believed that chemo (along with her ex-husband who was running the show and thought he knew it all and was in love with the poison that is chemo) was the way to go. I begged her to try RSO and immunotherapy even as an adjuvant to help with the chemo but she wouldn't do it. She believed her lying, greedy doctors and they killed her with the poison they were selling at a 20,000% markup. I didn't have any idea I'd be fighting the same cancer, I just desperately didn't want her to die because she was so important to so many people and to our parents as well, particularly my mother. Mom and Lori re-

MASS MURDERING DOCTORS: THE TRUTH ABOUT ONCOLOGISTS, CHEMOTHERAPY AND CANCER

attached the umbilical cord when she was a week old and they were inseparable—even as a child they had a bond no one could get between. It's a large part of why I have almost no relationship with my mother. The golden child just took every second of my mother's time—just they way they both wanted it. When I was about 25 I realized I'd never have anything like a close relationship with either of them so I pretty much went my own way. It wasn't worth the effort, and it was pretty obvious that neither of them were going to make any effort so I didn't see the point in killing myself to foment a closer relationship which no one apparently wanted and no one ever said a word about it to either of us.

Lori put up a good fight, I'll give her that. She never had a chance but she fought like a tiger. At the end she was tested for BRCA1 and sure enough she popped it and she told me to go get tested and I did and she doesn't know this but she may have saved my life by telling me to get tested. She died on November 18, 2015 and my husband John started nagging me THE NEXT DAY to get the hysterectomy so I did mostly to shut him up about it. His nagging is what saved my life if I beat this thing. I will literally owe him my life. I would not have gone in for at least another year because it was bad timing—right in the middle of a presidential campaign I desperately wanted to work on as one of the first supporters of the eventual nominee and now President Trump. Had I waited until summer 2017 I would have probably (possibly?) been showing symptoms by then and it would have been too late. I would have been almost stage 4, as a Stage 3C where Lori was, and I would not have had the chance to intervene to try and prevent the cancer. This cancer starts shedding cells when it reaches 3 centimeters in size AND DOUBLES IN SIZE EVERY FIVE WEEKS. Had I waited until summer 2017 which was my original plan, then I would have died for certain. I may still die, I don't know—but the surgery gave me a chance to save my own life. Lori and I had very little in common but we loved each other, albeit from a distance, and if I survive this, it will be ONLY because of her telling me to get tested and beloved husband John nagging me to get the surgery done. I am a BORN procrastinator, I would NEVER have gotten a hysterectomy to remove what I believed to be perfectly healthy organs if I hadn't found out how huge the risk if I didn't have the surgery but mostly it was the relentless nagging of my beloved husband that made me do it. My first surgeon, Dr. James DallaRiva of Maryville, IL, told me straight up that he removed perfectly healthy organs and said he loved doing that with BRCA1 people. Then he called me 5 days later to tell me I have ovarian cancer. Then I had to call my parents who buried my sister 90 days ago and tell them I have the same cancer that killed their other daughter. I think that's the hardest phone call I've ever made. I know I repeat things, but I write this as I think about what is to come and what has been. My friends have been wonderful and supportive. My family also supportive but I live far away from them. If this goes south and I go terminal, I'm going to see if I can go to Florida for the hospice to make it easy for the family to come see me if they want to. I'm so worried about John. I would be cracking under the pressure of what he's dealing with and he's doing his best to be brave. I hate to put him through this, it's killing me to see how upset he is. But that's another chapter. Thank you sis for trying to help me save my life—I wish I'd been smart enough to go make the appointment to have this done 3 months earlier, maybe I'd only have one cancer to fight instead of two. Statistically speaking, I have a 46% 5 year survival chance. It drops to 20% if I go to stage-III and there's also an 81% relapse rate within 6 months. This cancer is a motherfucker to kill—and I have to kill it or I die. It's really just that simple. I'm getting ready to gear up and fight aggressively with surgery and possibly chemo or I will definitely die. Pretty simple really.

CHAPTER 11: THE TEST RESULTS AND SECOND SURGERY

I had a mammogram Friday February 26th and it was sparkling clean—nothing even remotely wrong with the girls. I also got my CA-125 test results back as well. My CA-125 was 16 and normal is 0-35. Lori's first CA-125 was 964 (and went over 1100 later) so this is good news for me and I tell my friends and family. I'm not going to have to battle a THIRD cancer right now so I am one happy camper. It's a very encouraging sign and now I am praying to be 3 times lucky and have a good surgical outcome. John will be home tomorrow and I can't wait to see him! So much is riding on the labs on this surgery. I'm scared because all I am reading is how low the cure rate is, and how fast it recurs and how SO VERY FEW are totally cured, to where it never comes back. It's a frightening thing. I have so many plans for when we retire and so much to talk about and places to go and fun to have and I want to be around to enjoy it. John is everything in the world to me and the thought of being ANYWHERE he can't be with me is not one I want to entertain! No matter what; I am going to do my best to beat this cancer—I am not interested in a remission, I want a CURE—a forever cure where I live out my normal life span with John next to me in a rocking chair as we grow old.

SIDEBAR: STAGES OF OVARIAN CANCER

Once diagnosed with ovarian cancer, the stage of a tumor can be determined during surgery, when the doctor can tell if the cancer has spread outside the ovaries. There are four stages of ovarian cancer Stage I (early disease) to Stage IV (terminal disease). Your treatment plan and prognosis (the probable course and outcome of your disease) will be determined by the stage of cancer you have. Following is a description of the various stages of ovarian cancer:

Stage I- Growth of the cancer is limited to the ovary or ovaries.

Stage IA- Growth is limited to one ovary and the tumor is confined to the inside of the ovary. There is no cancer on the outer surface of the ovary. There are no ascites present containing malignant cells. The capsule is intact.

Stage IB- Growth is limited to both ovaries without any tumor on their outer surfaces. There are no ascites present containing malignant cells. The capsule is intact.

Stage IC- The tumor is classified as either Stage IA or IB and one or more of the following are present: (1) tumor is present on the outer surface of one or both ovaries; (2) the capsule has ruptured; and (3) there are ascites containing malignant cells or with positive peritoneal washings.

Stage II- Growth of the cancer involves one or both ovaries with pelvic extension.

Stage IIA- The cancer has extended to and/or involves the uterus or the Fallopian tubes, or both. This is where I believe I should have been staged.

Stage **IIB**- The cancer has extended to other pelvic organs.

MASS MURDERING DOCTORS: THE TRUTH ABOUT ONCOLOGISTS, CHEMOTHERAPY AND CANCER

Stage IIC- The tumor is classified as either Stage IIA or IIB and one or more of the following are present: (1) tumor is present on the outer surface of one or both ovaries; (2) the capsule has ruptured; and (3) there are ascites containing malignant cells or with positive peritoneal washings. **(This is where dr. Xynos staged me based on less than 20 "atypical" not cancerous cells.)**

Stage III- Growth of the cancer involves one or both ovaries, and one or both of the following are present: (1) the cancer has spread beyond the pelvis to the lining of the abdomen; and (2) the cancer has spread to lymph nodes. The tumor is limited to the true pelvis but with histologically proven malignant extension to the small bowel or omentum.

Stage IIIA- During the staging operation, the practitioner can see cancer involving one or both of the ovaries, but no cancer is grossly visible in the abdomen and it has not spread to lymph nodes. However, when biopsies are checked under a microscope, very small deposits of cancer are found in the abdominal peritoneal surfaces.

Stage IIIB- The tumor is in one or both ovaries, and deposits of cancer are present in the abdomen that are large enough for the surgeon to see but not exceeding 2 cm in diameter. The cancer has not spread to the lymph nodes.

Stage IIIC- The tumor is in one or both ovaries, and one or both of the following is present: (1) the cancer has spread to lymph nodes; and/or (2) the deposits of cancer exceed 2 cm in diameter and are found in the abdomen. **(Lori was at this stage when her cancer was discovered).**

Stage IV- This is the most advanced stage of ovarian cancer. Growth of the cancer involves one or both ovaries and distant metastases (spread of the cancer to organs located outside of the peritoneal cavity) have occurred. Finding ovarian cancer cells in pleural fluid (from the cavity which surrounds the lungs) is also evidence of stage IV disease. Ovarian cancer that spreads to the lungs is still ovarian cancer, it's never lung cancer which is a different type of cancer.

MASS MURDERING DOCTORS: THE TRUTH ABOUT ONCOLOGISTS, CHEMOTHERAPY AND CANCER

I arrive at the hospital and sign in and prepare for surgery. They tell me they haven't received the results of my CA-125 test and tell me they are going to do another one. I am cognizant that they will charge my insurance company several hundred dollars for a second test, so I refuse to have them do it and call to get the results of the original test sent over. It's ridiculous what they charge for these tests—plus we now have to pay 10% of the RETAIL price for labs, and my insurance company is very good to me when it comes to my healthcare so I am pretty stingy with their money because the cost of insurance could be brought down if people were not insulated from the cost of their decisions. 9 out of every 10 dollars spent on health care are paid by someone other than the patient.

I have prepped for this surgery and took a dose of Phenergan to prevent the vomiting I had last time and they wheel me away for surgery and I go into surgery more than an hour after my scheduled surgery time since Dr Xynos was extremely late getting to my surgery. I tell them that Demerol is what works best for me in a PCA pump and that Phenergan stops me from vomiting. You'd think after 34 surgeries the jackass Dr. Xynos would listen to me—but oh HELL no!! Waking up I am attached to a PCA pump that is squirting Dilaudid into my vein every 10 minutes on demand. Dilaudid doesn't work well for me for pain relief as it works on my like amphetamines—I was wired from head to toe and stayed up ALL NIGHT walking the halls of the hospital mashing that pain button to see if I could get some sleep but Dilaudid has no real effect on me, good old-fashioned Demerol is what works for me. I take a couple of 10mg Vicodin for pain since the PCA pump is woefully inadequate. I NEVER go to the hospital for surgery without some backup painkillers in my handbag—you never get sufficient pain meds in the hospital so I bring my own so that I am not at the mercy of Nurse Ratched's sorority sisters, although the nurses here were just as sweet as the ones at Anderson. Meghan was my primary nurse with Penny as her backup nurse and Dawattie was my CNA and they are all very competent, professional and very sweet. I'm in way more pain than the last surgery 2 weeks previous and I have 5 MORE stab wounds in my belly. I won't have any results on the labs until a week goes by. My beloved husband comes to my room and leaves my clothes and my purse and my iPad so that I can read if I feel like it. It's a bad night. I had TOLD (Dr. Know-It-All Xynos) the surgeon that Demerol works better for my pain but he gave me Dilaudid instead

MASS MURDERING DOCTORS: THE TRUTH ABOUT ONCOLOGISTS, CHEMOTHERAPY AND CANCER

so I cannot sleep at all and I am up all night long. Even the 20 mgs of Hydrocodone I sucked down from my personal stash didn't help much. Demerol controls my pain and puts me to sleep while Dilaudid amps me up and keeps me awake all night long. I've had over 30 surgeries in my life and I know what works on me, but they much prefer to give me newer and MORE EXPENSIVE drugs that don't work—including USELESS Zofran, an anti-emetic (anti-nausea & vomiting drug) that makes me puke constantly which baffles these morons. I take another Phenergan (I brought it with me as well, bringing my own meds is mandatory since no one listens to the patient) and the nausea stops, mercifully. The nurses, Meghan and Penny and Dawattie my CNA take very good care of me. My catheter is pulled around midnight, in the morning I eat and I am discharged with my husband waiting to take me home. It's a long and rough ride home, nearly 50 miles and I have the worst heartburn ever. We stop for gas and I hobble into the convenience store to get some Rolaids. John tries very hard to miss the bumps but his Prius doesn't have the pillow soft ride of my Lincoln Town Car but we get home and I go to bed. John makes me chicken noodle soup and I eat it and go to sleep. I'm home from my latest hospital adventure with five MORE stab wound in my belly. I look like Jack the Ripper had a go at me!! Waking up I can barely move because I am in so much pain and can barely get out of bed to go to the bathroom. I feel like I have been gutted like a common catfish. John calls my parents and close family and tells them I am home safe. Once again I am on bed rest with bathroom privileges and life is more painful. I am living on yogurt, blackberries, blueberries and chicken noodle soup with painkiller chasers. It's a miserable weekend with my poor husband trying to do anything to help me and me laying in the bed trying not to move at all—like the great white whale with red hair. I am grateful for my laptop which is my window to the world even though there's a great big TV in the room.

I start to research chemotherapies since I am fairly certain that I am going to have to have some chemo treatment of some type. I am shocked and STUNNED to see just how BAD my chances of survival are even WITH the miserable life experience known as chemo. The treatment my doctor, "the best gyno-oncologist in the Midwest" is advocating is almost FORTY YEARS OLD. Billions of dollars every year for FORTY f**king YEARS has been raised by the thieves known as the American Cancer Society and THIS ancient treatment is the best we've got? What are all those Komen bitches

MASS MURDERING DOCTORS: THE TRUTH ABOUT ONCOLOGISTS, CHEMOTHERAPY AND CANCER

running for?? Where's my CURE???? I am not interested in the FDA (owned by Big Pharma by the way) and their definition of an effective cancer treatment. Do you know what that is? I do. **If your cancer tumor shrinks by 50% for 28 days, the FDA considers it an EFFECTIVE CANCER TREATMENT.** What kind of total bullcrap is this???? Do you know what it does toward a cure to have your tumor halve in size for 28 days? **NOT A GODDAM f**king THING!!!!** I take that back—it nets 75-100 grand for your scumbag oncologist—but that is IT!! All these years and BILLIONS of dollars for research and THIS is ALL they have to show for it—a 40 year old treatment for the DEADLIEST women's reproductive cancer that exists? **As it turns out, it's the chemo that is used for every cancer as the first-line treatment.** WTF?? This is the best they've got and they really expect us to believe that they give a rat's rear end about curing cancer? They don't want to CURE cancer, they want to TREAT cancer—for a fuckton of money! All that American Cancer Society and Komen fundraising which is ALSO hundreds of millions EVERY YEAR would be GONE in a puff of smoke if there was a cure for cancer and they'd ALL be out of a job —oh and they spend 90% of their annual donations on everything EXCEPT research for a cure plus going out of their way to trash any kind of REAL cure no matter how scientifically sound. Wonder why THAT is? I don't. Job Security and MONEY. There's no money in a healthy population—we have to be sick so they can treat us with their ever more expensive procedures and medications.

These people are so totally full of crap—and they say: "Donate as we are SO CLOSE to a CURE!!" with a straight face when they KNOW they are lying sacks of crap. The head of the ACS makes 6 figures—GONE in the blink of an eye if they get a cure. Ditto for the head of the Susan G. Komen breast cancer foundation. I've spent 60K on cancer treatment so far, I've got a crappy plastic teal bracelet and a deadly cancer to show for it. I believe that Marijuana cures many forms of cancer and if it didn't, Big Pharma wouldn't be so desperate to keep it off the market while at the same time pulling every possible patent related to marijuana that they can get!! **They are not even REMOTELY interested in a cure, they are interested in keeping the 200 to 300 billion dollar a year cancer cash cow vomiting money while people suffer and die.** Immunotherapy also shows great promise but it's commonly in use in Europe, but not in America. I hate oncologists. Scumbags, every single one of

MASS MURDERING DOCTORS: THE TRUTH ABOUT ONCOLOGISTS, CHEMOTHERAPY AND CANCER

them. We owe a lot to pioneers and brave visionaries like Rick Simpson who experimented with homegrown marijuana and no lab to find the cure for their own cancer and use the power of the internet to get the word out; as marijuana becomes legal for medical and recreational use in more states every year. The genie is absolutely out of the bottle—in the USA, more states ALLOW medical and or recreational marijuana than don't. Florida will be the next state to legalize I think. I also believe that marijuana will help cure my cancer WITHOUT the chemotherapy I don't want to have. I hate to puke—I really hate it. I'd rather die—and so I'm leaning away from having chemotherapy as I don't want the terrible side effects and I am willing to risk my life to prove that Rick Simpson Oil (RSO) and immunotherapy will cure my stage 2-C (according to Dr. Xynos) ovarian cancer.

We won't know the test results until next week sometime. I don't know if there will be more surgery or chemo or what. It's a very aggressive—the MOST aggressive, most malignant and deadliest of all gynecological cancers with a very high recurrence rate, 89% to be exact which leave me with a dilemma: Chemo and all the side effects for a cancer I don't have OR no chemo and a recurrence that may or may not happen with or without the chemo since the oncologist flat out told me they don't know very much about early stage ovarian cancer since they ALMOST NEVER SEE IT. It's enough to make a statue scream—but not enough to make them think that chemo may NOT be the way to go in every case because they are so brainwashed by the medical community and the Big Pharma-owned FDA. It's beyond insanity, and all of America is clueless and continuing to allow themselves to be voluntarily poisoned for profit by their DOCTORS and Big Pharma.

The waiting for the lab results are the hardest part. I can't stand not knowing because what's left of my life is hinging on what these labs say. I am cautiously optimistic that they got all the cancer and that I might survive this. If they didn't, then there will be chemo and I have decided that I am going to go ahead and have the double mastectomy before the chemo starts IF there is going to be chemo. I'm not sure that I'm going to have chemo if they got all the cancer. I don't see any point in treating cancer I don't have any more and if they cut it all out, then it's GONE, right? The problem is that this cancer is like the red tide. It spews malignant cells all through the

MASS MURDERING DOCTORS: THE TRUTH ABOUT ONCOLOGISTS, CHEMOTHERAPY AND CANCER

pelvis and abdomen and then the cells stick to the pelvic wall and form tumors everywhere—it's like dandelions in your yard—they pop up everywhere. The only chance I have is that if the cancer was contained in the ovaries and the uterus and Dr. DallaRiva got it all with the first strike—before we knew there WAS any cancer and that the RSO will take care of any residual cancer cells and I will be CURED. If that's the case, then the peritoneal wash should be clean—and if it is then the omentum and the lymph nodes also should be clean theoretically. However, speculation does me no good. Clean labs are what I must have to have any kind of a chance to beat this. The anxiety of waiting for the lab reports to see what my future holds is the very hardest part and even though the asshole doctor knows the results, they are not going to reveal them without my driving 100 miles and billing me $40 co-pay and my insurance for an office visit—for info they could give me on the PHONE. What Assholes!!

The standard for care is simple: During primary surgery for advanced stage epithelial ovarian cancer all attempts should be made to achieve complete cytoreduction (get all of the cancerous tumor in lay terms). When this is not achievable, the surgical goal should be optimal (No residual tumors larger than 1 cm) residual disease. The findings that women with residual disease when the surgery cannot remove all the cancerous tumors, tumors smaller than 1 centimeter will still do better than women with residual disease of tumors larger than 1 centimeter (Ya think??). The biology of ovarian carcinoma differs from that of hematogenously (blood-borne) metastasizing tumors because ovarian cancer cells primarily disseminate (spread) within the peritoneal cavity and are only superficially invasive. **However, since the rapidly proliferating tumors compress visceral organs and are only temporarily chemo-sensitive, ovarian carcinoma is a deadly disease, with a cure rate at all stages of only 20% and 0% when it recurs, as chemo makes it immortal.** There are a number of genetic and epigenetic changes that lead to ovarian carcinoma cell transformation. Ovarian carcinoma could originate from any of three potential sites: the surfaces of the ovary, the Fallopian tube, or the mesothelium-lined peritoneal cavity. Ovarian carcinoma tumorigenesis either progresses along a stepwise mutation process from a slow growing borderline tumor to a well-differentiated carcinoma (type I) or involves a genetically unstable high-grade serous carcinoma that metastasizes rapidly (type II) which is of course the kind I have and

MASS MURDERING DOCTORS: THE TRUTH ABOUT ONCOLOGISTS, CHEMOTHERAPY AND CANCER

what MOST BRCA1s and BRCA2s get. During initial tumorigenesis, ovarian carcinoma cells undergo an epithelial to mesenchymal transition, which involves a change in cadherin and integrin expression and up-regulation of proteolytic pathways. Carried by the peritoneal fluid, cancer cell spheroids overcome anoikis and attach preferentially on the abdominal peritoneum or omentum, where the cancer cells revert to their epithelial phenotype. After the ovarian carcinoma cells have detached as single cells or clusters from the primary tumor, they spread to the peritoneum and omentum, carried by the physiological movement of peritoneal fluid. The initial steps of metastasis are regulated by a controlled interaction of adhesion receptors and proteases, and late metastasis is characterized by the oncogene-driven fast growth of tumor nodules on mesothelium covered surfaces, causing ascites, bowel obstruction, and tumor cachexia. It is not clear if ascites is present when tumor cells initially metastasize, or if ascites is a sign of a more advanced, high volume disease, as clinical studies and experience would suggest. ****Author's Note: Since ascites do not appear until at least stage 3-B in most cases, it has to be the number one symptom of advanced ovarian cancer. My sister saw a gastroenterologist who treated her with antacids for SIX MONTHS while her cancer progressed from possibly treatable to terminal and my niece is suing the gastroenterologist for malpractice and wrongful death.****

A combination of factors can contribute to ascites formation in ovarian carcinoma. Cancer cells can obstruct sub-peritoneal lymphatic channels and prevent the absorption of the physiologically produced peritoneal fluid (about 1 liter per day). Moreover, secretion of vascular endothelial growth factor (VEGF) by ovarian carcinoma cells increases vascular permeability and promotes the ascites formation. Once the cancer cells have detached from the primary tumor, they float in the ascites as single cells or as multicellular spheroids. It is not clear whether single cells detach and then aggregate to form spheroids, or if the cells detach as cell clumps that stay together while floating in ascites. Although ovarian carcinoma cells have the potential to metastasize throughout the peritoneal cavity, the organ distribution of ovarian carcinoma metastasis from the primary tumor is not completely random. Other than the Fallopian tube and the contra-lateral ovary, the most common secondary sites for distant metastasis are the omentum and the peritoneum Within the peritoneum, which covers the entire abdominal cavity the right diaphragm and small bowel mesentery are preferentially colonized. **We do not know if ovarian carcinoma cells arrive at the secondary site as single cells or as spheroids, or if the primary ovarian tumor prepares the omentum/peritoneum for successful colonization.**

IN MY OPINION I do not see what the tumor could POSSIBLY do that would cause the omentum/peritoneum to "prepare" for "successful colonization" as it could not possibly have any effect on the omentum OR peritoneum. I think that the cancer cells just like the omentum—yummy fat to eat, nice and warm—perfect for rogue cells to colonize. It's the environment that suits their pathology and effectively kills the host as the tumors progress. This is just MY opinion. Your mileage may vary.

The fact that most primary tumors and metastasis have similar genetic changes has several potential implications for the diagnosis and treatment of serous ovarian carcinomas. It suggests that serous ovarian carcinoma is able to metastasize quickly once completely transformed. This was confirmed by mathematic modeling based on clinical data from BRCA1-positive patients undergoing a prophylactic oophorectomy who had small, sub-clinical cancers. **Brown and Palmer showed that these occult tumors double every 2. 5 months and that serous tumors disseminate (shed cancer cells into the pelvic cavity) when they are only 3 cm in size.** During primary surgery for advanced stage epithelial ovarian cancer all attempts should be made to achieve complete cytoreduction. When this is not achievable, the surgical goal should be optimal (< 1 cm) residual disease. Due to the high risk of bias in the current evidence, randomized controlled trials should be performed to determine whether it is the surgical intervention or patient-related and disease-related factors that are associated with the improved survival in these groups of women. The findings of this review that women with residual disease (less than) < 1 cm still do better than women with residual disease (more than) > 1 cm should prompt the surgical community to retain this category and consider re-defining it as 'near optimal' cytoreduction (surgical tumor removal in English), reserving the term 'suboptimal' cytoreduction to cases where the residual disease is > 1 cm (optimal/near optimal/suboptimal instead of complete/optimal/suboptimal).

MASS MURDERING DOCTORS: THE TRUTH ABOUT ONCOLOGISTS, CHEMOTHERAPY AND CANCER

SIDEBAR: FROM MY HUSBAND:

Opossums are the only North American marsupial, and according to John, they have more teeth than any other mammal. Additionally, each and every one of their teeth are very sharp. Now, back to our regularly scheduled bits of wisdom about the cheery subject of cancer.

I'm not looking for "treatment", I am looking for a **cure** that allows me to live out my projected life span. I am not interested in battling this cancer over and over again. I am NOT going to put my husband, parents and friends through that for years to come. If I am in an un-winnable battle, then so be it—but I am not bankrupting my husband and put my family through another nightmare battle with ovarian cancer that I can't win but I am also going to get a second opinion from a different gyno-onco group.

CHAPTER 12: THE SECOND SURGERY FOLLOW-UP VISIT AND PROGNOSIS

I have made a list of questions I want Dr. Xynos to answer for me, and you should definitely make a list of your questions as well.

My Questions for the Gyno-Oncologist Surgeon (with answers):

Was the pelvic wash clean? (It had less than 20 "atypical" cells.)

Has the cancer spread anywhere else? (No.)

Why didn't you take out all the omentum? (Wasn't needed, there was no cancer)

What are the probabilities of the cancer spreading to my peritoneum, colon and bladder? (At this point is hasn't happened.)

How will you monitor me for a recurrence? (CA-125 and MRI scans.)

What are the chances of a recurrence in the omentum? (Chemo pushed hard here.)

How do we monitor for that? (CA-125 and MRI scans.)

Would you still recommend a double mastectomy to prevent breast cancer? (Yes.)

What are my chances for an expected 5 year survival? (None without chemo.)

MASS MURDERING DOCTORS: THE TRUTH ABOUT ONCOLOGISTS, CHEMOTHERAPY AND CANCER

Did you get all the tumor? (Yes, no residual tumor, got 100% of the cancer.)

Was there any omental cake? (No.)

How much? (None.)

Am I going to die from this cancer? (Again promised good results from chemo which was an out and out LIE. They will always say "No" but once this cancer recurs as peritoneal carcinomatosis you're going to DIE and sooner if you do chemo because chemo makes cancer cells IMMORTAL.)

Do I need chemotherapy? (Again chemo was pushed hard. This will ALWAYS be a yes since the oncologist will pocket at least a half million dollars from the horrendously ineffective chemo treatment.)

This cancer becomes chemo-resistant with the first round, if you got all the cancer and the wash is clean, why do I need chemotherapy? (Lots of stuttering here, he really didn't have an answer.)

What is your position on prescribing Medical Marijuana? (very helpful BTW Neutral.)

Are there any clinical trials you are aware of that would help me to be CURED? (No.)

May I get a copy of my records to take for a second opinion? (Took forever!)

I'd suggest you make a list of your own questions to ask your doctor as well, and don't be afraid to change doctors. I called their office for my surgical lab reports and they gave me the usual song and dance over "not releasing on the phone" and I explained to them it was more than 100 miles round trip from the Illinois home and that I actually live in Louisiana so hopefully I will get them over the phone, but of course that didn't happen so I had to go sit in his office again and submit to being chucked under the chin like a child. I was going to change doctors anyway, but their bullcrap on the phone sealed the deal as far as I'm concerned. The REAL reason they won't give them to you on the phone is because if they do, they can't bill my health insurance for an office visit—and God forbid they should miss ANY billing opportunity that might present itself. **HOWEVER, if you go to the hospital and ask for the surgical and lab reports, by law they HAVE to give them to you.**

MASS MURDERING DOCTORS: THE TRUTH ABOUT ONCOLOGISTS, CHEMOTHERAPY AND CANCER

SIDEBAR: MY PERSONAL OPINION OF ST. LOUIS UNIVERSITY MEDICAL

I hate this practice, this doctor, his staff, this hospital and the medical mill it's attached to. I don't want to go here any more after we see them on Weds of next week. I don't like them and I sure as hell don't TRUST them and I don't want to come back to this group or this scummy office filled with screaming brats and illegal aliens all over the place dropping anchor babies. **I ACTUALLY HAD TO CARRY A SIGN SAYING I DID NOT HAVE EBOLA!!** I don't know about you, but I am never EVER again going to a place in THE UNITED STATES OF AMERICA WHERE I HAVE TO CARRY A SIGN STATING I AM EBOLA-FREE. I am NEVER EVER going back to SLU-care FOR ANYTHING—it's without a doubt the WORST medical mill EVER!! St Louis University (SLU-Care) is nothing but a scummy medical mill in my opinion. It is poorly run by the front office group and they are only interested in pushing through as many patients as possible with insurance so they can over-bill and cost shift to make my insurance company pay for all the illegals they are running through the place. It's a medical factory, and my surgeon didn't even prescribe any pain medications for me after surgery, so he's one of THOSE—or at 71 he's forgetting the basic tenets. I thought he had decent bedside manner (and he was highly recommended by Dr. DallaRiva, whom I DID trust at the time, until I found out he left behind the papillary serous carcinoma tumor that recurred and is now trying to kill me), but he's not the doctor I want for this, my life is hanging in the balance. Don't get me wrong, I don't personally dislike the doctor, he's OK, but I wanted someone younger and more up to date on new treatments; until I discovered that there are NO new treatments—the useless 39 year old poison chemotherapy with it's 2.1% CURE rate (assuming NO recurrence) is the standard of care and so profitable that I can't wait to blow the whistle on their bullcrap lies! I also strongly dislike doctors who pat my hand or chuck me under the chin and don't TELL me anything about my care other than to "live in the now". What the f**k is that? Live in the now? REALLY?? I need to know what is going on so that I can be a proactive partner in my care and treatment so I can get working and try to save my life because sure as crap these scumbag doctors couldn't care less about anything but trying to force me to have chemotherapy. Being proactive is how I found the cancer to begin with, and while I did not expect to already have cancer at least I have something of a chance (I hope) since it was

MASS MURDERING DOCTORS: THE TRUTH ABOUT ONCOLOGISTS, CHEMOTHERAPY AND CANCER

discovered early-stage (even though it's still just as deadly and likely to kill me) I have time to try and fight back proactively and save my own life—but what do I fight with? I KNOW there must be a cure out there and I am going to find it. If it's medical marijuana, cool. If it's immunotherapy; I'll find a way to get into a trial—but I am NOT going to die vomiting, bald and miserable following months and months of being bald, vomiting and miserable from chemo until I can't wait to die because I've been so sick for so long that dying is a welcome respite from the nightmare of chemotherapy. That's bullcrap!!

I also DON'T want to be a patient at a practice where I'm just a billing number—this place is a medical mill and I don't trust them. I was in no position to be picky when I needed to get this surgery done and they were already approved, but I don't want to continue to see them. I am very uncomfortable with the office staff and not really comfortable with Dr. Xynos either—he may be the best surgeon and all that but I don't like his "tell the patient nothing" way of doing things. I'd have rather stayed with Dr. DallaRiva, I liked and (at the time) trusted him—way more than this medical mill. Maybe I'm too flipped out over this to see it correctly. I thought the office at SLU was the worst place I've ever been for medical care in my life and I never want to go back there again EVER. Dr. Xynos may be a brilliant doctor, without a doubt, but he is the wrong doctor for me because I don't want a doctor that doesn't keep me informed. I'm not the kind of person who goes in for hand patting, I want to be engaged in my healthcare decisions and treatments. I also want a doctor who is on the cutting edge of what is going with research and breakthroughs along with alternative treatments, not this walking testament to the utter fail that is chemo. I am not a one-size-fits-all patient and since the conventional treatments for my kind of cancer, according to my research are **not working and never work as a recurrence has ZERO survivability,** I want one that works. I don't consider a doctor who at age 71 HAS TO BE at the end of his career to be the best choice for me. I don't want a doctor who is about to retire to be in charge of my treatment. Great surgeons aren't generally good clinicians and I need a great clinician. Make a list of the questions you want answered so you don't forget to ask them all.

MASS MURDERING DOCTORS: THE TRUTH ABOUT ONCOLOGISTS, CHEMOTHERAPY AND CANCER

While the office is required to send your records to you doctor of choice, they ARE allowed to charge you for copies—but they are NOT allowed to gouge you for the copying costs. Usually they charge 25 cents per page or so of the records, and the law does not allow them to charge you more than the ACTUAL cost of copying the records. If you feel they gouged you, make a complaint to the state medical association and send a copy of your complaint to the practice as well and that should get them to comply quickly.

While I don't think chemo is necessary if they chopped out the entire cancer but from what I read about this cancer it's so virulent and aggressive that even at stage 1 you get chemo, but it's definitely for the profit, not to help the patient. The survival rate on this cancer is remarkably low as they don't know too much about it. The problem is that there's not accurate test for early detection of this cancer as most patients don't know they have it until it's too late for them to do anything. 90% of ovarian cancer is detected at stage 3 or 4 and, since they usually die shortly after discovery—but not before a half million in chemo, they don't really KNOW how to successfully treat it in the very early-stages of the disease, which is bad for me.

However, I'm seriously considering calling Cancer Center of America as they have one in Missouri and seeing what's up. They do chemo both intravenously and they also like to fill the pelvic cavity with cancer killing drugs as well. This cancer is deadly because of the WAY it spreads. The cancer cells get into the pelvic fluid and grab onto the surface of the peritoneum and form new cancerous tumors everywhere they stick. The key to this is to get it before it starts to spray cells into the pelvis but if my washes weren't clean then it has had the time to embed into the pelvis—that's what I'm afraid of more than anything—plus the fact that DallaRiva missed getting the whole tumor in the original surgery. My sister went in for a mastectomy and they found her cancer while she was there and she was stage 3C with tumors bigger than 2 cm all over her pelvic wall, and they told her when she had her hysterectomy that she was terminal and then chemo-ed her until they killed her. I watched my sister die a little more every day—believing in the doctors that murdered her when I begged her; crying and on my KNEES, to listen to me and stop the chemo and let me save her life. I'll never forgive myself for not kidnapping her and chaining her in my basement until she was cured. She didn't have to die—and the oncologist killed her just as sure as if he had put a gun to her head and pulled the trigger. Now I have my parents looking at me with the same cancer and with elephant in the room is: Do they blame me? Did I try hard enough to save her? I don't want anyone else to die needlessly. The reason I need to know the labs is because I need to make some arrangements, I can't just stop my life and say "OK-put me in a bed for 6 months—I've got nothing better to do"—It's a PRESIDENTIAL ELECTION YEAR!

Last night I had a horrible dream about this cancer—it was like that thing in the movie Prometheus that Dr. Shaw ripped out of her with the machine only much more horrible because NO ONE knew what they were supposed to be doing and they were running around like maniacs. It was like the 3 stooges meeting Dr. Kildare on the Prometheus ship with the machine—HORRIBLE!! I'm going bananas trying to cover all the angles and decide what to do. I am also considering alternative treatments such as medical marijuana which I have been researching and there are some amazing cures from it. Big Pharma has been very successful for the last 30 years keeping medical marijuana against the law and off the market because they can't reap obscene profits from it. I'm also going to go to see my own PCP Dr. Janet Alvarado and see what she thinks, I need to see her anyway. If we could enlist her help it would be helpful as all get out. Louisiana has approved medical marijuana too. I'm also leaning toward the alternative medicine that Sarah is wanting me to take. I was also going to seriously consider making DallaRiva my PCP for insurance purposes so that he can get me set up for baseline testing and a monitoring schedule, but the window wenches in his office are just too much to deal with on a regular basis, I'd rather pay cash to Dr. Janet since Obamacare cost me the insurance she accepted.

At the Doctor's Office with Dr. Xynos: While the second surgery proved that Dr. DallaRiva has apparently gotten every bit of the cancer; just as he said, Dr. Xynos is insisting that I do 6 rounds of both IP (intraperitoneal) AND IV (intravenous) chemotherapy. Clearly he's lost his f**king MIND. John and I agree that this is absolutely insane because we will be treating a cancer that is NO LONGER THERE. Of course at FIFTY TO A HUNDRED THOUSAND DOLLARS a pop, **chemo is an ENORMOUSLY profitable moneymaker for the cancer drug makers and the**

MASS MURDERING DOCTORS: THE TRUTH ABOUT ONCOLOGISTS, CHEMOTHERAPY AND CANCER

hospital AND THE DOCTORS WHO MARK UP THE CHEMOTHERAPY DRUGS 20,000% AND RE-SELL THEM TO THE PATIENT AND POCKET THE 500-750 THOUSAND DOLLAR DIFFERENCE. Cancer is the second leading cause of death in the United States. According to the National Institute of Health, around 1,658,370 new cases will be diagnosed and 589,430 people will die from cancer in 2015. While most conventional cancer treatments revolve around a mix of surgery, chemotherapy and radiation, some people question their efficacy—particularly chemotherapy. In these videos two naturopathic doctors make the argument that in many cases, chemo does more harm than good. Peter Glidden, BS, ND, brings up the relationship between cancer and monetary profit. Glidden, author of The MD Emperor Has No Clothes, cites a study published in the Journal of Clinical Oncology, which found that over a 12-year period, chemotherapy did not cure adult cancer 97 percent of the time. "Why is it still used? There's one reason, and one reason only," Glidden says in the video. "Money." "Chemotherapeutic drugs are the only classification of drugs that the prescribing doctor gets a direct cut of," Glidden says. "The only reason chemotherapy is used is because doctors make money from it—period. It doesn't work 97 percent of the time. If Ford Motor Company made an automobile that exploded 97 percent of the time, would they still be in business?" he asks. "No!"

An Australian study looking at the contribution of cytotoxic chemotherapy to 5-year survival rates in adults with malignancies found that the "overall contribution of curative and adjuvant cytotoxic chemotherapy to 5-year survival in adults was estimated to be 2.3% in Australia and 2.1% in the USA." In their conclusion, the researchers stated: "it is clear that cytotoxic chemotherapy only makes a minor contribution to cancer survival." He cites this issue as just one example of a so-called healthcare system that prioritizes profits over human wellness. "This is the tip of the iceberg of the control that the pharmaceutical industry has on us," says Glidden. "Medicine in the United States is a for-profit industry. Most people are unaware of this, and most people bow down to the altar of MD-directed high-tech medicine." Naturopathic doctor Leonard Coldwell shares a similar perspective, calling chemotherapy "The Agent Orange of the medical profession. If you have a garden with flowers and bushes and trees and grass, and some weeds, you come with Agent Orange and kill it all off, and now it's all dead, and you hope only the good stuff is

MASS MURDERING DOCTORS: THE TRUTH ABOUT ONCOLOGISTS, CHEMOTHERAPY AND CANCER

coming back," Coldwell says. "They bombard the entire system and then they say the cancer is in remission." He notes that statistics on the effectiveness of cancer cures refer to survival rates after five years. "You killed basically every bioelectrical and biochemical function in the body," he says. "Since nothing works anymore, for three years, you have no cancer, you're cured. You're just dead in five years." Coldwell claims that radiation can cause similar harm. "It's an assault with a deadly weapon," he says. "When you radiate someone, it's causing scars. A scar can never turn back into healthy tissue." The problem, he says, is the way doctors are trained. "No medical doctor ever learns about curing anything," says Coldwell. "They learn about chemical intervention or surgery to suppress symptoms. They don't go for the root cause."

He points out that doctors have high rates of suicide as well as alcohol and drug abuse. "These poor guys figure out over time that they have no tools and that they are murdering, and [have] murdered, their patients," Coldwell says. "You go into the medical profession, the first year, the first two years, you're really excited, you're really in it, you're giving your all, until you find out no matter what you do the patient gets worse, or they cure themselves. These poor doctors figure out they cannot help," he says. "The medical profession is a religion." Why so much use of chemotherapy if it does so little good? Well for one thing, drug companies provide huge economic incentives. In 1990, $3.53 billion was spent on chemotherapy. By 1994 that figure had more than doubled to $7.51 billion. This relentless increase in chemotherapy use was accompanied by a relentless increase in cancer deaths.

Oncologist Albert Braverman, MD, wrote in 1991 that "no disseminated neoplasm (cancer) incurable in 1975 is curable today...Many medical oncologists recommend chemotherapy for virtually any tumor, with a hopefulness not discouraged by almost invariable failure."

Why the growth in chemotherapy in the face of such failure? A look at the financial interrelationships between a large cancer center such as Memorial Sloan-Kettering Cancer Center (MSKCC) and the companies that make billions selling chemotherapy drugs is revealing. James Robinson III, Chairman of the MSKCC Board of Overseers and Managers, is a director of Bristol-Myers Squibb, the world's largest producer of chemotherapy drugs. Richard Gelb, Vice-Chairman of the MSKCC board is Chairman of

MASS MURDERING DOCTORS: THE TRUTH ABOUT ONCOLOGISTS, CHEMOTHERAPY AND CANCER

the Board at Bristol-Myers. Richard Furlaud, another MSKCC board member, recently retired as Bristol Myers' president. Paul Marks, MD, MSKCC's President and CEO, is a director. These incestuous relationships between BigPharma and the cancer centers is a clear conflict of interest as it gives the cancer centers a huge motive to push their over-priced and underperforming poison to desperate, frightened cancer victims. BigPharma is also responsible for having emails from First Immune BLOCKED so that they cannot respond to inquiries from people who have Email accounts from the following domains: att.net, sbcglobal.net, bellsouth.net, and live.com. If your internet service provider is any of these, you will need to communicate with First Immune through a different email account such as Gmail or Yahoo in order to make sure they get through. You can also call them as international calls are cheap these days.

While I don't **actively dislike** Dr. Xynos, the chemo protocols and drugs he wants to use are THIRTY-NINE YEARS OLD!! That is NOT my idea of cutting edge medicine from the top gyno-oncologist in the Midwest and I am shocked that he is recommending treatment this old. This is the same crap they gave to my sister for the same cancer and she's dead as fried chicken—from the chemo, not the cancer. He also wants to put two ports in my body to facilitate the chemo which is a deal breaker from the get-go. The office wouldn't tell my results on the phone, apparently it's necessary for me to get up, get dressed, drive 140 miles, and pay a $40 co-pay so they can bill my insurance $550 for an office visit so you can bet your ass I will not be continuing to see this doctor. I like the doctor well enough, he's OK, but JUST OK, and I want someone younger and more up to date on newer treatments like immunotherapy which I have **ALWAYS** believed is the key to all cures. I am not comfortable with a doctor that is 71 years old in a field where cutting edge new treatments are what's saving lives, not ancient chemotherapy protocols that are God only knows how many years old. I have a very aggressive cancer with a very high recurrence rate and I need the best treatment I can get with someone up-to-date. He's a good surgeon but I am going somewhere else for follow-up care because I hate his office staff—a computer terminal where I could input information and scan my insurance card would be just as good as his office staff along with being nicer and more compassionate. The real calling for his office help should be checking people in for euthanasia, they'd enjoy the crap out of that, it suits their assembly-line medical mill operation perfectly: patients check in but they DON'T check out. I was in no position to be picky when I needed to get this surgery done and they were already approved by my insurance, but I don't want to continue to see them. I am very uncomfortable with the office staff and not comfortable with Dr. Xynos as a clinician either—he may have the reputation of being the best surgeon and all that but I don't like his "tell the patient nothing" way of doing things. I'd have rather stayed with Dr. DallaRiva, I liked and had trusted him-way more than this SLU-care medical mill. I thought that office at SLU-care (St. Louis University) was the worst place I've ever been for medical care in my life and I never want to go back there again EVER. Short version: Excellent SURGEON as far as I can tell. Office at SLU-care is godawful-the worst place I've ever been in MY LIFE. I made my follow-up appointment to go to his Chesterfield office which is 30 miles FARTHER away just to keep from having to go to SLU again. His office staff are horrible and the entire place is a medical mill designed to bill your insurance company for every possible penny. I am having serious misgivings about chemo, it did NOTHING for poor Lori and was the real reason she died, so I'll be damned if I'm going to just sign up for a treatment I may not need and even if I do, I don't want to spend what may be my last 6 months of life sick and miserable from the chemo. I'm going to seek a second opinion and I am also going to try some alternative therapies and medicine in the interim. I have just ordered 7 grams of RSO (Rick Simpson Oil) and I will start using that as soon as it gets here. These people are here for the MONEY; they do NOT CARE about their patients at all; and that attitude comes shining through from EVERYONE other than Dr. Xynos who is a sweet old guy and if handholding and chin-chucking were the level of care I need, this would be where I'd go. However, I want to live out my lifespan, not be another ovarian cancer death statistic an I'm absolutely certain that if I listen to Dr. Xynos that I will die before 2017 and this is NOT acceptable to me. He's in love with chemo and that spells certain death for me and 97.9% of his patients, so there's NO WAY I'm having ANY chemo.

I am thrilled to discover that I have NO ADDITIONAL CANCER. Dr. DallaRiva—God love him—apparently got it ALL just like he said he did. If they had just cut them out and tossed them we'd be in blissful ignorance, but I am having serious doubts about having any chemo. However, if it comes back we can fight it tooth and nail with

MASS MURDERING DOCTORS: THE TRUTH ABOUT ONCOLOGISTS, CHEMOTHERAPY AND CANCER

chemo then—and they can take out the rest of the omentum which apparently is just about all still there. In all likelihood it is going to come back anyway, statistically speaking and ANY recurrence will be stage 3 from the get-go. I just don't see the benefit to doing this because if it comes back I'm really no worse off because it will start in the omentum which is removable because it's STILL THERE. I'm not about to pay ANYONE a million bucks for chemotherapy that has such an abysmally low success rate and has left millions of corpses in its wake.

As I research the tremendous and HORRIFIC damage that cisplatin and carboplatin (with taxanes) chemo does to the human body and I am really more and more uncomfortable with the oncologist wanting to do SIX ROUNDS of high-powered cisplatin chemo over a few ATYPICAL cells that were surrounded by white cells in a still-healing-from-surgery pelvic cavity. These people are in love with chemotherapy and obviously out of their f**king minds if they think I'm signing up for this bullcrap chemo for a few cells that aren't even cancerous Because of the extreme toxicity of this kind of chemo, you can only do 6 rounds of it in your LIFE and this cancer becomes chemo-resistant almost immediately because chemo is totally ineffective anyway. The oncologist told me that they had enlarged nuclei which cancer cells always do HOWEVER while all cancer cells have enlarged nuclei—not all cells with enlarged nuclei are cancerous. I just cannot justify this level of chemo for a few cells that are not even malignant—especially when I know that chemo is a huge moneymaker for the medical industry at 75-100K a pop—so filling me with poison may not be medically necessary but they have $500,000 to $750,000 reasons to do it anyway "to be sure". That's not just a no, it's a HELL NO! While I could possibly learn to trust Dr. Xynos, he's still 71 years old and, in my opinion, clearly not up to date with the latest and best treatments if he is recommending a 39 year-old treatment for a deadly cancer and never even mentions immunotherapy which I believe is the very best way to treat cancer or anything else for that matter. Throughout history, disease has not been a huge mystery, HEALTH is what they don't understand. Immune systems are powerful weapons and when your immune system can be manipulated to fight tumors and kill them, it HAS to be the way to go and I believe the future of ALL cancer treatment. It also needs to be the front-line treatment rather than the useless but very profitable poison that is chemotherapy. I'm going to do my best to stay alive

MASS MURDERING DOCTORS: THE TRUTH ABOUT ONCOLOGISTS, CHEMOTHERAPY AND CANCER

until immunotherapy is is use in the next 2-5 years and then I'm going use that to fight this cancer. Right now I am essentially cancer free, but this cancer is aggressive and virulent and it comes back in more than 88% of the people who have it once EVEN WITH CHEMO. I believe the RSO (Rick Simpson Oil) will cure it once and for all but I am going to cover my bases and try everything. Both John and I are convinced that chemo is a bad idea and I am going to get a second opinion and talk to my PCP Dr. Janet Alvarado as well. However, if the cancer comes back we can fight it tooth and nail with chemo then—maybe—and they can take out the rest of the omentum which apparently is just about all still there. In all likelihood it is going to come back anyway, statistically speaking and ANY recurrence will be stage 3 minimum from the get-go JUST because it would be in the omentum and/or peritoneum and would then be called extra-ovarian adenocarcinoma and peritoneal carcinomatosis. I just don't see the benefit to doing this because if it comes back I'm really no worse off because it will start in the omentum which is removable because it's STILL THERE. However, if it does recur, intravenous chemotherapy is totally ineffective (although the oncologists still try to coerce you into paying hundreds of thousands of thousand of dollars for chemo to make you sick and miserable when they KNOW it can't help you). This is why oncologists are the scum of the universe—they are perfectly willing to poison me for profit while lying to me and selling me false hope—like they did to my poor doomed sister who NEVER had a chance but believed their lies. Sadly (for them anyway) I don't believe a word they say. Maybe it's the way their eyes light up when they scream "chemo chemo chemo!!!" at the thought of a new boat for poisoning me and the memory of how they lied to my sister when they KNEW—had to know—that they couldn't help her. They chemo-ed her AFTER she went to hospice and it was the final chemo (God forbid they should let her die in piece after poisoning her for nearly a year but they wanted every single penny they could get for killing her) that resulted in the ruptured esophagus from the chemo-induced vomiting.

Also, I won't have used up my big gun chemo weapons—I'll still be able to use them if I should change my mind about being poisoned and no one really knows what they'll do when there are no other options when it's a life and death choice. My cancer is a rare and aggressive cancer—but it has been definitively and completely removed-there is NO RESIDUAL TUMOR LEFT and there was NO CANCER found ANYWHERE during

MASS MURDERING DOCTORS: THE TRUTH ABOUT ONCOLOGISTS, CHEMOTHERAPY AND CANCER

the second surgery—every single lymph node was clean and they took a LOT of them because in the lymph nodes is a bump to stage 3. Dr. Xynos took 12 extras to be sure and that's fine with me. I can do chemo down the road if this comes back and that will be AFTER they take out the omentum. My oncologist flat out told me he didn't know much about this cancer at early stages because he never sees it this early, he sees it in late stage 3 and 4 and they have poor outcomes because it's too late which translates to "they all die". I have circumstances he and MOST of the oncologist in America are NOT familiar with and therefore are acting very conservatively in order to A. Not get sued and B. It's very lucrative. I don't trust the medical establishment since all they want is MONEY and they are getting billions every year. I'm not paying anyone 50-100K a pop to poison me with chemicals if I can help it. The second surgery revealed no spread of the cancer but the doctors are pushing me hard to start big-gun chemo—even though all the cancer was surgically removed. Really? Seriously? NO WAY José!! I'm not inclined to put the ungodly amount of poison they want to pump through my veins AND into my pelvic cavity (which they say is FOUR HUNDRED TIMES the amount they will give me IV) for a cancer that has been totally surgically removed. John and I agree that's crazy—but I am getting a second opinion from another oncologist and my PCP and I am looking into alternative treatments as well. The incredible amount of damage caused by chemo seems unnecessary at this point and this cancer returns AFTER CHEMO in 80% of people who have it, as it is aggressive and virulent but the chemo damages my heart, lungs, kidneys, liver, nerves and brain and I am NOT doing it at this point. I'm more in favor of monitoring it and alternative treatments and save the big gun weapons-grade chemo for when it returns—and it may NEVER return which is why I am NOT doing chemo. I hate to barf more than ANYTHING so chemo will NEVER work for me.

I look at it like this: I am a professional dragon-slayer (call me Big Pharma) and I go to kill the only dragon (cancer) in the kingdom. It's a lose-lose for both of us. If I kill the dragon, I'm unemployed if the dragon kills me I'm dead. However if I start a foundation to study HOW TO KILL DRAGONS (American Cancer Society) I can make in millions in donations and equipment sales every year. I can also sell swords, poison and other dragon fighting weapons (Surgery Chemotherapy and Radiation), Big Pharma can't let cancer be cured—they make 300 BILLION DOLLARS A YEAR—EVERY

MASS MURDERING DOCTORS: THE TRUTH ABOUT ONCOLOGISTS, CHEMOTHERAPY AND CANCER

YEAR—on Cancer treatments and drugs that would vanish in a puff of smoke if they let a cure happen. Since our corrupt government gave them control of the FDA as a thank you for their bribes—er—CAMPAIGN DONATIONS, the effective alternative treatments remain unapproved and people keep dying. Big Pharma is not about to allow the killing the goose that keeps laying 300 BILLION DOLLARS worth of golden eggs every single year. I am also NOT going to let another dragon-slayer (RSO oil and/or GcMAF immunotherapy) sell a product that will kill this dragon either and I will bribe the corrupt, greedy King (US Government) to keep it off the market which the King is delighted to do in return for campaign donations that keep the king and his jokers in office. Thus endeth the story.

Treating cancer is BIG business in America; in fact, it's a $200 billion a year business. Yet 98 percent of conventional cancer treatments not only FAIL miserably, but are also almost guaranteed to make cancer patients sicker. What's worse: The powers are suppressing natural cancer cures like GcMAF/Goleic that could help tens of thousands of people get well and live cancer free with little or no dependence on drugs, surgery and chemotherapy. The treatment of cancer in the U.S. is one of the most bald-faced cover-ups in medical history. Enough is enough! You deserve to know the truth about the criminality of oncologists and about the dangers of chemotherapy, conventional cancer treatments and the cancer "business." Chemotherapy kills more than cancer. Want proof? Did you know that 9 out of 10 oncologists would refuse chemotherapy if they had cancer? That's up to 91% -- a huge percentage that clearly shines a light on the truth: chemotherapy kills. Conventional oncologists are not only allowing this to happen, but they're also bullying many patients into chemotherapy and surgery right after their diagnoses. Why would that large percentage of oncologists—the ones telling so many patients to get chemotherapy—refuse to do it themselves? Because they know it's not just ineffective, but extremely toxic. Regardless, 75% of cancer patients are directed to receive chemotherapy. Not shocked enough yet? A rigorous review of chemotherapy revealed that it fails for 98% of people. And when chemotherapy was tested against no treatment, no treatment proved the better option. What's more is only two to four percent of cancers respond well to chemotherapy. In a German study of women over age 80 with breast cancer, those who received no treatment lived 11 months longer on average than those who received conventional cancer treatments. A 14-year study by two oncologists in

MASS MURDERING DOCTORS: THE TRUTH ABOUT ONCOLOGISTS, CHEMOTHERAPY AND CANCER

Australia reported in the film "A Shocking Look at Cancer Studies" that conventional treatment such as chemotherapy for all of our major cancers is totally ineffective--far below a 10% success rate. Chemotherapy is a barbaric and pointless procedure. It attacks and kills not just cancer, but also all the living, healthy cells in the body and completely cripples the body's immune system. While this extreme treatment has been called effective against testicular cancers and lymphocytic leukemia, in many cases it's hard to tell which the supposed "therapy" will kill first—the cancer or the patient. In fact, it wouldn't be a stretch to say most people, who die from cancer, actually die from cancer TREATMENTS. From a major medical journal, here's a paper from Feb 2017 that demonstrates that the standard of six chemotherapies KILLS THE PATIENT SOONER than four chemotherapy treatments which is obvious since chemo drugs are nothing but poison. Here's the report from PubMed, a major medical journal:

Arch Gynecol Obstet. 2017 Feb;295(2):451-458. doi: 10.1007/s00404-016-4256-x. Epub 2016 Dec 3.**The number of cycles of neoadjuvant chemotherapy is associated with prognosis of stage IIIc-IV high-grade serous ovarian cancer. (*LESS chemo=longer survival, but they ALL died anyway--TDN*)**
Xu X1, Deng F2, Lv M2, Chen X3.

OBJECTIVE:
No consensus exists on the number of chemotherapy cycles to be administered before and after interval debulking surgery (IDS) in patients with advanced stage epithelial ovarian cancer. (*So these "doctors" don't EVEN KNOW how many times to poison you—TDN*) The present study **aims to explore the optimal number of cycles of neoadjuvant chemotherapy** (NAC) and post-operation chemotherapy to treat the International Federation of Gynecology and Obstetrics stage IIIc-IV high-grade serous ovarian cancer (HG-SOC). (*When you are stage IIIC-4 you are going to die—soon. They can't help you-TDN*)
MATERIALS AND METHODS:
A total of 129 IIIc-IV stage HG-SOC (*High Grade Serous Ovarian Cancer--TDN*) cases were retrospectively analyzed. Cases were comprised of patients who underwent NAC (*neoadjuvent chemotherapy—which means BEFORE surgery*) followed by IDS (*Interval Debulking Surgery*) and who achieved clinical complete response at the end of primary therapy. Patients were recruited from the Jiangsu Institute of Cancer Research between 1993 and 2013. Optimal IDS-associated factors were explored with logistic regression (*cancer came back*). The association between progression-free survival (PFS), overall survival (OS) duration, and covariates was assessed by Cox proportional hazards model and log-rank test.

MASS MURDERING DOCTORS: THE TRUTH ABOUT ONCOLOGISTS, CHEMOTHERAPY AND CANCER

RESULTS:

The median number of NAC cycle (*Pre-surgery chemo*) was 3 (range 1-8) (*Women in the study had between one and eight chemos*). CA-125 decreasing kinetics (p=0.01) was independently associated with optimal IDS. CA-125 decreasing kinetics, optimal IDS, and NAC cycles was independently associated with OS (p <0.01, p <0.01, p=0.03, respectively) and PFS (p<0.01, p<0.01, p=0.04, respectively). **The PFS of patients who underwent ≥5 NAC cycles was shorter than those of patients who underwent<5 NAC cycles (12.3 versus 17.2 months).** (*The more chemo they had THE SOONER THEY DIED*) The PFS (*Progression-Free Survival*) and OS (*Overall Survival—total time they lived after chemo*) of patients who underwent<5 cycles (*Less than 5 treatments*) of adjuvant chemotherapy post-IDS were shorter than those of patients who underwent ≥5 cycles (*MORE than 5 treatments*) (14.2 (*shortest survival time Months NOT years*) and 20.3 versus 21.2 and 28.8 months)

CONCLUSION:

NAC cycles, CA-125 decreasing kinetics, and optimal debulking are independently associated with the prognosis of patients with advanced stage HG-SOC who underwent NAC/IDS and achieved CCR. The number of administered NAC cycles should not exceed 4. (*So the authors of this paper are saying that four rounds OR LESS of chemo is less deadly than FIVE or MORE. I'm giving them today's "NO SHIT, SHERLOCK!" Award*

KEYWORDS:

CA-125; Clinical complete response (CCR); High-grade serous ovarian cancer (HG-SOC); Interval debulking surgery (IDS); Neoadjuvant chemotherapy (NAC)

PMID: 27913927 DOI: 10.1007/s00404-016-4256-x
[Indexed for MEDLINE]

The date of this paper is February 2017. FORTY YEARS of killing people by pumping poison chemo into them and they FINALLY admit that the chemo killed them faster and the more they gave them, THE FASTER THEY DIED. These are the same mass murdering doctors that are telling YOU that you have to have chemo, so do the smart thing and WALK AWAY and get in touch with a REAL doctor who will help you.

Mammograms do more damage than good (and preventive mastectomies are pointless)The $4 billion-a-year mammogram industry urges women to rely on these x-ray tests to "protect" their health. However, what they don't tell you is mammograms are a highly unnecessary and harmful treatment. In fact, mammograms harm ten women for every one the procedure helps. A study by researchers from the Nordic Cochrane Center in Demark reviewed both the benefits and negative effects of seven

MASS MURDERING DOCTORS: THE TRUTH ABOUT ONCOLOGISTS, CHEMOTHERAPY AND CANCER

breast cancer screening programs on 500,000 women. **For every 2,000 women who received mammograms over a 10-year period, only one would have her life prolonged, but ten would be harmed. This is because mammograms can actually INCREASE a woman's risk of developing breast cancer by as much as 3% a year by irradiating the breast cells and triggering breast cancer.** One alternative cancer treatment expert says someday people will look back and wonder "what kind of Neanderthals we were" for practicing surgery, radiation and chemotherapy (or cut, burn and poison). He also calls the conventional approach to cancer treatment "medieval." Statistics show that there is no proof preventive mastectomy (removal of the whole breast) extends the life of breast cancer patients, yet oncologists go right on doing it on a regular basis. Preventative mastectomies are pointless procedures, and many patients are led to believe they have cancer due to false positive cancer screenings. This means they are pressured into having breasts removed for no reason whatsoever. The women undergoing these treatments are scarred for life. **CT scans, or computed tomographies, are a common testing procedure for most cancer types, but the irony is that this CT scan radiation is highly dangerous and can lead to cancer itself. The radiation from a CT scan actually has been shown to cause a substantial amount of cancer. A recent report published in the New England Journal of Medicine suggests that the radiation from current CT-scan use (estimated at more than 62 million CT scans per year in the US) may cause as many as 1 in 50 future cases of cancer. This is nothing to be taken lightly.** Radiation from medical devices is a huge and under-estimated contribution to the growing incidence of breast and other forms of cancer. According to an article in Time Health, other studies prove doctors are performing too many unwarranted CT scans, exposing a countless amount of patients to cancer-causing radiation. **Many mammogram machines are also mis-calibrated, so they end up churning out far too much radiation to be safe. If a woman begins getting routine mammograms at age 40, then by age 60 it is almost certain she will have breast cancer. It's no wonder so many women end up with this form of cancer—they begin getting frequent screenings starting in middle age at the urging of doctors everywhere. The health and cancer industries know about the connection between CT scan radiation and mammograms and cancer statistics, yet they keep pushing**

MASS MURDERING DOCTORS: THE TRUTH ABOUT ONCOLOGISTS, CHEMOTHERAPY AND CANCER

patients to perform these "preventive" procedures. The outrageous truth is frequent mammograms purposely bring repeat business to the corrupt cancer industry by creating cancer tumors over time.

Speaking of lies, virtually NONE of Komen's donation money goes toward funding actual cancer research. Up to 95% of the donation money at Komen goes to provide "free mammograms" to African American women and low income women—after all, they wouldn't want them to be left out from all this unnecessary radiation. Better ensure they get cancer, as well. Komen's money is almost entirely contributed toward doing more mammograms and pumping more radiation into women. There is actually a little-known test for breast cancer that exists, and this method yields no false positive or negatives: a saliva test. Researchers from the University of Texas Health Science Center in Houston discovered that women with breast cancer carry different proteins than women with no cancer; this can be tested by a saliva test so simple a dentist could do it. Big Pharma lies to convince us that their so-called cancer "cures" work. Oncologists and Big Pharma use clever tricks to promote their cancer treatments such as using relative numbers to supposedly prove the effectiveness of their cancer treatments. For example, if you or a loved one has breast cancer, doctors will likely recommend the drug Tamoxifen. They'll tell you it reduces the chances of breast cancer recurring by 49%, which sounds fairly impressive. However, based on absolute numbers, Tamoxifen reduces the risk of breast cancer returning by 1.6% -- 30 times less than advertised. Relative numbers instead of cold, hard statistics are often used by oncologists because relative numbers can be manipulated in many ways. Any relative statistic that allows the percentages to be spun in a false positive light could be used in these situations. Perhaps you have heard through the major media that treating early stage breast cancer creates a 91% cure rate over five years. This statement is absolutely ridiculous—you could get the same cure rate by doing nothing at all (breast cancer is a very slow growing cancer).The point is: Don't be fooled by ambiguous "relative" numbers. Get the real facts!

Drug companies pay oncologists to promote (expensive) ineffective and toxic cancer drugs. **Most oncologists don't make their money by treating patients, but by selling cancer drugs. In fact, according to the Journal of the American Medical Association, as much as 75% of the average oncologist's earnings come from selling chemotherapy drugs in his or her office—and at a**

MASS MURDERING DOCTORS: THE TRUTH ABOUT ONCOLOGISTS, CHEMOTHERAPY AND CANCER

substantially marked-up price. Pharmaceutical companies not only hire charismatic people to charm doctors, exaggerate drug benefits and underplay side effects, but they also pay oncologists kickbacks to push their drugs. For example, Astra Zeneca, Inc. had to pay $280 million in civil penalties and $63 million in criminal penalties to the federal government after it paid kickbacks to doctors for promoting its prostate cancer drug. Many oncologists are criminals and bullies, not doctors. (I can attest to this!!) **Oncologists not only bully patients into taking the destructive route of chemotherapy, toxic drugs and surgery, but they also don't tell their patients the whole truth about the danger of these treatments, other available options, cancer survival statistics, and much more. An innumerable number of cancer patients have suffered needlessly at the hands of these so-called doctors, who are often really corrupt and immoral human beings that could not care less about the healing process of their patients. Many of these shameless oncologists deserve to be arrested and prosecuted immediately for the crimes they commit, yet they keep on sending patients down the same treacherous and painful road that has resulted in too many deaths to keep track of.** More and more patients are waking up to the truth about cancer treatment and educating themselves on the power of whole food nutrition and supplements they are choosing doctors that educate and heal them rather than bully them into surgery and chemotherapy. The staggering documentary **Cancer is Curable** mentioned earlier interviews doctors who tell you how patients are often pressured by conventional oncologists; sometimes they're even hustled onto the operating table the day after their diagnosis without having any of their other choices explained to them. What's worse is that no matter how effective a treatment could be, conventional patients are still being killed by the food they are fed in hospitals. All the doctors in Cancer is Curable unanimously explain that sugar is the No. 1 killer for every cancer patient and although every medical doctor should know that fact, they still continue to give their patients tootsie rolls and candies in the chemotherapy room. Many oncologists are also telling their cancer patients to stop taking antioxidant supplements while they're undergoing treatment. Why? Because they're saying there is a possibility that antioxidants could be lowering the effectiveness of cancer treatments like radiation treatment and chemotherapy. In spite of what you might have been told or led to believe, chemo is hardly the exact

MASS MURDERING DOCTORS: THE TRUTH ABOUT ONCOLOGISTS, CHEMOTHERAPY AND CANCER

science that it pretends to be. And yet, on the mere hunch that antioxidants could be protecting the cancer cells that chemotherapy seeks to destroy, oncologists feel justified in telling their patients to forfeit antioxidant supplements. There are a ridiculous number of false positives in cancer screenings. Among 1,087 individuals participating in a cancer screening trial who received a battery of tests for prostate, ovarian, colo-rectal and lung cancer, 43 % had at least one false positive test result, according to a study published in an issue of Cancer Epidemiology, Biomarkers & Prevention That's almost half of the patients who were tested!

One of the obvious downfalls of this is the needlessly expensive medical care costs associated with false positive cancer screenings. Considering the high cost of testing and treatments, the economic consequences of false-positive screening results are significant. Let's not neglect to mention the pointless emotional and physical suffering inflicted upon thousands of patients who are led to believe they have cancer. In the study mentioned above, men that specifically were given a false positive result for either prostate, lung or colo-rectal cancer averaged almost $2,000 in additional medical care expenditures compared to men with all negative screens. More than half or 51% of the men in the study had at least one false positive test. The lesson to take home from all this. These cancer cover-ups and myths are just a few basic examples of how corrupt and dishonest the cancer industry really is. This especially pertains to the oncologists, who are treating patients regardless of knowing the disturbing truth about the procedures, testing and treatment processes they so frequently push upon their patients. While not all oncologists should be placed into the same category, a large majority of these criminal "doctors" should be held accountable and properly punished for the needless struggle they are inflicting upon thousands of cancer sufferers. If you know anyone who is being pushed into chemotherapy and other deadly and unnecessary "treatments," share the truth with them today and you could save a life. Fortunately, more and more people are waking up to these cancer lies and are looking into safer and more effective alternative treatment protocols and therapies.

Chemotherapy will damage my heart, brain, liver, kidneys. It will cause irreparable painful neuropathy in my hands and feet and legs for the rest of my life. It could damage my kidneys to the point of having to being dialyzed every 3 days for the rest of my life. I could get brain damage and go BLIND from the chemo as well. Dr. Xynos

MASS MURDERING DOCTORS: THE TRUTH ABOUT ONCOLOGISTS, CHEMOTHERAPY AND CANCER

thinks I'm going to risk that bullcrap FOR A FEW ATYPICAL CELLS? Are you f**king KIDDING ME? Doctors are the handmaidens of big Pharma and I don't trust them.

Just for your amusement, here's the opinion of the American Cancer Society (millions in donations every year) about alternative medicines: "Mainstream cancer treatments such as radiation, chemotherapy and surgery can be unpleasant (THERE'S the understatement of a lifetime—the side effects KILL HALF OF THE CANCER VICTIMS before the cancer does), but they have been scientifically tested and proven to work (nope it's 2% CURE rate) for treating cancer. Even though the side effects of mainstream cancer treatment can be serious, these treatments help you fight a life-threatening disease. People with cancer who choose alternative medicine instead of mainstream cancer treatments may be putting themselves at serious risk. They are giving up the only proven methods of treating their disease. Delays or interruptions in standard treatment can give the cancer more time to grow. Even early stage cancers can become impossible to treat successfully if effective treatment is delayed long enough. And even when cancer reaches a stage where cure is not possible, it's important to remember that mainstream care can still offer a lot in the way of cancer control and comfort." -American Cancer Society.

(Of course they have a vested interest in keeping the millions in donations rolling in, so I have to call that a huge conflict of interest.)

The drugs they want to use on me are ANCIENT—first approved in 1979 and the last new chemotherapy drug for ovarian cancer was 2006—ELEVEN YEARS AGO—which in this technological day and age is a VERY long time. I am not confident at all in this treatment although there have since been some new drugs approved. Two new agents have recently been approved by the FDA for patients with recurrent ovarian cancer. Bevacizumab, a humanized antibody that blocks vascular endothelial growth factor (VEGF), in combination with one of three chemotherapy regimens (i. e. dose-dense paclitaxel, liposomal doxorubicin, and topotecan), is now approved for the treatment of patients with platinum-resistant ovarian cancers. Olaparib, a PARP inhibitor, has been approved as a mono-therapy for BRCA mutation–positive, recurrent ovarian cancer patients who have had three prior chemotherapy treatments. **Despite the high response rate to aggressive initial treatments, most (88%) women diagnosed with advanced ovarian cancer will eventually have an always**

MASS MURDERING DOCTORS: THE TRUTH ABOUT ONCOLOGISTS, CHEMOTHERAPY AND CANCER

fatal recurrence. The rate of relapse in ovarian cancers is highly dependent upon the initial stage at diagnosis, the histologic type, and the presence of residual disease at the time of primary or interval debulking. Women with Type II ovarian cancers HGSC (mine, naturally) are also likely to have higher rates of recurrence. High-grade serous carcinoma is UNSURVIVABLE which chemotherapy when it recurs/relapses. Game over. The other 4 kinds are OCCASIONALLY cured (until the metachronous cancer shows up from the chemo) but **I am the ONLY known long-term survivor of High-grade Serous-cell Carcinoma—there are NO others—and I have never had ANY chemo. I've lived longer with NO chemo than people who HAVE chemo.** I've lived longer than anyone with no treatment than virtually ALL of the chemo-ed victims of killer oncologists. I am also in NO danger of dying, I am not depressed and no one who has fought as hard to stay alive as I have is SUICIDAL. Remember that if Big Pharma goons get lucky and manage to kill me to silence me from telling the truth about how they are murdering about a million cancer victims a year worldwide. They murdered Jeff Bradstreet and 60 more doctors who were using GcMAF and medical marijuana among all the other EFFECTIVE medications to cure cancer. Because it could cost them their blood money from pushing the poison that is chemo with a double side of false hope for the huge profits of chemotherapy. If you can't trust your DOCTOR not to murder you for money, what's the point of letting them keep their medical licenses?

I have contacted people in California for some Rick Simpson Oil (RSO) and the protocol for the cure is 60 grams of RSO ingested within 90 days. It's supposed to kill the cancer but it sure isn't cheap and naturally my insurance isn't going to pay for it. I can afford the 5k it's going to cost so I'm going to do this. I am not afraid of the cancer, nor am I afraid to die, but I'm going to have quality of life. I've made my decision not to have chemotherapy and if I die because of it, then that's God's will and I will accept that. I'd rather die young in my 50s than live to 100 and die alone and forgotten like so many elderly—even those with children. I have no children, just 7 surviving nieces and nephews. My oldest nephew, Justin, is the one I have the closest relationship with, the others I barely know. It's the penalty for being the family gypsy and not wanting to live my life in Jupiter, Florida—which, ironically is a pretty good-size place these days. I've been around the world, lived overseas and I've seen many things that most people only read about. I've been married 5 times. I've met people I

MASS MURDERING DOCTORS: THE TRUTH ABOUT ONCOLOGISTS, CHEMOTHERAPY AND CANCER

never dreamed I'd meet and done things that I never thought I'd do. I ran for Congress in 2010 and actually won the Republican primary but lost the general. It's been a hell of a life and if it's check out time, then so be it—and I will die still thinking I am the LUCKIEST person that ever drew breath! However, this isn't about my battle with cancer and a lovely description of how I suffered through chemotherapy to save my life from ovarian and uterine cancer.

When I started writing, it was about BRCA1 and to raise awareness of the risks of the genetic defect that is a killer for so many women who don't even know the danger they face including my sister who didn't find out she was BRCA1+ until she was in the last weeks of her battle with ovarian cancer. I wanted to write about her and raise awareness of this killer gene and what I did to PREVENT cancer. However, my attempt to prevent cancer was too late and I already have it. I watched her die from the cancer—radiated, poisoned and chopped up. It's become about both of us. She chose conventional medicine and lost. I'm not going to do that—I believe I will be cured by medical marijuana and immunotherapy and I am documenting the trip along the way for several reasons:

1. As a tribute to my sister who like me was BRCA1+

2. To raise awareness of the danger of the BRCA1+ genetic defect.

3. To raise awareness of the effectiveness of medical marijuana and immunotherapy that is available outside of conventional medicine (GcMAF/Goleic) to cure some cancers.

4. To blow the whistle on Big Pharma and our totally CORRUPT government that tailors laws to be financially beneficial to their donors.

5. To prove that immunotherapy is the way of the future. I will be taking GcMAF/Goleic if I have a recurrence, I'm ready to pull the trigger on that one as well. I was able to get some of it from a biotech called First Immune in Guernsey, England. I hope not to need it because it's expensive but it's still a tenth of what chemo would cost. I refused chemotherapeutic cancer treatment and I am literally betting my LIFE on the biochemists that make GcMAF/Goleic and the RSO that has cured so many cancers.

MASS MURDERING DOCTORS: THE TRUTH ABOUT ONCOLOGISTS, CHEMOTHERAPY AND CANCER

People can be helped and deserve to be helped as well. Big Pharma doesn't want a cure—they would lose 200 billion a year from Cancer, Inc. The American Cancer Society doesn't want a cure either as they have millions of dollars coming in every year and if there was a cure, they'd have to lock their doors and they spend their money—not on research, but on DISCREDITING REAL CURES. Susan G. Komen will continue being dead from breast cancer. The hundreds of millions of dollars her foundation gets every year (very little of it is left after admin costs at either "charity") would be gone with the wind. Oncologists would be out of business as well. I'm going to push hard for medical marijuana and GcMAF/Goleic if it saves my life—so that other people can be saved as well. Big Pharma has kept marijuana illegal for years because a cure for cancer would cost them so much money and the corrupt politicians have joined them in lockstep causing millions of unnecessary deaths in order to keep cancer profitable. However, BigPharma is happily pulling every possible patent they can on marijuana so that they can charge a bloody fortune for their new lifesaving cancer drugs. I call bullcrap on that as well.

I called a second oncologist, Dr. Alfred Grecco in Belleville, IL for a second opinion as I wanted to get the thoughts of another MD about my plans to see alternative treatment for my cancer. His incredibly rude staff informed me that he "doesn't do second opinions" and that he wouldn't see me. Of course they did say I could send all my records and then they would decide but when one has a virulent and aggressive cancer like HGSC (High-grade Serous Carcinoma) time is of the essence. I filed a complaint with my health insurance provider as he is the only medical oncologist on my HMO so if I can't see him, I can't get a second opinion so I will go see my PCP, Dr. Janet Alvarado and have a talk with her about my treatment and go from there. I have already decided that I will try RSO (cannabis extract) that I can purchase from a dispensary or make on my own. It's $60-$100 a gram and the protocol for the cure is to ingest 60 grams in 90 days which is what is recommended for cancer treatment and I am going to put the recipe for the oil and the RSO protocol in the book so that you can seek the same treatment that I believe is going to help save my life. This is a high-grade THC oil and I have asked for and received permission to include the recipe from the creator, Rick Simpson, who is an American hero who has helped so many. I am definitely not going to do chemo. I believe that my cancer has been totally resected and is no longer there. Since the return rate of this cancer is astronomical

MASS MURDERING DOCTORS: THE TRUTH ABOUT ONCOLOGISTS, CHEMOTHERAPY AND CANCER

(88% even WITH chemo) and the #1 factor affecting Long-Term Survival is getting as much of the tumor as possible with the surgery and in my case the FIRST surgeon got every bit of it—and not a minute too soon. Should I survive this and not end up dying of cancer, I will know that it was because Rick Simpson and Dr. Yamamoto saved my life with RSO and GcMAF/Goleic and because the second surgery turned out to be totally unnecessary. They pulled 30 pelvic area lymph nodes which is 12 more than the gold standard of care. Every single one of them showed NO sign of malignancy-crystal clear. They took samples from all over the omentum and examined the whole thing internally under magnification and nothing—no cancer there either. They didn't even take it out because it had NO cancer. The pelvic wash had "inflammation" in the wash which is white cells and of course it did, it's still healing from having the uterus, ovaries, cervix, tubes ripped out of it 19 days previous. It had less than 20 "atypical" cells—and they were LOOKING HARD FOR CANCER. A diagnosis of cancer means 500K plus in chemotherapy billings for the hospital so they WANT to find cancer. If they didn't know they'd get caught for lying about it if I went for a second opinion, they might even be tempted to fudge the results—and they look really close because if they MISS the cancer it's a big malpractice/wrongful death award. I see NO reason to do 6 rounds of nuclear weapons-grade chemotherapy for a few atypical cells. Also, that sample was time stamped when they pulled it out of me and when they analyzed it NINETEEN HOURS later. Think it might have degraded a bit?? I'm doing the Rick Simpson protocol as a follow up. I know several people personally who swear it killed their stage 4 cancer AFTER they had been sent home to die—after surgery, chemo and radiation to go home and die to protect Big Pharma's profits. Nauseating. I begged Lori to do it but she wouldn't and she's dead from the chemo—not her cancer. EVERYONE including my dad is agreeing with my decision not to go for chemo. It's scary because I'm betting my life—but I can fight off the first recurrence with more surgery if I monitor closely which means I'm not looking at chemo till the third recurrence—and that may never happen. High stakes—scary high. I got a lot of my courage from this article:

SIDEBAR: Can You Trust Chemotherapy to Cure Your Cancer? A. Moritz

The research covered data from the Cancer Registry in Australia and the Surveillance Epidemiology and End Results in the USA for the year 1998. The current 5-year relative adult survival rate for cancer in Australia is over 60%, and no less than that in

MASS MURDERING DOCTORS: THE TRUTH ABOUT ONCOLOGISTS, CHEMOTHERAPY AND CANCER

the USA. By comparison, a mere 2.3% contribution of chemotherapy to cancer survival does not justify the massive expense involved and the tremendous suffering patients experience because of severe, toxic side effects resulting from this treatment. With a meager success rate of 2.3%, selling chemotherapy as a medical treatment (instead of a scam), is one of the greatest fraudulent acts ever committed. The average chemotherapy earns the medical establishment a whopping $500,000 to $1,000,000 per patient, and **80% of EVERY oncologist's income is from FAILED chemotherapies** and has so far earned those who promote this pseudo-medication (poison) over 1 trillion dollars. It's no surprise that the medical establishment tries to keep this scam alive for as long as possible. In 1990, the highly respected German epidemiologist, Dr. Ulrich Abel from the Tumor Clinic of the University of Heidelberg, conducted the most comprehensive investigation of every major clinical study on chemotherapy drugs ever done. Abel contacted 350 medical centers and asked them to send him anything they had ever published on chemotherapy. He also reviewed and analyzed thousands of scientific articles published in the most prestigious medical journals. It took Abel several years to collect and evaluate the data. Abel's epidemiological study, which was published on August 10, 1991 in The Lancet, should have alerted every doctor and cancer patient about the risks of one of the most common treatments used for cancer and other diseases. **In his paper, Abel came to the conclusion that the overall success rate of chemotherapy was "appalling." According to this report, there was no scientific evidence available in any existing study to show that chemotherapy can "extend in any appreciable way the lives of patients suffering from the most common organic cancers."** Abel points out that chemotherapy rarely improves the quality of life. **He describes chemotherapy as "a scientific wasteland"** and states that even though there is **no scientific evidence that chemotherapy works,** neither doctor nor patient is willing to give up on it. The mainstream media has never reported on this hugely important study, which is hardly surprising, given the enormous vested interests of the groups that sponsor the media, that is, the pharmaceutical companies. A recent search turned up exactly zero reviews of Abel's work in American journals, even though it was published in 1991. I believe this is not because his work was unimportant—but because it is irrefutable.

MASS MURDERING DOCTORS: THE TRUTH ABOUT ONCOLOGISTS, CHEMOTHERAPY AND CANCER

Consider the following statement from cancer specialist professor Charles Mathe: "If I contracted cancer, I would never go to a standard cancer treatment center. Cancer victims who live far from such centers have a chance."

Walter Last, writing in The Ecologist, reported, "After analyzing cancer survival statistics for several decades, Dr. Hardin Jones, professor at the University of California, concluded '... patients are as well, or better off untreated.' Jones' disturbing assessment has never been refuted."

Or what about this? "Many medical oncologists recommend chemotherapy for virtually any tumor, with a hopefulness not discouraged by almost invariable failure."— Albert Braverman, MD —Medical Oncology in the 90s, 1991 Lancet 1991 337 p901

Or this "Most cancer patients in this country die of chemotherapy. Chemotherapy does not eliminate breast, colon, or lung cancers. This fact has been documented for over a decade, yet doctors still use chemotherapy for these tumors." — Allen Levin, MD, UCSF — The Healing of Cancer

Or even this? "Despite widespread use of chemotherapies, breast cancer mortality has not changed in the last 70 years." — Thomas Dao, MD — NEJM Mar 1975 292 p 707

Chemotherapy is an invasive and toxic treatment able supposedly to eliminate cancer cells. Unfortunately, though, its ferocious chemistry is not able to differentiate between the cancerous cell or the healthy cell and surrounding healthy tissue. Put simply, chemotherapy is an intravenously administered poison that kills all living matter. Repeated chemotherapy and repeated radiation treatments kill the whole body by degrees. The immune system is hit particularly hard by chemotherapy and often does not recuperate enough to adequately protect from common illnesses, which can then lead to death. Some 67 percent of people who die during cancer treatment do so through opportunistic infections arising as a direct result of the immune system failing because of the aggressive and toxic nature of the drugs. What is this if it is not death by doctoring?

The side effects from both chemotherapy and radiation itself are extensive. They can include dizziness, skin discoloration, sensory loss, audio-visual impairment, nausea, diarrhea, loss of hair, loss of appetite leading to malnutrition, loss of sex drive, loss of

MASS MURDERING DOCTORS: THE TRUTH ABOUT ONCOLOGISTS, CHEMOTHERAPY AND CANCER

white blood cells, permanent organ damage, organ failure, internal bleeding, tissue loss, cardiovascular leakage (artery deterioration) to name but a few. Vincristine is a commonly applied chemotherapy agent. Its side effects include rapid heartbeat, wheezing or difficulty breathing, skin rash or swelling fever or chills, infection, unusual bleeding or bruising, abdominal or stomach cramps, loss of movement or coordination, muscle spasms, seizures, or convulsions. Another common drug is Actinomycin-D. The side-effects again are horrendous. They include hair loss, anemia, low white platelet count, nausea, sickness, diarrhea, and liver failure. Here's the experience of Jane who was diagnosed with breast cancer. She described her chemotherapy as the worst experience of her life. "This highly toxic fluid was being injected into my veins. The nurse administering it was wearing protective gloves because it would burn her skin if just a tiny drip came into contact with it. I couldn't help asking myself, If such precautions are needed to be taken on the outside, what is it doing to me on the inside? From 7 p.m. that evening, I vomited solidly for two and a half days. During my treatment, I lost my hair by the handful, I lost my appetite, my skin color, my zest for life. I was death on legs." For a graphic visual account of the dangers posed by chemotherapy when making contact with bare skin, google chemo spill. This page is not for the faint-hearted. It seems though that with chemotherapy, we have once again been visited by King Charles' ammonia treatment, and again being administered by the highest, most learned physicians in the land. Similarly, on the toxicity of radiation "therapy," John Diamond noted that it was only when he began his radiation treatment that he began to feel really ill. Senior cancer physician Dr. Charles Moertal of the Mayo Clinic in the U.S. stated, "Our most effective regimens are fraught with risks and side effects and practical problems, and after this price is paid by all the patients we have treated, only a small fraction are rewarded with a transient period of usually incomplete tumor regressions ..."

Dr. Ralph Moss is the author of The Cancer Industry, a shocking expose of the world of conventional cancer politics and practice. Interviewed live on the Laurie Lee show in 1994, Moss stated: "In the end, there is no proof that chemotherapy actually extends life in the vast majority of cases, and this is the great lie about chemotherapy, that somehow there is a correlation between shrinking a tumor and extending the life of a patient." Scientists based at McGill Cancer Center sent a questionnaire to 118 lung cancer doctors to determine what degree of faith these practicing cancer physicians placed in the therapies they administered. They were asked to imagine that they had cancer and were asked which of six current trials they would choose. Seventy-nine doctors responded, of which 64 (81 percent) would not consent to be in any trial containing Cisplatin — one of the common chemotherapy drugs they were using, (currently achieving worldwide sales of about $110,000,000 a year). Fifty-eight of the 79 (73 percent) found that all the trials in question were unacceptable due to the ineffectiveness of chemotherapy and the unacceptably high degree of toxicity.

"The success of most chemotherapies is appalling. There is no scientific evidence for its ability to extend in any appreciable way the lives of patients suffering from the most common organic cancer. Chemotherapy for malignancies too advanced for surgery, which accounts for 80 percent of all cancers, is a scientific wasteland."

–Dr. Ulrich Abel, Stuttgart, 1990

Chemotherapy can cause cancer An amazing admission is made by the U.S. National Cancer Institute. Giving the reader information on the treatment of Wilm's Tumor (a children's cancer which affects the kidney) the site goes on to state: "When very high doses of chemotherapy are used to kill cancer cells, these high doses can destroy the blood-forming tissue in the bones (the bone marrow). If very high doses of chemotherapy are needed to treat cancer, bone marrow may be taken from the bones before therapy and frozen until it is needed. Following chemotherapy, the bone marrow is given back through a needle in a vein. This is called autologous bone marrow reinfusion. "Radiation therapy uses x-rays or other high-energy rays to kill cancer cells and shrink tumors. Radiation for Wilms' tumor usually comes from a machine outside the body (external radiation therapy). Radiation may be used before or after surgery and/or chemotherapy. "After several years, some patients develop another form of cancer as a result of their treatment with chemotherapy and radiation. Clinical trials are ongoing to determine if lower doses of chemotherapy and radiation can be used." The truth of the matter would be far too costly for the pharmaceutical industry to bear, thus making it unacceptable. **If the mass media reported the truth that medical drugs, including chemotherapy drugs, are used to practically commit genocide in the U. S. and the world, their best sponsors (the pharmaceutical companies) would have to withdraw their misleading advertisements from the television media, radio stations,**

MASS MURDERING DOCTORS: THE TRUTH ABOUT ONCOLOGISTS, CHEMOTHERAPY AND CANCER

magazines, and newspapers. But neither group wants to go bankrupt. **Many doctors go as far as prescribing chemotherapy drugs to patients for malignancies that are far too advanced for surgery, with the full knowledge that there are no benefits at all.** This is what Brian Slomowitz, MD and Karuna Murray, MD tried to do to me as a condition of surgically removing my tumors. Yet they claim chemotherapy to be an effective cancer treatment, and their unsuspecting patients believe that "effective" equals "cure. " The doctors, of course, refer to the **FDA's definition of an "effective" drug, one which achieves a 50% or more reduction in tumor size for 28 days.** They neglect to tell their patients that there is no correlation whatsoever between shrinking tumors for 28 days and curing the cancer or extending life. **Temporary tumor shrinkage through chemotherapy has never been shown to cure cancer or to extend life.** In other words, **you can live with an untreated tumor for just as long as you would with one that has been shrunken or been eliminated by chemotherapy** (or radiation). **Chemotherapy has never been shown to have curative effects for cancer. By contrast, the body can still cure itself,** which it actually tries to do by developing cancer. Cancer is an immuno-defficiency disease. Unfortunately, as the previously mentioned research has demonstrated, **the chances for a real cure are greatly reduced when patients are treated with chemotherapy drugs**. It is my belief (and I am betting my LIFE to prove it) that cancer is a disease of immuno-defficiency and can be cured by reactivating the immune system. The side effects of the treatment can be horrendous and heartbreaking for both patients and their loved ones, all in the name of trustworthy medical treatment. Although the drug treatment comes with the promise to improve the patient's quality of life, it is just common sense that a drug that makes them vomit for days and lose their hair, while wrecking their immune system, is doing the exact opposite. Chemotherapy can give the patient life-threatening mouth sores. It attacks the immune system by destroying billions of immune cells (white blood cells). It's deadly poisons inflame every part of the body. The drugs can slough off the entire lining of their intestines. The most common side effect experienced among chemo patients is their complete lack of energy because they are so anemic from being poisoned that the red cells are now insufficient to carry oxygen through the body. The new additional drugs now given to many chemo patients may prevent the patient from noticing some of the side effects, but they

MASS MURDERING DOCTORS: THE TRUTH ABOUT ONCOLOGISTS, CHEMOTHERAPY AND CANCER

hardly reduce the immensely destructive and suppressive effect of the chemotherapy itself. Remember, the reason chemotherapy can shrink some tumors is because it causes massive destruction in the body. If you have cancer, you may think that feeling tired is just part of the disease. This rarely is the case. Feeling unusually tired is more likely due to anemia, a common side effect of most chemotherapy drugs. **Chemo drugs can dramatically decrease your red blood cell levels, and this reduces oxygen availability to the 60-100 trillion cells of your body. You can literally feel the energy being zapped from every cell of your body—a physical death without dying.** Chemo-caused fatigue has a negative impact on day-to-day activities in 89% of all patients. With no energy, there can be no joy and no hope, and all bodily functions become subdued. **One long-term side effect is that these patients' bodies can no longer respond to nutritional or immune-strengthening approaches to cancerous tumors.** All of this may explain why cancer patients who **do not** receive any treatment at all, have an up to four times higher remission rate than those who receive treatment.

The sad thing is that chemotherapy does not cure 98% of all cancers anyway. Conclusive evidence (for the majority of cancers) that chemo has any positive influence on survival or quality of life does not exist. To promote chemotherapy as a treatment for cancer is misleading, to say the least. **By permanently damaging the body's immune system and other important parts, chemo has become the leading cause of treatment-caused diseases such as heart disease, liver disease, intestinal diseases, diseases of the immune system, infections, brain diseases, pain disorders, and rapid aging.** Before committing themselves to being poisoned, cancer patients need to question their doctors and ask them to produce the research or evidence that shrinking a tumor actually translates to any increase in survival. If they tell you that chemotherapy is your best chance of surviving, (**which is exactly what Dr. Xynos told me),** you will know **they are lying** or are simply misinformed. **As Abel's research clearly demonstrated, there is no such evidence anywhere to be found in the medical literature. "Subjecting patients to chemotherapy robs them of a fair chance of finding or responding to a real cure and deserves criminal prosecution."**

MASS MURDERING DOCTORS: THE TRUTH ABOUT ONCOLOGISTS, CHEMOTHERAPY AND CANCER

Whoa!! HOLY crap!!

After reading THAT and deciding to share it with you, I've decided I am going to get a second opinion on chemo as I am already strongly opposed to chemo for a cancer that has been surgically removed to the point of nothing left other than a few "atypical cells" that they could barely find and they were not malignant. I am not about to sign up for 6 rounds of high-powered chemo for less than 50 "atypical" cells that came from a pelvic wash of a still-healing from surgery pelvic cavity. NO WAY. I am going to seek alternative treatment because I just cannot justify the incredible amount of DAMAGE that chemo does to my heart, lungs, kidneys, liver, and brain to kill off some ATYPICAL cells that were surrounded by white cells in a healing-from-surgery pelvic cavity—especially when I know that chemo is a huge moneymaker for the medical industry at 50-100K a pop and a "round of chemo" is 6 treatments—so filling me with poison may not be medically necessary but they have five hundred thousand to a million reasons to do it anyway "to be sure" and every one of them is money. While I arrived based on Dr. DallaRiva's glowing recommendation, I don't think I trust Dr. Xynos, he's still 71 years old and clearly not up to date (I had NO idea at the time that an almost 40 year old treatment was STILL the best and ALL they had to offer!) with the latest and best treatments if he is recommending a 39 year-old treatment for a deadly cancer and never even mentions immunotherapy which I believe is the very best way to treat cancer or anything else for that matter. In all likelihood it is going to come back anyway, statistically speaking and ANY recurrence will be stage 3 from the get-go JUST because it would be in the omentum. I just don't see the benefit to doing this because if it comes back (and it comes back in 80% of people after chemo), I will have used up my big gun chemo and this cancer gets resistant to chemo immediately. I don't trust the medical establishment since all they want is MONEY and they are getting billions every year—the cancer industry makes **WAY** too much money from cancer to want a cure—that would kill their hundreds of billions of dollars of ANNUAL revenue. I'm not paying anyone 50-100K a pop to poison me with chemicals if I can help it. I'm not inclined to put the ungodly amount of poison they want to pump through my veins AND into my pelvic cavity (which they say is FOUR HUNDRED TIMES the amount they will give me IV) for a cancer that has been totally surgically removed. John and I agree that's crazy.

MASS MURDERING DOCTORS: THE TRUTH ABOUT ONCOLOGISTS, CHEMOTHERAPY AND CANCER

I BEGGED my sister not to do chemo and to do the RSO and immunotherapy because it was her only chance but she believed—or more likely her ex-husband believed—in conventional medicine and it killed her—of course giving her idiot ex-husband the authority to direct her care and be her medical surrogate was the second dumbest thing she ever did in her too-short life, marrying that jackass was the dumbest. Her best friend, Gerilyn, is an RN and should have been her surrogate and care plan provider, but she let ex-husband run her medical care even though he was totally unqualified to do it. Personally I think she did it just so she wouldn't have to put up with his bullcrap if she didn't. She was doing Chemo and this asshat would bring his stupid Purse-DOG to the house when her immune system was non-existent. What a jackass he is—and it broke my heart to discover how hurt Geri was over the whole thing when it was too late for me to say anything to poor doomed Lori. I don't trust them at all. I made an appointment with my PCP to see what she had to say about all of this and I have started on the RSO protocol and will be seeing my PCP in a few days.

CHAPTER 13: MY VISIT WITH DR. JANET, MY PCP FOR 11 YEARS.

I have a great relationship with my PCP as she and I go back for ten years. We have discussed medical marijuana in the past as I have a chronic pain condition and have had a meeting of the minds so to speak and cancer is definitely a qualifying condition in Illinois which approved medical marijuana in 2013 but while happily charging people $150 a year for a dispensary card ever since 2013 without bothering to open any dispensaries until 2015, typical of the way the corrupt state is run by the corrupt scumbag Mike Madigan—but remembering to bill $150 a year like clockwork for a dispensary card (WITH NO DISPENSARIES available to use the card until 2015) made it a giant pain in the ass of paperwork that I wouldn't even bother with. It would also have cost me my CCF permit which is the main reason I didn't get the card. I am having no issues ordering the RSO oil from a California dispensary and they are shipping to Illinois and Louisiana with no issues, thank GOD for the Internet! The state of Illinois wonders why their medical marijuana program hasn't been the roaring success it is in every other state. I don't wonder for a second, as Illinois has the Jonah touch—everything they touch turns to whale crap.

MASS MURDERING DOCTORS: THE TRUTH ABOUT ONCOLOGISTS, CHEMOTHERAPY AND CANCER

I talk with Dr. Janet for a while and we discuss medical marijuana I don't ask her for a recommendation (since I don't need one at the moment) and I can get whatever I need via mail order or the internet without having to deal with the insane bureaucracy of the state of Illinois and give them money for nothing. We also discuss olaparib which is a brand-new drug for BRCA1+ ovarian cancer patients and it's an oral chemotherapy drug that is for after the THIRD recurrence of this cancer after chemo which is nuts—why would ANYONE WAIT TILL THEN?? I told her I'd be willing to do 30 days of this oral chemo if I could tolerate it, but she wants to research it since it's an off-label use. She says she will call me, writes my prescriptions for my ongoing medically necessary prescription medications and we part ways. She seems to be on board with what I am going to do and didn't try to convince me that chemo was the way to go. We are also looking at a high-def MRI of my pelvis every three months for 18 months and after that every 6 months until 3 years have passed and monitor my CA-125 and if the cancer comes back we will know soon enough to surgically intervene. What is the worst part of this is that ANY recurrence will be Stage III-B or HIGHER which is right where baby sister was when they got her diagnosis and she died from the chemo shortly thereafter, so it's a wait and see and hope because the TERMINAL complication of ovarian cancer after the ovaries et al. are long gone and is called peritoneal carcinomatosis and it is invariably fatal as IV chemo is ineffective and the peritoneum cannot be surgically removed and you cannot RADIATE your intestines, so you die.

SIDEBAR: NO CALL FROM DR XYNOS?? Here's something else about the chemo. Don't you think that if Dr. Xynos was so convinced that this chemo was so needed to save my life and that I would die without it, that he would have AT LEAST called me PERSONALLY to talk to me about it? He didn't. I guess they really ARE the medical mill I thought they were for all his bullcrap about "It's about YOU and the right treatment for YOU" which is apparently only true if you want to spend 6-7 figures plus on chemo and oncologists BUY the drugs they use and mark them UP and re-sell them to the patient and pocket THOUSANDS OF DOLLARS for a treatment that won't help their patients. Yep. It's "ALL about me" isn't it Francisco? As much as I dislike doctors, oncologists now occupy a special place on the list of the world's scumbags.

SIDEBAR: PUSHING A FAKE CURE AND SELLING FALSE HOPE: One study showed chemotherapy only contributed to 2% of the reported 5-year cancer

MASS MURDERING DOCTORS: THE TRUTH ABOUT ONCOLOGISTS, CHEMOTHERAPY AND CANCER

remissions—not even a cure because there's now a lot of evidence that the chemo causes SUBSEQUENT cancers 5 years down the road (called metachronous cancers) which of course means MORE MONEY for Big Pharma and their scumbag oncologists. Clinical Oncology 2004 **"These failed chemotherapies generate 80% of every oncologist's income."** Integrated Health Strategies 2013 Another study shows that cancer cells regrow in between treatment sessions and are a major cause of treatment failure. Nature Reviews Cancer 2005. A long-term study in Canada showed that patients who elected to undergo cancer treatment achieved a median survival of only 9-months over patients who refused to undergo radiation, surgery or chemotherapy.

Also, the lab that checked the fluid in the wash on the second surgery was LOOKING HARD for cancer cells AND DID NOT FIND ANYTHING BUT LESS THAN 20 "ATYPICAL" CELLS. They are trained to LOOK HARD for cancer for two reasons. 1. If they find cancer, it's 500K to 1 million in chemo treatment billings for the hospital so they don't want and can't afford a CURE for cancer. 2. If they MISS finding cancer that was present then they are looking at a million-dollar medical malpractice case for missing it which could go into multi-millions if negligence is proven and also if I die would be upgraded to wrongful death and shouldn't be a stretch since they look for cancer every day.

Anyway, they didn't find one single cancer cell and this oncologist is so sure I have to have all this chemo that he can't be bothered to call me and ask why I decided against chemo which he is so certain I will die without. I'm glad I followed my instincts and didn't sign up for the chemo and I think I'm going to be OK without it. I'm going with Rick Simpson Oil (RSO) and their protocol. I will fight the good fight, but not with Big Pharma's weapons and drugs because their 2.1% cure rate just doesn't get it. I reached out personally to Rick Simpson for permission to use his protocol and recipe to make the now-famous Rick Simpson Oil (RSO) along with his treatment protocol and he graciously has given permission for the recipe and protocol to be included in the book, so it is included in the next chapter.

Dr. Janet isn't OK with me not seeing an oncologist for the olaparib chemo but she writes the order for the high-def MRI and I'm having that on Wednesday as we need a baseline MRI so we will know when/if the cancer returns. I am hoping that the RSO protocol prevents the return of the cancer and I have been taking it for more than 2 weeks and I hope it's doing what it's supposed to be doing since I am losing weight and have zero appetite. I want to go back to Louisiana and my kitchen and such so I can go back to cooking the stuff Mom and I like to eat!! I will go into the RSO protocol with the recipe and methodology of the RSO cancer cure.

CHAPTER 14: RICK SIMPSON OIL (RSO) RECIPE AND PROTOCOL

Rick Simpson's Hash Oil Recipe

To make the Rick Simpson's hash oil, start with one ounce of high quality dried bud. One ounce will typically produce 3-4 grams of oil, although the amount of oil produced per ounce will vary strain to strain. A pound of dried marijuana will yield about two ounces of high quality oil.

IMPORTANT: These instructions are directly summarized from Rick Simpson's website with his written permission. Be VERY careful when boiling solvent off, the fumes are extremely flammable. **AVOID** smoking, sparks, stove-tops, and red hot heating elements. Set up a fan to blow fumes away from the pot, and set up in a well-ventilated area for whole process. I recommend virgin-grade acetone for the solvent since it cooks off 100% clean and your body produces acetone naturally anyway, so it's safe to use and MUCH less expensive than other solvents.

1. Place the completely dry material in a plastic bucket.
2. Dampen the material with the solvent you are using. Many solvents can be used. You can use pure naphtha, ether, butane, 99% isopropyl alcohol, or virgin grade acetone. Two gallons of solvent is required to extract the THC from one pound, and 500 ml is enough for an ounce.
3. Crush the plant material using a stick of clean, untreated wood or any other similar device, (I've found a potato masher works very well). Although the material will be damp, it will still be relatively easy to crush up because it is so dry.
4. Continue to crush the material with the stick, while adding solvent until the plant material is completely covered and soaked. Remain stirring the mixture for about three minutes. As you do this, the THC is dissolved off the material into the solvent.
5. Pour the solvent oil mixture off the plant material into another bucket. At this point you have stripped the material of about 80% of its THC.

6. Second wash: again add solvent to the mixture and work for another three minutes to extract the remaining THC.

7. Pour this solvent oil mix into the bucket containing the first mix that was previously poured out.

8. Discard the twice washed plant material.

9. Pour the solvent oil mixture through a coffee filter into a clean container.

10. Boil the solvent off: a rice cooker will boil the solvent off nicely, and will hold over a half gallon of solvent mixture. **CAUTION: avoid stove-tops, red hot elements, sparks, cigarettes, and open flames as the fumes are extremely flammable.**

11. Add solvent to rice cooker until it is about ¾ full and turn on HIGH heat. Make sure you are in a well-ventilated area and set up a fan to carry the solvent fumes away. Continue to add mixture to cooker as solvent evaporates until you have added it all to the cooker.

12. As the level in the rice cooker decreases for the last time, add a few drops of water (about 10 drops of water for a pound of dry material). This will help to release the solvent residue, and protect the oil from too much heat.

13. When there is about one inch of solvent-water mixture in the rice cooker, put on your oven mitts and pick the unit up and swirl the contents until the solvent has finished boiling off.

14. When the solvent has been boiled off, turn the cooker to LOW heat. At no point should the oil ever reach over 290° F or 140° C.

15. Keep your oven mitts on and remove the pot containing the oil from the rice cooker. Gently pour the oil into a stainless steel container

16. Place the stainless steel container in a dehydrator, or put it on a gentle heating device such as a coffee warmer. It may take a few hours but the water and volatile terpenes will be evaporated from the oil. When there is no longer any surface activity on the oil, it is ready for use.

17. Suck the oil up in a plastic syringe, or in any other container you see fit. A syringe will make the oil easy to dispense. When the oil cools completely it will have the consistency of thick grease.

In order to get the cure, you must ingest 60 grams of RSO in 90 days so you have to build a tolerance FAST so that you won't be on a 60-day sofa lock. Start with a dose the size of a half a grain of rice every 4-6 hours for the first 4 days, then double the dosage every 4 days until you are up to a gram a day which means it should take about 90 days to complete the protocol. You also should not eat sugar or carbohydrates such as potatoes, rice, cereal, flour, pasta or oat meal. Try to stick to lean proteins and leafy green vegetables. Fish, chicken, leafy green veggies, cauliflower, cabbage, lean pork, lean beef, beans, cheese, berries and fruit. A modified Atkins or standard diabetic diet are the best choices when battling cancer and the one I try to maintain, although I am not the best for sticking to a diet my life depends on sticking to this one. In addition to the RSO oil I was also eating 10 apricot seeds a day for a therapeutic dose of laetrile. I am hoping and praying that this protocol along with eating more fruits and vegetables and doing my very best NOT to eat sugar and minimal carbs I hope will be the right protocol to prevent the return of the deadly serous cell carcinoma in my ovaries and my uterus. I can only wait and see. I just took my first laetrile apricot seed. Yuck. It tastes like crap!

The Rick Simpson Oil has me in an ongoing buzz most of the time but I'm oddly almost totally functional, which is weird but pleasant. I'm doing OK and my protocols are to prevent a recurrence more than to be cured and seems to be working since I just got my 3 month MRI which has shown no cancer, so it seems to be working. The RSO (Rick Simpson Oil) has more of a sedative effect than I like, I would much prefer something that amped me up a bit more, but one is supposed to rest with cancer so I suppose this is one way to make sure I rest. I must go to Costco and stock up, I've just returned to Louisiana and of course there's nothing much here to eat although I could put off going for a few more days—which I am going to do.

Chemo has a 2.1% cure rate I did a ton of research and discovered that marijuana extract has a 71% cure rate with people who have been sent home to die, and I spoke to a number of people who swore that the extract commonly referred to as "Rick Simpson Oil" from the first guy who made the extract for his cancer. Just to see if it really works, I smeared a tiny bit on my little skin cancer and it is GONE, so that gave me some faith. I'm supposed to take a gram a day but I can't—in 3 weeks I've only managed to eat 7 grams of it—because it puts you in a 6 hour sofa lock if you eat too much—it's wicked potent. I am trying to eat 9 apricot kernels a day for the laetrile which is Vitamin B-17 and they taste like bitter rose water so I will try to chew them just enough to break them up but not enough to get them caught in my teeth where they taste nasty for a WHILE. Unfortunately I simply cannot tolerate the

MASS MURDERING DOCTORS: THE TRUTH ABOUT ONCOLOGISTS, CHEMOTHERAPY AND CANCER

apricot seeds as I keep vomiting them back up so I won't be taking them any more. I also have to take a fish oil supplement and a flax oil supplement. I don't know why I feel like crap. I keep barfing and I'm losing weight and I feel terrible when the RSO wears off. My baseline MRI was spotless for cancer though, so that's a plus—and it needs to stay spotless as I will be having it repeated at 3 months. (I have since stopped eating the seeds/taking laetrile as I kept vomiting it back up so I realized my body will not tolerate the laetrile.) However, I'm backing off the Rick Simpson oil and cutting down to 2 doses a day because that's the maintenance dose and it's expensive as hell, $100 a gram, and my insurance company that couldn't wait to pay a million bucks for a 39-year old chemotherapy treatment to poison me to death won't cough up a dime for RSO that has an exponentially hugely higher cure rate. No wonder big Pharma is fighting legalization while pulling every patent they can on cannabis. The reason I am writing this book about my little adventure—if one person forgoes chemo and their life is saved by using the RSO GcMAF/Goleic immunotherapy protocol and/or reading the book it will all be worth it. Anyway I am lounging around the house in Louisiana living off the fat of the land doing some consulting and telecommuting and looking after mama G. I decided that I was NOT going to go ahead and do the mastectomies and reconstruction since I currently have no breast cancer. It's easier to prevent that to treat. I think I'm going to be OK for all that the oncologist told me I'd die "vomiting feces" from this cancer, but so far so good, and the clean MRI was a good sign. If it was all contained in the ovaries and uterus and wasn't spraying cells through the peritoneum, I may very well survive this. I got lucky because John nagged me to DEATH over having this surgery. I was just so darn sure I didn't have and wasn't going to GET cancer that I came very close to standing up to John and telling him that I was going to wait until summer 2017 to have the surgery—and had I waited until then, this would be a definite death sentence rather than a probable one. This is a very aggressive cancer with an 88% recurrence rate WITH chemo so I am taking a big chance not having chemo, or maybe not—I hope not, but even though I feel that I am making the right choice, it's still a pretty high-stakes gamble. If I am right, I get to live out my life span. If I am wrong then I pay for it with my life. High stakes for a woman who isn't a gambler by nature, but I hate puking (and probably being bald) more than I'd hate to die. My first cancer protocol is this: 9 apricot kernels

MASS MURDERING DOCTORS: THE TRUTH ABOUT ONCOLOGISTS, CHEMOTHERAPY AND CANCER

a day for the laetrile (that I could not tolerate), 1200 mg fish oil capsule every day. 1400 mg flax seed oil capsule per day. As much RSO oil as I can get down which is about ¼ gram a day right now. I hope to work up to more but the maintenance dose is about a gram a month or a 30th of a gram a day, so the fact that I can't get a gram a day right is not concerning me at the moment. I am also eating fresh fruits and vegetables and drinking Earl Grey tea instead of soda and keeping my sugar and carbohydrates to an absolute minimum. This is hard for me because my diet isn't what it should be, but I'm trying hard to cure this cancer once and for all. No wonder I'm losing weight eating this stuff—but I wish I liked it, that would make it so much easier to consume. Last night it was roasted chicken breast with broccoli and the night before it was a yummy NY strip steak, juicy and rare. I don't eat very much these days because it's not that interesting to eat this stuff. I miss my sugar and junk food, but I'd miss not being alive even more. I had an almond poppy seed muffin and blackberries for lunch plus my laetrile apricot pits which haven't gotten any better tasting by the way. They are still disgusting and I keep vomiting every evening after dinner. My California dispensary is amazing at getting my RSO oil to me. I have been taking it for 4 weeks and have only managed to get down 7 grams in 28 days or about a quarter of a gram a day. I'm supposed to work up to a tolerance of a gram a day and then get down 60 grams of this oil in 90 days, but I don't see that happening. On a quarter gram a day, I've been literally stoned as crap for a month and have accomplished a lot around the house and at work although I'm not really working very much right now. I have to get well before I can do anything else and it would be unfair to my clients to take on a new project that I might not be able to complete if I happen to die from this pesky cancer. My clean MRI made me happy, and if I get another clear one in 3 months, then I am hoping to go to a bi-annual MRI rather than a quarterly study although if that's what I need to do to keep tabs on the cancer, then obviously that's what I am going to do. I am losing weight, but I think it's more due to the boring food choices and disinterest in the food at the moment. Ingesting RSO doesn't bring on the munchies the way smoking weed will do, it's way more of an appetite suppressant than a hunger/appetite stimulant. Maybe it's just me. I was starting to shop around for plastic surgeons on my plan, while I am NOT looking forward to more surgeries, I have decided that I will not be getting new boobs

MASS MURDERING DOCTORS: THE TRUTH ABOUT ONCOLOGISTS, CHEMOTHERAPY AND CANCER

courtesy of Ms. BRCA1+ germline defect and Blue Cross/Blue Shield of Missouri at the moment. I can't bother with it right now, but my cancer risk for breast cancer is ALSO huge—higher than my risk was for the ovarian and uterine cancer I already have, so I am going to proceed with the double mastectomies with immediate reconstruction somewhere down the road if I survive this other cancer, and hopefully I will get to do this at Anderson Hospital and Kathi and Irene will take care of me like last time. I hate that I'm going to be doing this since I LIKE my boobs but I have learned firsthand how much better it is to PREVENT cancer than to TREAT cancer. I don't really want to have the double mastectomies but I am too frightened about getting another cancer to battle not to do it down the road. Oddly enough, I have zero fear of surgery as I've had almost 30 surgeries in my life—surgery to me is about like getting my teeth cleaned at the dentist, but am terrified of chemotherapy. I've had enough bouts of food poisoning in my life to know that I hate vomiting more than anything. I had the MRI with and without contrast so I am confident in the results of the study. I lost my faith in medical doctors with the Heliobacter Pylori (H. pylori) bacteria scandal. Google it and you will be STUNNED at the mendacity and ruthlessness with which BigPharma shuts down anything that might affect their blood money. There's NO MONEY in a healthy population. NONE. They have to keep us sick.

The H.pylori fiasco told me everything I needed to know about doctors and Big Pharma needing to keep America sick and on drugs—they must be crapting bricks with the DEA cracking down on them for creating drug addicts who have to pay for an office visit every 30 days; so they are guaranteed income and they pay in CASH. The Heliobacter Pylori scandal came about when an Australian doctor discovered that his patient's ulcers were being caused by a bacterial infection. He further discovered that a course of simple, cheap (uh-oh) antibiotics would PERMANENTLY CURE (double uh-oh) the gastric and duodenal ulcers of his patients and promptly published a paper about the miracle cure for ulcers which he expected to be met with acclaim from his peers. Instead, they tried to run him out of medicine, buried his results and continued to treat their patients with milk, antacids and bland diets that didn't work to cure the ulcers TO KEEP THEIR REVENUE STREAM HIGH. Unconscionable and criminal. The Australian doctor had discovered that 97% ulcers were caused by an Heliobacter pylori INFECTION and were wiped out **permanently** with a course of antibiotics. This

MASS MURDERING DOCTORS: THE TRUTH ABOUT ONCOLOGISTS, CHEMOTHERAPY AND CANCER

meant that the millions of patients would no longer be filling expensive Tagamet prescriptions (which was the BEST-SELLING and most profitable prescription medication at the time) and making monthly visits to check on the healing of ulcers THAT WERE NEVER GOING TO HEAL. This had the very profitable effect of making these poor suffering people cash cows for gastroenterologists. These same doctors who have ALL taken an OATH to DO NO HARM fought like banshees to SILENCE the truth about the H. pylori infections causing ulcers from coming out. Unfortunately for the MD cartel, antibiotics aren't illegal (unlike medical marijuana). With people talking to each other about their ulcers being cured with antibiotic, the word to spread **pre-internet** with such speed that the gastroenterologists knew the jig was up. They actually had to CURE their ulcer patients with antibiotics and, in doing so, cut their incomes so drastically that they had to get into the cancer game by finding a way to troll for patients. It was later calculated that the cure for ulcers cost every gastroenterologists in America 28% of their annual income. Almost as good as being able to put up billboards trolling for litigation plaintiffs. 1-800-WhoCanISue.Com is another way that lawyers are trolling NATIONWIDE for plaintiffs. My mother in law's pain management doctor made her get a Narcan "save shot" kit in case she overdoses on her narcotic painkillers which doctor are now being forced to to prescribe. It's a 30 year old drug, LONG out of patent and the kit was $4500.00 at the drugstore. That's not a typo, it was FOUR THOUSAND FIVE HUNDRED DOLLARS for a kit that didn't cost $10 for the drug, 2 needles and 2 syringes. I called the doctor's office to complain about the cost of this—had I known it was this much, I would NOT have filled the prescription. I am also getting rid of this doctor, half the time he sends his nurse practitioner to see my mother in law but bills the same for it. If her insurance is paying to see the DOCTOR then by God she's going to SEE the doctor, not the nurse practitioner—no insult to ARNPs. It's absolutely ridiculous that Big Pharma is raping us for charging Americans 100 times as much as they charge everyone else in the world for medications because NO ONE knows what their meds cost because someone OTHER THAN THE PATIENT pays 9 out of every 10 dollars of medical bills. When people are shielded from the cost of their health care and don't have to reach into their pockets to PAY for this healthcare will continue to skyrocket. However, that's another book for another day. I can't decide who the worst scumbags are—BigPharma or their doctor handmaidens. It's also nefarious that Big Pharma has spent hundreds

MASS MURDERING DOCTORS: THE TRUTH ABOUT ONCOLOGISTS, CHEMOTHERAPY AND CANCER

of millions of dollars to keep medical marijuana **off the market** and **on the list of Schedule 1 drugs** while in the interim they are pulling patents on every aspect of the drug that they can legally pull. The reason medical marijuana is legal in 30 states is a testament to it's efficacy since the pressure to legalize medical marijuana came from millions of people cured by it. Even Big Pharma could no longer keep it off the market as a cancer treatment but they do their very best to marginalize it to protect their blood money for failed chemotherapies. It's really sickening that this is being allowed happen in America because of the greed of Big Pharma and the corruption of our elected officials, but it is and we need to fight for our rights. However, the genie is out of the bottle and marijuana and/or medical marijuana will be legal nationwide in ten years. By 2025 the discussion on MMJ (Medical Mary Jane) will be over and Big Pharma will be scrambling to prevent cures for other diseases from going mainstream and cutting into their profits. No one is really aware of the huge risk of being BRCA1+ or BRCA2+ since it hasn't gone mainstream yet—there's no dead Susan G. Komen equivalent for a sympathetic figure. I had NO IDEA that I had a genetic time bomb ticking away in me and had never even heard of it until Angelina Jolie who is also BRCA1+ had all her surgery because her mother died of breast cancer and so she also had to be BRCA1+ as well. They didn't test my sister until October 2015—and I already had the cancer but I didn't know it. I was totally clueless and just so smug when my husband was insisting I get the surgery ASAP. I was stage 2 or so probably and so I went and got tested—in no particular hurry either—and it takes almost a month to get the results and the cancer I have doubles in size EVERY 6 WEEKS and begins shedding cells when it is only 3 cm in size (how it metastasizes) and then it's like tossing a handful of grass seed on a bed of top soil and then every new tumor starts shedding cells at 3 cm and in a shortly thereafter they've filled your pelvis and abdomen with cancerous tumors that are eating the serous cell lining that protects the organs and then you usually die when the mushrooming growth of the cancer crushes your colon and other visceral organ function with explosively growing tumors. If it hadn't been for my husband's insistence that I do something ASAP, I would have put it off for a year or so and then I would have been stage 4 when they opened me up as well—and died shortly thereafter in all likelihood as I might have been too afraid to stand up and refuse chemo as I am doing now. Even if I die from this now, (although I am hoping that won't happen) I am content and calm with my decision. I've never

MASS MURDERING DOCTORS: THE TRUTH ABOUT ONCOLOGISTS, CHEMOTHERAPY AND CANCER

met anyone who had a positive experience with chemotherapy, but I've met a lot who swear by RSO and are convinced it saved their lives. I am literally being a lab rat for cannabis oil and betting my life that it will help me, and the stakes are pretty high. However, I am feeling much better these days and I've gotten used to the hemp oil's effects. The first couple of weeks were tough, I slept a LOT and I was unbelievably mega-wasted almost all the time and ate too much RSO a couple of times which resulted in a 4 hour sofa lock dozing off and a little dizziness, but nothing terrible. I like it MUCH better dispensed into the gelatin caps, it's easy to regulate the dose and there's no issues with the taste although my surviving sister Sarah says vaping RSO is the best. You can't vape or smoke it with cancer though, you HAVE to eat it. You could smoke/vape on top of it but I'm already fairly buzzed. This has to be one of the more pleasant medical treatments I have ever experienced although I do puke once in a while, but I'm like a cat in that respect—I just barf occasionally and have all my life. John is here in Baton Rouge for Mother's Day weekend, Trump has locked up the Republican nomination and I'm taking John to New Orleans in the morning and I don't want him to go!! However, he has to go and then in 3 weeks I am going to take Gloria back to Illinois and look for a surgeon to consult about the double mastectomies and immediate reconstruction. I'm starting the doctor hunt when I get back from New Orleans. It's much easier to prevent cancer than it is to treat it, and I know this first-hand—but I already HAD ovarian cancer when I found out I was BRCA1+ so I never really had the chance to prevent it, I wasn't even a previvor (that's the new term for BRCA1/2s that haven't had cancer YET) when I found out I was going to have to step it up to survivor, assuming I live through all of this. I am shocked every day by the people who have no idea of the potential risk they face when I tell them I have ovarian cancer and they tell me of all their cancer-stricken relatives and then I tell them about BRCA1/2and their risk and they go pale. It's frightening how huge the risk is and how many people are at risk and have no idea. **That's why I'm writing this book!** It's already longer than I thought it would be!

I'm almost through with the RSO protocol and I have another MRI (every 90 days for the next 3 years) coming up in July. If it is clean that will go a really really long way toward settling me down. I have to admit the RSO has a very calming and mildly euphoric effect and I am sleeping better and usually through the night. I've noticed

MASS MURDERING DOCTORS: THE TRUTH ABOUT ONCOLOGISTS, CHEMOTHERAPY AND CANCER

my appetite (which has been dismal) is perking up as well but I still don't feel good and I'm not sure why—maybe just minor blues from all of this stress. The recurrence rate is about 80% within 6-18 months even WITH chemo; so if I get to 24 months without a recurrence after doing the protocol and the maintenance (which is a gram a month at bedtime) then I would venture to opine that would speak to at least some sort of efficacy of the medicine, don't you think? At that point I may discontinue the maintenance dose, or maybe continue to take it as a sleep aid and John has always said he would much prefer I eat my recreational MMJ than to smoke it. It's really pleasant and is effective for so MANY things. It has helped my back pain tremendously and, even though I am more flipped out and more crazy scared than I have ever been in my LIFE, it also gives me enough serenity that I am functional. I am certain that without it I would be spending my days curled in a ball; alternating between passing out from exhaustion and screaming until I pass out from exhaustion and start screaming again as soon as I wake up. I'm scared—really scared—and this is a path I have to walk alone no matter how much my friends and family are trying to be supportive. No one who hasn't had this understands the terror of the disease— because while I am sure there is an afterlife, I am not sure it will be as interesting or as much fun as this one, so what happens if I don't like it? Am I recycled right away as another soul? Will I know anyone? Will they know me? It's the unknown that is the most terrifying part and in changes you in weird ways. I wanted to get a new car, maybe next year, but now I'm wondering if I would die before it was paid off. Would God find my financing a car for 5 years be arrogant enough to incur His wrath? It is insane questions like this that race through your head at night when you have an unusual pain for a few moments; you panic for a few seconds. Is it another cancer? Did they miss something? For the first time in my life, my destiny is out of my hands and beyond my influence or control. There is literally nothing I can do but wait and see—and hope I don't get hit by a bus after going through all this!

SIDEBAR: THE DIFFERENCE BETWEEN DOCTORS AND LAWYERS: LAWYERS MERELY ROB YOU; DOCTORS ROB YOU—AND THEN THEY KILL YOU.

Dr. Barbara Starfield was the author of A JAMA study, published in 2000, and her research documented how a staggering **225,000 Americans die from iatrogenic**

MASS MURDERING DOCTORS: THE TRUTH ABOUT ONCOLOGISTS, CHEMOTHERAPY AND CANCER

causes, meaning their death is caused by a physician's or hospital's activity, manner, or therapy. Her statistics showed that each year:

- •12,000 die from unnecessary surgery

- •7,000 die from medication errors in hospitals

- •20,000 die from other errors in hospitals

- •80,000 die from hospital-acquired infections

- •106,000 die from the negative side effects of drugs taken as prescribed

Back then, few people believed it, but in recent days, headlines echoing the original 2000 article have made the rounds in many of the major media outlets. One of the reasons why many are still surprised by these statistics is due to fundamental flaws in the tracking of medical errors, which has shielded the reality of the situation and kept it out of the public eye.

Medical Errors Are STILL the Third Leading Cause of Death!

Dr. Starfield's findings 16 years ago still stand today. In fact, recent research suggests matters have only gotten worse, and the reason for this is because no affirmative action was ever taken to address and correct the situation.

According to a new study published in the British Medical Journal, **medical errors now kill an estimated 250,000 Americans each year, an increase of about 25,000 people annually** from Dr. Starfield's estimates.

That means medical errors are STILL **the third leading cause of death**, right after heart disease and **cancer. These numbers may actually be vastly underestimated, as deaths occurring at home or in nursing homes are not included.** Isn't that a cheery thought. As shown by Dr. Starfield's research, side effects from drugs, taken as prescribed, account for the vast majority of iatrogenic deaths. Research published in 2013 estimated that preventable hospital errors kill 210,000 Americans each year—a figure that is very close to the latest statistics in 2016.

MASS MURDERING DOCTORS: THE TRUTH ABOUT ONCOLOGISTS, CHEMOTHERAPY AND CANCER

However, when they included deaths related to diagnostic errors, errors of omission, and failure to follow guidelines, the number skyrocketed to 440,000 preventable hospital deaths each year. This too hints at the true enormity of the problem. According to Centers for Disease Control and Prevention (CDC) statistics, the third leading cause of death is respiratory disease, which claims 150,000 lives each year, not iatrogenic causes. In fact, the CDC doesn't publish any information relating to medical errors at all. As reported by Newsweek:

"The researchers for the study from Johns Hopkins say their findings suggest the CDC's method for collecting data on causes of death is flawed, leading to inaccurate estimates on just how dangerous a visit to your local hospital has become.

Death certificates currently don't have a separate coding classification for medical errors, which means estimates are not accurate.

The medical coding system used by the CDC was originally developed for physicians and hospitals to determine what to bill health insurance companies for individualized patient care. The authors recommend an overhaul of how cause of death data is collected." The researchers suggest adding an extra field to the death certificate, asking whether a preventable complication or medical error contributed to the death. At present, no such check box exists. **Instead, when a patient dies from a medical error, the original complaint is listed as the cause of death.** This is why my sister's death certificate says cancer and not chemotherapy!

They also recommend a number of strategies to reduce the number of deaths from iatrogenic causes (medical errors not reaching the level of malpractice for some unknown reason), including increased transparency and communication. As long as health care providers and hospital administrators remain in the dark about the severity of the problem, few course corrections are likely to be made.

Iatrogenic deaths are a global problem in addition to being a huge American one. Bob Anderson, chief of the mortality statistics branch for the CDC, claims there *are* codes that capture iatrogenic causes of death. However, the published mortality statistics do not take them into account. They only look at the condition that led the individual to seek medical treatment in the first place. As a result, even if a doctor lists medical errors in the death certificate, they are not included in the CDC's mortality statistics. Anderson defends the agency's approach, saying it's "consistent with international guidelines". In essence, most countries tally their deaths in a similar fashion, in order to be able to compare mortality statistics internationally. All that really means is that this is a global problem, and all nations really need to take a closer look at how deaths are recorded and counted. According to Anderson, the CDC is unlikely to change the recording of deaths unless there's a really compelling reason to do so. **But what could be more compelling than the fact that modern medicine is a *leading cause* of preventable deaths!?**

I've got the surgeons under my thumb, right where I want them; as I continue to ignore their pleas to submit to chemotherapy which are now becoming tinged with desperation and becoming ominous. It's almost amusing to see how far their little pink tongues are hanging out to sodomize my health insurance for a 39 year old treatment with a 2.1% cure rate. Where's all that research money going anyway? Where's all that Komen money going? They make those Komen gals run for it every year, but the best they have for the deadliest female cancer going is a 39 year-old chemo protocol? Does this seem right to you? Additionally, since 80% of every oncologist's income is failed chemotherapy treatments yet as I type, Big Pharma is patenting everything about cannabis they can—which has a much larger cancer cure rate. I did a TON of research on this by the way as I'm writing this book about it. There's no money in a cure, so people continue to suffer and die because the government—that could stop this—lets Big Pharma and their lobbyists own the FDA in our government by bribe—which is JUST what it is. Anyone still wondering why I refused chemo to do my own protocol? I have NEVER trusted doctors with the exception of plastic surgeons who avoid my contempt because unlike other specialties who have the shame of taking money from the very sick, Plastic Surgeons take money from the very vain. Like me. I've had some plastic work and I got lovely, natural looking results. Now I want new boobs. I let Blue Cross off the hook for a million dollars worth of useless chemotherapy. They can buy me some new boobs to keep from having to shell out for more cancer surgery and chemotherapy (they'll think) down the road. I'm tired of these huge 38DDDs, a single D or solid C works for me!

CHAPTER 15: RETURN TO ILLINOIS FOR MORE SURGERY

I have an appointment with the plastic surgeon on June 1 at 10 am and I am looking forward to getting up to Illinois to see John and the "kids" (we have 9 cats) and live in

MASS MURDERING DOCTORS: THE TRUTH ABOUT ONCOLOGISTS, CHEMOTHERAPY AND CANCER

my OWN house for a while. I'm wanting to get the surgery over with and I also have to have my next MRI as well. A clean MRI is what I want to see more than anything because it will show that I am managing to keep my very aggressive cancer at bay with the RSO protocol. I have an MRI every 90 days for the next year and every 6 months for the next 4 years after that and then maybe once a year for the rest of my life. When you consider that this cancer is the single most virulent, aggressive reproductive cancer that there is, every clean test and clear MRI tells me I made the right decision. The waiting is always the hardest part because you just don't know and you're holding your breath with every test, with every exam you know you could hear that the cancer is back so you live from appointment to appointment knowing that the next one might be the one where your whole world comes crashing down—and then you realize it's never going to end—the rest of your life is going to be lived in 6 month segments. Each clean test gives you 5. 5 months of life, 2 weeks of worrying about the test, a week of worrying about the results of the test and then, hopefully, another cancer-free 6 months of life. When you get to 2 years, you can go once a year—if you can stand it—and then 5 years is the cure, but I don't think I'll be able to breathe again until 2021 and every recurrence starts the 5 year clock all over again. I'm still scared but I am coping with it better. One of the side effects of RSO is that you feel calmer because you're semi-buzzed most of the time but it does reduce your stress and keeps you calm and not in a state of semi-panic all the time.

I may have to do a maintenance dose of RSO for the rest of my life as well, I'm OK with that too, it can be my sleeping pill. Take it at dinner and sleep like a rock—in addition to it's life-saving cancer-killing miracle drug status, it's also the best sleeping pill EVER. I sleep like a rock. I take my last dose at dinner around 7 pm and by 9:30 I am passing out in the chair. I am never groggy in the morning either, so that's a huge plus as well. I sure hope Florida passes medical marijuana in November. I also bought a vaporizer which I find gives me a bit more energy than just eating the RSO although I have to admit to having been in couch-lock a few times. I just went to sleep (no problems there) and woke up and was fine. RSO is one of the least toxic substances known to man but you CAN take too much and be rewarded with room spins and some dizziness and possibly barf it back up. You have to be conservative and build your resistance which does happen quickly. I find that I have energy to work and get things done when I take an RSO pill (I squeeze 1/10th of a gram into

MASS MURDERING DOCTORS: THE TRUTH ABOUT ONCOLOGISTS, CHEMOTHERAPY AND CANCER

empty gelatin capsules, 10 capsules a gram) I am supposed to be taking a half gram a day until the end of May when I will drop to a maintenance dose of 1/10th of a gram a day until I reach the 5 year cure point.

The appointment with the plastic surgeon went well but unfortunately he is going to have to bring in one of his buddies to do the mastectomies and then he will do the reconstruction right behind him. It means his practice gets paid twice for the same surgery, but there's not a lot I can do about it even though I hate seeing my insurance company take it in the shorts, they are getting off the hook for a million bucks worth of chemo, not to mention 5K worth of RSO I paid for out of pocket. We are now waiting on a mutually convenient time for me to meet with BOTH doctors to plan the new breasts. I'd like to have them a few sizes smaller—38DDD is just too much to lug around at the age of 58! I've also decided to get my back fixed if I survive the cancer. I am going to get my life back, get OFF painkillers and make the most of my remaining time on this mortal coil. I'm fine with being a C or D cup, I've been in underwire since third grade. I have also finished the RSO protocol and am due for my 6 month MRI in a few week. I'm not feeling great though. Nothing major but just not feeling like I should—can't put a finger on it.

SIDEBAR: AN ARTICLE: HOW BIG PHARMA CONTROLS WASHINGTON

Leaks Show Senate Aide Threatened Colombia Over Cheap Cancer Drug

Zaid Jilani

May 14 2016, 9:30 a. m.

LEAKED DIPLOMATIC LETTERS sent from Colombia's Embassy in Washington describe how a staffer with the Senate Finance Committee, which is led by Sen. Orrin Hatch, R-Utah, warned of repercussions if Colombia moves forward on approving the cheaper, generic form of a cancer drug.

The drug is called imatinib. Its manufacturer, Novartis, markets the drug in Colombia as Glivec. The World Health Organization's List of Essential Medicines last year suggested it as treatment not only for chronic myeloid leukemia, but also gastrointestinal tumors. Currently, the cost of an annual supply is over $15,000, or about two times the average Colombian's income.

MASS MURDERING DOCTORS: THE TRUTH ABOUT ONCOLOGISTS, CHEMOTHERAPY AND CANCER

On April 26, Colombian Minister of Health Alejandro Gaviria announced plans to take the first step in a multi-step process that could eventually result in allowing generic production of the drug. A generic version of the drug that recently began production in India is expected to cost 30 percent less than the brand-name version.

Andrés Flórez, deputy chief of mission at the Colombian Embassy in Washington, D. C. wrote letters on April 27 and April 28 to Maria Angela Holguin of Colombia's Ministry of Foreign Affairs, detailing concerns he had about possible congressional retaliation for such a move. The letters were obtained by the nonprofit group Knowledge Ecology International, which works on drug patent issues. They were also leaked to Colombian media outlets El Espectador and NoticiasUno.

In the second letter, after a meeting with Senate Finance Committee International Trade Counsel Everett Eissenstat, Flórez wrote that Eissenstat said that authorizing the generic version would "violate the intellectual property rights" of Novartis. Eissenstat also said that if "the Ministry of Health did not correct this situation, the pharmaceutical industry in the United States and related interest groups could become very vocal and interfere with other interests that Colombia could have in the United States," according to the letter.

In particular, Flórez expressed a worry that "this case could jeopardize the approval of the financing of the new initiative 'Peace Colombia. '"

The Obama administration has pledged $450 million for Peace Colombia, which seeks to bring together rebels and the government to end decades of fighting that has resulted in hundreds of thousands of deaths and a shattered civil society. These funds will be used for, among other things, removing land mines. The country has the second-highest number of land-mine fatalities in the world, behind only Afghanistan.

Hatch has close ties to the pharmaceutical industry. Pharmaceutical and health product manufacturers form the second-largest pool of donors to his campaigns. The industry's main trade association, the Pharmaceutical Research and Manufacturers of America, spent $750,000 funding an outside nonprofit that backed Hatch's re-election in 2012. The lobbying group also employed Scott Hatch, one of the senator's sons, as a lobbyist, while donating to his family charity, the Utah Families Foundation.

TELL ME HOW THIS ISN'T BLATANT BRIBERY AND INFLUENCE PEDDLING!!

For his part, Eissenstat has won the "Lighthouse Award" at the annual dinner of the Washington International Trade Association. WITA's board of directors is composed largely of government relations staff from major corporations who help shape trade and intellectual property policy in their favor: WalMart, Microsoft, and Gap all have representatives. In bestowing the award on Eissenstat, WITA board member Bill Lane said the award is given to a "shining light of the trade community." The same year, his boss Hatch received the dinner's Congressional Leadership Award. Andrea Carolina Reyes, a pharmacist who works with the Colombia-based medical nonprofit Misión Salud, called the pressure to suppress the cheaper drug harmful. "I would ... ask Hatch to consider that we're talking about people's lives, and this needs to mean something to him," she told The Intercept. "In Colombia, we really have health constraints. There's people, they have no access to anything. They live hours from health institutions, and they don't have even the cheapest medicines. "Neither Eissenstat nor Hatch responded to multiple requests for comment. "We do not comment on internal correspondence," Olga Acosta, press officer at the Colombian Embassy, told The Intercept.

See? They don't care about lives in other countries either, it's all bullcrap. All Big Pharma cares about is keeping control of their lobbyist bought and paid for politicians. Total scumbags—there's no other word for them. These are the jagoffs making your prescriptions cost about 100 times what they should be priced. Greed and corruption. What a piece of crap Orrin Hatch is as well.

SIDEBAR: Article about Big Pharma is preventing a cancer cure.

We Can't Afford To Cure Cancer

https://www. lewrockwell. com/2016/06/bill-sardi/cant-afford-cure-cancer/

June 7, 2016

MASS MURDERING DOCTORS: THE TRUTH ABOUT ONCOLOGISTS, CHEMOTHERAPY AND CANCER

Someone has said there are just too many jobs in the pursuit of a cancer cure to allow any therapy to be proven and put into practice. Recognize the nation is dotted with cancer research centers that hold billions of dollars of debt. For example, the Fred Hutchinson Cancer Research Center in Seattle, Washington holds $176 million of debt. Moody's Investor Service Sloan-Kettering Cancer Center in New York, the nation's cancer research center, holds $1.9 billion of debt. A cancer cure would leave research centers like these on the hook for loans that could not possibly be paid back. Better for cancer research centers to live off the $4.95 billion of research grants that get divvied out by the National Institutes of Health each year than to find a cure. In light of this revelation, the public may be better served by private enterprise that is not reliant on public funding to find a cure for cancer. While Facebook co-founder Sean Parker has pledged $250 million towards a "moon shot" attempt to cure cancer, donating his money to six cancer research centers another entrepreneur operating clinics he founded in Austria and Germany is way ahead of the pack having successfully treated thousands of patients, though he had to resurrect a dismissed cancer therapy from its grave, undergo closure of his company by health authorities and incur severe criticism in order to do it. (I am certain this is First Immune)

CHAPTER 16: THE RISE OF IMMUNOTHERAPY PROTOCOLS AND GcMAF/Goleic

Before I get to that compelling story, let me say cancer therapy is undergoing a massive change. The slash-burn-poison era of cancer therapy may be over. The age of cancer immunotherapy has begun. And I'm not the person saying this. Many cancer researchers are saying immunotherapy is already replacing chemo. Just how much longer conventional oncologists can continue to subject their patients to harsh of cancer treatments is unknown.

An article entitled: "Cancer Immunotherapy: The Beginning Of The End Of Cancer," says: "the tide has finally changed and immunotherapy has become a clinically validated treatment for cancer cancers. ————-BMC Medicine

The futility of chemotherapy is revealed by the very fact toxic anti-cancer drugs impair a type of white blood cell known as natural killer cells, thus limiting the cancer patient's chances for a cure altogether. —————— Molecular Cancer Therapy

MASS MURDERING DOCTORS: THE TRUTH ABOUT ONCOLOGISTS, CHEMOTHERAPY AND CANCER

SIDEBAR GcMAF/Goleic: ENTER STAGE LEFT!

The clock is counting down on chemotherapy as immunotherapy is already producing long-term remissions for some types of cancer, particularly non-solid tumors. Toxic chemotherapy finally comes to the end of its product life cycle. The goal of cancer immunotherapy is to stimulate a patient's immune system to recognize cancer cells as foreign and attack them. The four white blood cells that kill cancer. Cancer immunologists are presently unleashing four types of white blood cells against cancer:

1. Neutrophils, which produced "cancer-proof mice" at Duke University. Neutrophils track down, dock up next to tumor cells and blow them up with a burst of oxygen free radicals. However, a trial was proposed to glean activated neutrophils from healthy patients and instill them in cancer patients, but it never materialized. It became apparent healthy young subjects exhibit the same immunity from cancer in summer months as laboratory mice bred for their ability to produce neutrophils. This strongly suggests sunlight exposure in summer produces sufficient amounts of vitamin D to reduce cancer risk. However, instead of launching a vitamin D trial, vitamin-averse researchers ludicrously proposed the removal of activated neutrophils from healthy subjects and instillation in cancer patients because it needed a profitable business model to be successful. What can be concluded is that any natural and inexpensive cancer therapy will be summarily dismissed.

2. T-cells are successfully being harvested from cancer patients, grown in numbers and then activated and instilled back into the patient to produce long-lasting cures for non-solid tumors like leukemia (cancer of the blood) and lymphoma (cancer of the lymph system).

3. Natural killer cell therapy involves NK cells that inject toxins directly into cancer cells. This is considered the most direct way to conquer cancer because NK cells do not depend on the development of antibodies like T-cells do.

4. Macrophages that literally digest or engulf roaming cancer cells and are abundant in the environment surrounding solid tumors have long been considered for use in cancer therapy. Since most immunotherapies for cancer have had limited success in solid tumors, focus on macrophages has been intense.

MASS MURDERING DOCTORS: THE TRUTH ABOUT ONCOLOGISTS, CHEMOTHERAPY AND CANCER

Macrophages are not all beneficial. There is a Janus face to macrophages. One type of macrophage actually induces biological chaos at tumor sites –uncontrolled inflammation and suppression of tumor-fighting white blood cells. Tumor cells escape what is called "immune surveillance" via inflammation and produce immune suppressors. Out-of-control macrophages even facilitate the spread (metastasis) of cancer. Reckless macrophages via their ability to wreak havoc by inducing uncontrolled inflammation not only interfere with the immune system's ability to ward off cancer but also can, for example, induce inflammation in the lungs due to a viral infection that fills the lungs with fluid, with a potentially deadly outcome. Out of control macrophages are also a major cause of morbidity and mortality in childhood arthritis. These uncontrolled macrophages are responsible for legal blindness induced by wet macular degeneration, a condition where the visual center of the eye (macula) leaks fluid or produces new blood vessels (angiogenesis) in an attempt to deliver oxygen to eye tissues. Knowledge of Health One group of cancer researchers describe macrophages as "unwitting accomplices in cancer malignancy." Another report characterizes macrophages as "corrupt policemen in cancer-related inflammation."

A damning revelation here is that conventional chemotherapy can in many instances inhibit the anti-tumor properties of macrophages.

Dietary factors control macrophage-induced inflammation

Dietary factors may determine whether macrophages are cancer killing or not. For example, it has been demonstrated that high intake of salt converts macrophages into devilish villains that impair the ability of T-cells to control cancer. Salt is highly alkaline (so much for the alkaline theory of cancer). A high-fat diet also predisposes macrophages to become inflammatory.

What can train macrophages to seek out and eradicate tumor cells without inducing inflammation and suppression of the very immune system that is attempting to do the same thing? Enter vitamin D binding protein! Vitamin D binding protein, a molecule that facilitates the transport of vitamin D throughout the body. When two enzymes (galactosidase and sialidase) knock off two sugar-like molecules off of vitamin D binding protein, this becomes a unique molecular entity called Gc protein-macrophage activating factor, or GcMAF/Goleic. The discovery of the process by which GcMAF/Goleic is produced was published in 1991 and 1993 by Nobuto Yamamoto,

MASS MURDERING DOCTORS: THE TRUTH ABOUT ONCOLOGISTS, CHEMOTHERAPY AND CANCER

then a noted immunologist at Temple University in Philadelphia. Dr. Yamamoto comes from a prestigious background having been appointed a full professor of microbiology and immunology at Hahnemann University School of Medicine. It was Dr. Yamamoto who noted that GcMAF/Goleic greatly enhances the cancer ingesting properties of macrophages by 3-7 fold.   In 2003 Dr. Yamamoto also noted that GcMAF/Goleic increased tumoricidal activity without releasing two known activators of inflammation-tumor necrosis factor (TNF) and nitric oxide (NO). GcMAF/Goleic was like taking wild horses and saddling them to work together as a team against cancer. Were cancer biologists paying attention? Just 10-50 picograms (a trillionth of a gram) of GcMAF/Goleic was demonstrated to stimulate the activity of macrophages by 7-9 fold in laboratory mice.

Dr. Yamamoto fails to carry the torch for GcMAF/Goleic

Dr. Yamamoto advanced further into his research with GcMAF/Goleic by administering this blood protein in minuscule amounts to laboratory mice that had tumor cells implanted. A single injection of GcMAF/Goleic resulted in an average survival time of 21 days (one mouse survived beyond 60 days) whereas untreated mice survived an average of 13 days. Dr. Yamamoto described this curative therapy as "a consequence of sustained macrophage activation by inflammation resulting from the macrophage tumoricidal process."

Are nagalase enzyme levels a marker of GcMAF/Goleic activity?

Dr. Yamamoto took another step forward in 1996 by instilling GcMAF/Goleic into a lab dish with macrophages taken from cancer patients. Dr. Yamamoto reported that an enzyme is known as nagalase (akaalpha-N-acetylgalactosaminidase) was blocking the conversion of vitamin D binding protein to GcMAF/Goleic. Later Dr. Yamamoto reported **nagalase enzyme levels correlate with the size of tumors.** Here was Dr. Yamamoto pioneering cancer immunotherapy two decades before it is now being given the spotlight in cancer therapy. Dr. Yamamoto's work was also validated by other researchers in the field; yet there was no impetus to advance it from the laboratory bench to the bedside of cancer patients. Then Dr. Yamamoto embarked upon a series of published human studies conducted in Japan and published in 2008 to demonstrate GcMAF/Goleic had remarkable ability to inhibit nagalase and reduce the size of tumors and produce tumor-free individuals. Dr. Yamamoto's GcMAF/Goleic

MASS MURDERING DOCTORS: THE TRUTH ABOUT ONCOLOGISTS, CHEMOTHERAPY AND CANCER

was positively reported to rescue patients battling prostate, breast, lung and colon cancer. It was then, in 2008 that I was alerted by a laboratory researcher, Timothy Hubbell, that I should examine the published works of Dr. Yamamoto dealing with GcMAF/Goleic and cancer. I published an online report about Dr. Yamamoto's seemingly remarkable discoveries and wondered why the research community wasn't paying attention. My report drew worldwide attention and broke the story to the public. ---LewRockwell.com

Unexpectedly, Dr. Yamamoto was not pleased with issuance of the report. He claimed only his GcMAF was safe to use. But when asked what plans he had to market it, he provided nebulous answers. I arranged for a major worldwide Fortune-500 company to enter into discussions about licensing his GcMAF/Goleic, but he never responded to that offer. Cancer patients called him frantically begging for GcMAF/Goleic, to no avail. Dr. Yamamoto advised me to get a job writing about other topics. By 2014 the editors of a cancer journal retracted Dr. Yamamoto's report involving GcMAF/Goleic and nagalase in breast cancer patients citing irregularities in documentation for institutional review board approval.

Retraction Watch pilloried Dr. Yamamoto, discrediting his work completely. Inexplicably, the 90+ year old researcher did not respond or comment about the retraction. Was Dr. Yamamoto guilty of fabricating or was he being silenced? But, as it is pointed out by the besmirched clinic in Europe that is administering GcMAF/Goleic to cancer patients, there are 142 scientists that have penned research papers regarding GcMAF/Goleic. If Dr. Yamamoto produced fraudulent research, then what are all these other research scientists doing studying it Since 1998 Dr. Yamamoto works at a tax-exempt foundation he established, the Socrates Institute in Philadelphia, which appears to be a very modest operation. From 1993 thru 2015 he filed for 13 patents involving GcMAF/Goleic.

Yamamoto's studies questioned

In 2014 The Anticancer Fund pf Belgium delved into the human GcMAF/Goleic studies conducted under Dr. Yamamoto. **They have a Big Pharma director on their board, appear to be funded by Big Pharma, and put forward entirely fraudulent science to get two of Yamamoto's papers retracted.** They report that institutional review boards for these trials "do not exist." Dr. Yamamoto's co-

MASS MURDERING DOCTORS: THE TRUTH ABOUT ONCOLOGISTS, CHEMOTHERAPY AND CANCER

authors "could not be found." They claim naturally occurring GcMAF/Goleic in cancer patients is about 4 milligrams/liter of blood, "making the 100 nanograms (used by Yamamoto) meaningless." But were researchers in Japan clamming up, cowering from pressure that would surely come and ruin their careers? These Belgian researchers demanded "adequate randomized controlled trials," full well knowing they would be unethical. You can't ethically leave cancer patients to take placebos and die. GcMAF/Goleic must be compared against existing conventional therapy, and not chemo that degrades it. ----Cancer Immunology Immunotherapy

I often remind skeptics that insulin, penicillin, aspirin, nitroglycerin, digoxin and most vaccines came into common use without long-term double-blind placebo-controlled studies. In the modern pharmaceutical world, drugs are approved if they marginally improve markers of disease, not the disease itself. For example, statin drugs are widely prescribed for cholesterol reduction but have never been shown to significantly reduce mortality, though they do marginally reduce the risk for a non-mortal heart attack (by 3% over 5 years). **Cancer drugs are approved if they reduce the size of a tumor by 50% in 28 days regardless of whether they improve survival or not.**

This means they are useless—but profitable which is ALL Big Pharma and the oncologists care about. A cure puts them out of business so, first they rob you and when they kill you, and you're glad to die after the miserable chemo poisoning. TDN

Searching for an alternative hypothesis

Another troubling report published in 2009 probed into the mechanism that converts vitamin D binding protein to GcMAF/Goleic. The claim is that an enzyme, nagalase, degrades GcMAF/Goleic in cancer patients. In fact, these researchers show there is a significant amount of the precursor for GcMAF/Goleic in blood serum of cancer patients (~4 milligrams/liter), which "makes it unlikely there is a depleted GcMAF or Goleic precursor in cancer patients." These researchers say "alternative hypotheses must be considered to explain the relative inability of patient serum to activate macrophages." But then again, we refer to the previously mentioned paper published in 2010 where it was shown that GcMAF/Goleic exhibits "a direct and potent effect upon tumor cells in the absence of macrophages." GcMAF/Goleic is taking us on a scientific roller coaster. GcMAF/Goleic exhibits very potent ability to inhibit tumor cell growth directly. Was this the alternative hypothesis GcMAF/Goleic researchers were searching for? Another research study, authored by researchers at Harvard Medical School and the University of Kentucky, showed GcMAF/Goleic produces "strong inhibitory activity on prostate tumor cells independent of macrophage activation." By the way, that study was funded by a Department of Defense grant.

Should GcMAF/Goleic be renamed DNMAF — direct non-macrophage activating factor? The unexpected occurred in another recent study. Macrophages were instilled into a dish of breast cancer cells and nothing happened. Tumor cells were unaltered. But when human breast cancer cells were cultured with macrophages that had been previously activated by GcMAF/Goleic, these macrophages surrounded the breast cancer cells and induced their death. This was anticipated, but the following experiment wasn't

Even more striking was when GcMAF/Goleic was added to a lab dish with breast cancer cells only (no macrophages). Researchers at the University of Firenze, Italy, showed GcMAF/Goleic treated tumor cells reverted back to healthy cells! This direct reversion of tumor cells to a healthy state without macrophages should have provoked a top-to-bottom re-think on the dynamic mechanisms exhibited by GcMAF/Goleic. Maybe GcMAF/Goleic had little to do with nagalase levels. But researchers could not rule out that the dramatic reduction in breast cancer cells observed in a lab dish emanated from the ability of GcMAF/Goleic to inhibit angiogenesis.

GcMAF/Goleic and angiogenesis

Angiogenesis is a biological phenomenon where blood vessels near oxygen-starved tissues develop new tributaries to nourish tissues with oxygen and other nutrients. In this case, angiogenesis facilitates tumor growth by provision of nutrients. GcMAF/Goleic has been shown to inhibit the sprouting of new blood vessels that feed tumors. Researchers also demonstrated vitamin D3, the natural form of D, works synergistically with GcMAF/Goleic.   These researchers showed GcMAF/Goleic has multiple biological activities, notably its interaction with the cell surface receptor for vitamin D, that could be responsible for its seven anti-cancer effects." GcMAF/Goleic's ability to activate macrophages may be overemphasized. It exerts other powerful biological actions to quell cancer. This compelling experiment involving the vitamin D cell surface receptor was performed by the very same researchers affiliated with

MASS MURDERING DOCTORS: THE TRUTH ABOUT ONCOLOGISTS, CHEMOTHERAPY AND CANCER

Immuno Biotech Ltd, the maligned company in Europe that makes GcMAF/Goleic. Let's not overlook the fact that vitamin D itself, a synergistic co-factor with GcMAF/Goleic, activate two other classes of cancer-killing white blood cells – neutrophils and natural killer cells.

Attempts to make a synthetic GcMAF/Goleic

If GcMAF/Goleic were an outright fraud, then why are research centers attempting to develop look-alike molecules (analogues) to make into patentable drugs? Efforts to synthetically produce molecular mimics of GcMAF/Goleic date back to 2002. Other researchers reported their attempt to produce a patentable GcMAF/Goleic synthetic in 2006.

Author's Note: Big Pharma can't patent the original under current FDA rules because it's a human-derived protein and therefore not patentable so there's no pot of gold at the end of the rainbow for them if they can't patent it and gouge people for it. If they do manage to do this then presumably insurance would pay for it. I will have to pay out of pocket for it, just like the RSO, but I may not need it unless I have a recurrence.

David Noakes, uncloaked

That businessman mentioned in the opening page of this report, who has founded the GcMAF/Goleic clinics in Europe, is tech entrepreneur David Noakes. His broad-based team of researchers has, like Dr. Yamamoto, shown that GcMAF/Goleic decreases nagalase levels in patients with advanced-stage cancer. As nagalase activity diminished with weekly GcMAF/Goleic injections, patients experienced improvement. Mr. Noakes' company, Immuno Biotech, sponsored another study that demonstrated how GcMAF/Goleic complexes with olive oil (oleic acid) to further stimulate its immune-therapeutic effect. This curative effect was visibly observed in ultrasound images of human cancer that confirmed reduction in tumor size from 8.7 to 4.9 1-4 weeks of GcMAF/Goleic/oleic acid treatment among humans with stage-4 cancer. This answers the criticism lodged at Dr. Yamamoto that he never provided evidence of tumor shrinkage, only evidence of reduced nagalase activity, and he only chose patients with early-stage cancer. David Noakes finally provided the evidence Dr.

MASS MURDERING DOCTORS: THE TRUTH ABOUT ONCOLOGISTS, CHEMOTHERAPY AND CANCER

Yamamoto couldn't produce. The absence of side effects was also noted. Is it the cure for cancer that the patients have been begging for?

Immuno Biotech provides evidence for examination

Immuno Biotech has 33 scientific research papers currently published on the mechanisms and results of GcMAF/Goleic therapy for cancer, autism and other disorders. There are now over 200 scientists who have published over 120 research papers on GcMAF/Goleic. Immuno Biotech's website cites an 80% response rate (reduction in tumor size for Stage 1 and Stage II cancer). In their experience at Immuno Biotech, late-stage cancer may require up to 18 months of treatment to become cancer free. Immuno Biotech asks all of its cancer patients to adhere to a no-added sugar/ low carbohydrate diet and to supplement their diet with 10,000 units of vitamin D3 and 200 mcg K2 daily. According to information obtained online, Immuno Biotech currently employs five doctors at its clinics. GcMAF/Goleic is injected directly into the tumor using ultrasound imaging. Mr. Noakes clinics generally provide GcMAF/Goleic for a period of 3-4 weeks and then patients are sent home to receive it on their own. In general by the first week a 25% reduction in tumor size is achieved (range 8-40% reduction). He says his company has supplied GcMAF/Goleic now to 11,000 patients. He also supplies 100 clinics and 250 doctors around the world with genuine GcMAF/Goleic. His company also offers an improved dropper form of GcMAF/Goleic. Recognize, it is difficult for a company like Immuno Biotech to provide data on cure rates since 5-year survival is the gold standard.

Is this a health quack?

A distant assessment does not reveal David Noakes to be acting like the health quack he is portrayed to be online. In fact, all of the evidence demanded of Dr. Nobuto Yamamoto, David Noakes seems to have provided – mechanism studies, survival data, ultrasound images of shrinking tumor volume that correlate with GcMAF/Goleic therapy. Despite his transparency, David Noakes has undergone considerable scrutiny by authorities. Shamefully, that oversight was coming from a country whose cancer survival rate is the worst in western Europe.

Where are the dead bodies?

MASS MURDERING DOCTORS: THE TRUTH ABOUT ONCOLOGISTS, CHEMOTHERAPY AND CANCER

As we ask in the natural medicine business, "where are the dead bodies?" With all of the clamor about GcMAF/Goleic being branded as an unlicensed health product that poses "a significant risk to health," **it is difficult to find a cancer patient who feels he was bilked by Mr. Noakes.**

While the Medicine and Healthcare products Regulatory Agency (MHRA), an agency bereft with corruption itself MHRA Corrupt, raised concerns whether the GcMAF/Goleic product is sterile and free from contamination, no product-related infections were reported. Mr. Noakes explains his company's GcMAF/Goleic product goes through 22 steps of purification. Batch testing for sterility by an independent laboratory are reported to show perfect sterility for 5 years. Hundreds of people in Guernsey applied pressure on their doctors and politicians to maintain GcMAF/Goleic therapy but it was banned on the isle Guernsey in February of 2015 anyway. Health authorities demand GcMAF/Goleic be synthetically produced and undergo drug testing, something that would, according to Mr. Noakes, cost around $20 million and take 5 years to gain approval. Immuno Biotech's laboratories have made two forms of a synthetic GcMAF/Goleic, but human drug trials are not likely to happen, says Mr. Noakes.

In The Guernsey Press, a letter (abridged) **(author: not by me!)** to the editor read: Up until recently I was a bit skeptical about GcMAF/Goleic, however events in the last few weeks have made me reconsider my position. I have recently met with several people who have been told that they have terminal cancer and there were no avenues left for their treatment. These people have taken GcMAF/Goleic and also have changed their lifestyle and have fantastic results. One lady who was diagnosed as terminal is now completely clear, whilst another gentleman has had his tumor shrunk by over 50%. I was at David Noakes' house two weeks ago along with over 80 other people there, deputies from the local cancer charities and people who were currently receiving treatment. *What strikes me about this treatment is the conspiracy of silence about it.* For example I know of a local cancer charity whose board members will not actively talk about it for fear of upsetting certain other board members. I am also aware that the local clinicians refuse to acknowledge this treatment for fear of upsetting Health & Social Services Department (HSSD). People who are in hospices are not made aware of this potential treatment and let's be brutal about this if you are dying what have you got to lose. I urge the cancer charities to acknowledge this is your job is to promote treatments to get rid of this disease. If charities fail to acknowledge this, the question begs to be asked "WHY?," and what are they hiding from?----Guernsey Press July 18, 2014

Deaths of researchers surrounds GcMAF/Goleic

This report will not delve into the unexplained deaths of clinicians and researchers associated with GcMAF/Goleic Global Research except to say that early on in 2009, Narasimha Swamy PhD of Brown University, who had knowledge how to produce GcMAF/Goleic, died suddenly at age 39 without a history of any health problems. He authored and co-authored papers on GcMAF/Goleic. It was an untimely if not a suspicious death. Did Dr. Swamy plan to bring GcMAF/Goleic back to his homeland of India where generic drug makers would distribute it globally without regulatory approvals? Who knows? Health product licensing and manufacturing oversight have become roadblocks to innovation, not assurances a product is safe and effective. The public can see through this now. **Author:** I fully expect Big Pharma to come after me when this book comes out. I have NO other health issues except a genetic defect that gives me cancer. I don't drink or smoke and I have a spotless driving record—so ask questions if I have an accident!

SIDEBAR: CULLING THE POPULATION

In the UK the National Health Service is billions of dollars in debt. Hospitals there have resorted to withdrawing drinking water from bedridden patients, which is the perfect way to cull this patient population, as it leaves no fingerprints. According to one news report, 12,000 are "killed" annually in British hospitals due to dehydration. Elderly patients report they have averted dehydration by drinking water from flower vases. A more horrific report delivered to the Royal Society of Medicine in London by a leading professor of medicine claims 130,000 patients annually in the National Health Service system have been placed on a "death pathway" instead of a "care pathway." ----

It's not **just** physician greed nor Big Pharma profiteering, it's something much more ghastly that keeps cancer from being cured. Health systems worldwide are underfunded. Health systems can't afford a cancer cure. For the good of insolvent retirement and health trust funds and life insurance companies the elderly must die on time. That is the hidden determinant that blocks adoption of any cancer cure.

SIDEBAR: NICE TO KNOW IT'S NOT JUST GREED

MASS MURDERING DOCTORS: THE TRUTH ABOUT ONCOLOGISTS, CHEMOTHERAPY AND CANCER

It's not very reassuring to discover that it's not just Big Pharma greed that is keeping a cure off the market. Apparently our totally corrupt governments were so busy handing out taxpayer dollars so their cronies could make money that they forgot basic accounting and laws of supply and demand. Essentially we have been fucked over by the duly elected ruling class—instead of the inherited ruling class.

By Steven Vasilev, MD
Source: National Cancer Institute. Ovarian Epithelial, Fallopian Tube, and Primary Peritoneal Cancer Treatment–for health professionals (PDQ®). Recurrent or Persistent Ovarian Epithelial, Fallopian Tube, and Primary Peritoneal Cancer Treatment. Updated 08/21/15. http://www. cancer. gov/types/ovarian/hp/ovarian-epithelial-treatment-pdq#section/_82 Updated January 30, 2016 This is a study that shows exactly how useless and detrimental to the patient—not that it mattes because they all die anyway with the chemo—and chemo causes cancer down the road which is of course treated with MORE chemo. Talk about protecting profits by insuring repeat customers who were ALREADY willing to pay hundreds of thousands of dollars be voluntarily poisoned come back to be re-poisoned for the greed of their "doctors".

Ovarian cancer recurrence: WHAT HAPPENS WHEN IT COMES BACK?

What treatments are available for ovarian cancer recurrence? My ovarian cancer is back or it never went away after the first set of treatments. What should I do now? That is the question asked by most ovarian cancer patients at some point in time. Unfortunately, for roughly **85% of people who undergo first-line chemotherapy, the cancer comes back.** Chemotherapy does not work. It has a 2.1% cure rate. When it comes back it is renamed peritoneal carcinomatosis and it's terminal. Every time. **THERE ARE NO KNOW SURVIVORS OF THIS CANCER.** The answer to this question depends on how the diagnosis of recurrence was made and how long after the end of initial treatment this happened.

Generally, there are three separate categories which carry three different prognoses and usually lead to three general different treatment plans. However, beyond that, please be aware that while there is a pretty standard approach to initial treatment options, treatment for recurrence is highly individualized. While there are pretty good guidelines, there are no universally agreed upon standards of practice. In general, the more time passes before a recurrence the better the chances for a possible cure or long second remission. Also, more options are available in this scenario.

Recurrence In Six Months (After Chemotherapy)

If the recurrence is diagnosed at least 6 months after initial treatment (preferably closer to a year), the tumor is deemed to be "platinum sensitive" if the initial treatment contained a platinum drug (Carboplatin or Cisplatin).

Author's note: These 'LIFESAVING CHEMOTHERAPY" drugs are almost 40 years old—and that's the best they've got after all those Komen gals ran all over hell's half acre to raise money? The American Cancer Society—where's all their money gone? A trillion dollars and 40 years—WHERE'S MY CURE?? We're getting hosed folks!!

The later the recurrence after this point, the more it might be reasonable to perform a "secondary cytoreduction" surgery to once again remove as much cancer as possible. Most gynecologic oncologists would strongly consider this if the cancer recurs at least two years after initial treatment and a mass or masses is/are seen on scan or felt on examination. However, it may be a very good option prior to this time frame too, depending upon your specific situation. Whether or not repeat secondary cytoreduction surgery is performed, many oncologists would suggest treating with the same drugs that were used the first time, especially if the recurrence is found more than a year after initial treatment. If it is found between 6 months and a year after treatment, options might include re-treatment with Taxol and cisplatin or carboplatin, or using new drugs as discussed below. Most oncologists would favor new drugs within this time frame.

Recurrence Within Six Months

If the recurrence is diagnosed 6 months or less after the initial treatment, the tumor is deemed to be "platinum resistant". The tumor likely grew back at some point toward the end or after the initial chemotherapy. **In these situations, repeat surgery is rarely recommended as it is highly unlikely to improve length of life or quality of life.** There are three main chemotherapy drugs available today which most oncologists use interchangeably. (50-100 THOUSAND DOLLARS per treatment for a 39 year old drug protocol—and you thought that donation to the American Cancer Society (of Thieves) was a good idea!) All work just about equally well and can be used in sequence, one at a time, as one drug or the other stops working. These

MASS MURDERING DOCTORS: THE TRUTH ABOUT ONCOLOGISTS, CHEMOTHERAPY AND CANCER

are: Doxil, Topotecan and Gemzar. Combination therapies have also been tried, but generally without dramatically better success and with higher toxicity side effects. However, each situation is different, so please ask your doctor about all possible options. While aggressive chemotherapy with these drugs can still be ongoing, you should keep in mind that the chances for cure are very small and keeping quality of life in mind is very important. Again, this is a risk/benefit discussion with your physician(s).

Recurrence During Or Immediately After Treatment

If the recurrence is actually cancer growth during initial treatment, this is called "platinum refractory", or an extreme case of resistance to chemotherapy. Additional chemotherapy can be given, mainly using the drugs discussed about, but the chances of response are quite low. Also, keep in mind that the drugs mentioned above are NOT the only ones available for treatment, they are just regarded as the best ones to try first. (Not to mention only 40 years old—and this is the BEST we've got?) Ask your doctor(s) about others and what the chances are that they might help in your particular case. This may also be a good time to inquire about promising but unproven options through clinical trials, or you can just go home to die because after the chemo, you have no chance to survive—and there are NO known survivors.

Clinical Trials

There are many clinical trials in progress for ovarian cancer that has recurred, and research looking at some of these options is encouraging but I don't know anything about them so I can't really give an educated. Some of these options include targeted therapy medications that are designed to specifically target cancer cells, and one medication of a new class of drugs called PARP inhibitors was just approved for use in 2015 called oleparib but you can't get it until you have had 2 recurrences which is stupid and makes no sense.

Palliative vs. Curative Treatment Intent

A word about "palliative surgery" and "palliative radiation". Even if surgery is no longer a curative option at some point in treatment, there may be surgical options which "palliate" or help resolve or calm symptoms. In rare cases this might be an intestinal bypass surgery, or removal of one blocked area of intestine (usually many segments are blocked) in order to allow someone to eat food for at least a number of months. In other cases, this might mean placing a tube directly into the stomach through the skin (gastrostomy) so that vomiting is relieved and a tube in the nose (NG tube) does not have to be in place for weeks or months.

Sometimes in advanced cancer, fluid accumulates in the chest. Various procedures to drain the fluid, including tubes and scarring procedures (pleurodesis) can help eliminate or reduce this fluid and help with breathing problems. These are just several examples, but on a case by case basis, some type of surgery or radiologically guided invasive procedure might be helpful to you. If you are suffering from a particular symptom, ask whether or not some type of surgical or invasive procedure might be helpful. Finally, although rare, ovarian cancer may involve your bones, often producing severe pain. Also rarely it can spread to the brain and produce seizures. In both of these situations, radiation therapy to that area might be very helpful to reduce or eliminate symptoms. Source: National Cancer Institute. It's nice that instead of finding a CURE, the NCI is willing to help you die comfortably. That's pretty white of them don't you think?

CHAPTER 17: MEANWHILE BACK IN ILLINOIS...

My first MRI post surgery was crystal clear and I hope the second one at 6 months is as well, it would show that the RSO protocol is everything it is supposed to be although it's not 100%. I finished the RSO protocol about 2 weeks before my 1st MRI and now all that is left is for me to monitor for a recurrence. This means I have a date with the MRI machine every 3 months for the next 15 months and then I can breathe again. 88% of HGSC BRCA1+ patients have a recurrence—with or without chemotherapy within 6-18 months of original diagnosis and treatment. My next MRI is July 9th 2016 and I am scared and nervous but I feel OK I guess. My CA-125 is 19 though—slightly elevated from the first CA-125 which was 16 but still in the normal range of 0-35 but it went UP and that worries me after my July 11th doctor's appointment but the MRI isn't back yet so I don't know that anything is wrong. I'm not too worried but Dr. Janet informs me I've dropped 29 pounds. That was disturbing as I knew I had lost a bit of weight as my size 12 jeans were a little loose but upon closer inspection I discovered it was my size 10 jeans that were getting loose. Now I'm somewhat worried, but I'll know for sure soon enough and I feel pretty OK, but not as good as I did after the surgery, but I think it's probably just stress. I had a bad time on a business trip to Chicago last week and I am worried that I only eat a few bites of food and I'm full and that coupled with the blah feelings, and nausea and occasional barfing which is more frequent than I am used to, but I chalk it up to mild depression, losing my sister and having the same cancer and so on and John keeps telling me that they got it ALL in the surgery and to think positive but until I get the 6 month clear MRI, I will be wound up—not that I'm not wound up anyway. The recurrence rate is SO high and I am terrified. I call Dr. Janet's office to ask if they have my MRI, and could the nurse read it to me and she does. It's the worst possible news. My cancer is back and the doctors agree on one thing: I am going to die. Soon. 6 months give or take according to them. I'm stunned: in 3 months I went from cancer free to TERMINAL?? Really? REALLY?? Are you f**king KIDDING ME?? TERMINAL??? What the...??

CHAPTER 18: IT'S BAAAAAAACKKKK....AND I'M OFFICIALLY TERMINAL

So, my 6 month MRI showed a return of my cancer with several small tumors and a 2.8 cm "mass" that the MRI radiologist diagnosed instantly as ovarian serous carcinoma and Peritoneal carcinomatosis which is medical speak for: "You are going to die". I make a conscious decision, due to the research I have done that I am NOT going to die from this and I am NOT going to do chemo. If I DO have chemo, it will only be because I am forced via COURT ORDER which in this day and age is entirely possible unless Trump is elected and we get our America back!! The takeaway here is that even very early stage HGSC is deadly. My CA-125 took a jump to 19 from the last time when it was 16. 0-35 is normal so just the CA-125 test would have sent me out the door of the lab, ignorant that the killer in my belly was back. This cancer came to kill me—but I don't die so easily.

Here's the official skinny on the cancer that I looked up so I could see what I was up against. This is bad—very bad. I am up against a killer with nothing left with which I can fight back. I have NO REMOVABLE tissue left after the two surgeries to cut out the bastard and I don't know if my 3 month MRI was clean because I did the RSO protocol or because the cancer was too small to see. Either way, this means I have to step up to the plate big time and got for some experimental immunotherapy. I'm scared to death and I am really, really mad now. I am unleashing all of the power of the legendary redhead DNA-coded rage and fury at this cancer, so I almost feel sorry

MASS MURDERING DOCTORS: THE TRUTH ABOUT ONCOLOGISTS, CHEMOTHERAPY AND CANCER

for it. Almost. However, it came to kill me, so as far as I am concerned, it assumes the risk that I will kill it and I will! I will kill this cancer and become cancer-free or die trying. Literally. The takeaway from this is simple: Early detection doesn't always mean cure. It means you get to fight for your life for an additional 6-12 months. Here's the official scoop on this bastard:

Peritoneal carcinomatosis is the **most common terminal (oh no no no!!) feature of abdominal cancers.** For gastrointestinal surgeons and medical oncologists, it is a vexing condition because, **although the disease is limited to the peritoneal surface, complete surgical removal is impossible and systemic chemotherapy is powerless.** Peritoneal carcinomatosis is **generally considered to be an untreatable condition** that makes clinicians abandon further aggressive treatments. Why so much use of chemotherapy if it does so little good? Well for one thing, drug companies provide huge economic incentives. In 1990, $3.53 billion was spent on chemotherapy. By 1994 that figure had more than doubled to $7.51 billion. This relentless increase in chemotherapy use was accompanied by a relentless increase in cancer deaths.

Oncologist Albert Braverman, MD, wrote in 1991 that "no disseminated neoplasm (cancer) incurable in 1975 is curable today... Many medical oncologists recommend chemotherapy for virtually any tumor, with a hopefulness undiscouraged by almost invariable failure."

Why the growth in chemotherapy in the face of such failure? A look at the financial interrelationships between a large cancer center such as Memorial Sloan-Kettering Cancer Center (MSKCC) and the companies that make billions selling chemotherapy drugs is revealing. James Robinson III, Chairman of the MSKCC Board of Overseers and Managers, is a director of Bristol-Myers Squibb, the world's largest producer of chemotherapy drugs. Richard Gelb, Vice-Chairman of the MSKCC board is Chairman of the Board at Bristol-Myers. Richard Furlaud, another MSKCC board member, recently retired as Bristol Myers' president. Paul Marks, MD, MSKCC's President and CEO, is a director

Gynecologists have some different views on ovarian cancer. They have tried extensive debulking surgery for the peritoneal disease followed by intraperitoneal (i.p.) cisplatin-based chemotherapy. A large, randomized controlled trial has recently

MASS MURDERING DOCTORS: THE TRUTH ABOUT ONCOLOGISTS, CHEMOTHERAPY AND CANCER

shown significant survival benefit of heated intra-abdominal cisplatin as compared with intravenous cisplatin in patients with stage III ovarian cancer and residual tumor masses of 2 cm or less This treatment strategy for ovarian cancer is, needless to say, based on the high sensitivity of the tumor to the agents. In such situations, cytoreductive surgery may even be regarded as neoadjuvant treatment to chemotherapy. In gastrointestinal cancers, however, no chemotherapeutic regimen has shown the same effectiveness. The study doesn't say what the survival rate is, but THEORETICALLY they could triple the survival rate and still save less than 10% so I'm not too impressed with the results of the new way of poisoning people by surgically implanting a tube and then pumping their bellies full of poison 400 times stronger than the intravenous (IV) chemotherapy. **Also, oncologists make money from the drugs—they buy them from the pharmaceutical companies, mark them up tens thousands of dollars and resell them to the patients.** The more I learn about oncologists, the more useless I think they are and the less respect I have for them as medical professionals—and as human beings, they are beneath contempt. They're just pushing high-priced poison and selling false hope—like they did to my sister. Those scumbag oncologists robbed her of nearly seven hundred fifty thousand dollars in chemo treatments that they knew had no chance of helping her and they were literally doing more treatments on her almost to the day she died and, as I later found out, it was the ruptured esophagus causing her to bleed to death, NOT THE CANCER that killed her. They are beneath contempt are is the ones I saw, like Dr. Francisco Xynos, who told me I'd die vomiting feces if I didn't take his horrendously overpriced poison—a choice I do NOT regret even if I die. If it really comes down to it and I am going to die, I will wait until it starts getting painful and I will check into hospice in Florida (everyone I know and am related to lives in Florida) and die there in a Demerol-induced coma.

Life without the things I love would be meaningless to me and I wouldn't do it. I am not about to spend the last few months of my life as a bald, puking, starving, miserable sack of bones in a Florida hospice with my friends and family having to watch me slowly die a little bit at a time. My husband needs me and my mother-in-law has Alzheimer's and I take care of her because I will never put someone I love in a nursing home, and she needs me, so I can't die right now, it's just not an option, I have to much I have to get done. I do political consulting and it's killing me to be in

MASS MURDERING DOCTORS: THE TRUTH ABOUT ONCOLOGISTS, CHEMOTHERAPY AND CANCER

bed sick during the BEST and most exciting election of my lifetime and I'm MISSING IT! ARRGH!!! I've told my husband that if I am on life support he's not to pull the plug until after midnight on November 8th 2016 so my vote for Trump via absentee ballot will count, it's the last thing I can do for the America I love so much and the utterly corrupt government that I despise with every fiber in my being and if America goes down I won't live to see it. If the cancer doesn't kill me, the memory of America and seeing her demise certainly will so please vote Trump—or I hope you did!

This is, however, the worst possible scenario with this recurrence as there's no way to treat this cancer again with surgery or chemotherapy (which I won't have) other than the intra-peritoneal chemo which I consider certifiable insanity. This essentially means that my chances of survival with "conventional medicine" are zero. My chances of survival if I do nothing are also zero. I have a recurrence of the deadliest, most aggressive, most malignant cancer that there is and it kills 95% of the women who contract it within 12 months; the rest in less than 2 years, and when you are BRCA1+ you are genetically programmed to get this cancer—and the fact that I am a lifetime baby powder user doesn't help either because THAT could have caused my cancer as well. My sister had 3 risks of ovarian cancer, she took Clomid which is widely believed to cause ovarian cancer, she was also a life-long baby powder user in addition to being BRCA1+ but I never took Clomid but I have the "childless" risk factor. I am also a life-long baby powder user, so I don't know if it was the BRCA1 defect or the baby powder but it doesn't matter now. All that matters now is that I have to find a way to survive an unsurvivable cancer and I'll be just fine as a frog hair and live out my life with my beloved husband and watch the grands grow up and have kids of their own. These are the thoughts racing through my head while I try to get a grip on myself and I realize Dr. Janet is talking to me but I can't hear her because I can't hear anything over the screaming in my head.

Meanwhile, Back at the Doctor's Office

I don't know know what to think—I'm so freaked out my hands are shaking. My second surgery with a gyno/onco 3 weeks after the surgery (that revealed the sub-clinical cancer), called a "staging surgery" showed NO spread, 30 crystal clear lymph nodes, no cancer, no NOTHING! The tissue samples were all clean and the pelvic wash had less than 20 "atypical" NOT cancerous cells. I had a 100% resection of the tumor. **THEY SAID THEY GOT IT ALL and it didn't f**king matter.** I refused

MASS MURDERING DOCTORS: THE TRUTH ABOUT ONCOLOGISTS, CHEMOTHERAPY AND CANCER

chemo because I wasn't about to destroy my immune system and all the other stuff that comes with chemo; including leukemia, painful neuropathy in my hands and feet and worst of all, my sense of taste would be gone, and I have been a chef my whole life. I went to Le Cordon Bleu in Tokyo and owned a restaurant—and grew up in them, so that alone would destroy my quality of life. Last, it won't help me. I believe the immunotherapy is my best chance for survival and since I didn't blow out my immune system with the useless poison they call chemo, there's every reason to think this might work. Fully 40% of the women with this cancer are BRCA1+ or 2+ it is how we die and no amount of chemo or radiation or surgery will stop it. I've been studying and researching this cancer for hours every day, 7 days a week since the day I found out I had cancer and my sister died November 18th 2015. My parents are nearly crazy with worry and I had considered not telling them to spare them the suffering and just tell them at the end since I live 1500 miles away, but my husband said they had the right to know and so did all my friends. I still wasn't going to tell them but my husband said if I didn't he would. He had to call them to tell them it was terminal though, I couldn't do it. Right now sitting in Dr. Janet's office, all I can hear is the roaring in my head and that the walls in the office are closing in on me and I can't even BREATHE.

I have to do something but right now all I feel is the horrible panicked gasping for air and I want to talk to my husband and I am certain that if I stay one more second in the office the walls will crush me and I have to get out of there before I start screaming. I babbled something to my doctor and ran out the door to my car where I read the MRI report again with the paper rattling in my shaking hands. I'm scared to death and I have to get enough of a grip to call my husband which I do and he says he's leaving work and wants to talk to Dr. Janet. I go home and put on a brave face for my Mother-in-Law who is suffering from Alzheimer's disease and is in the mid-stage where her memory issues are painfully obvious and I've been looking after her for 2 years in Baton Rouge, Louisiana but brought her up to Illinois with me for the original surgeries. My husband gets home and we go to lunch at the Rail Shake and talk about what we are going to do and I had already made contact First Immune in Europe and they had shipped me 10 vials of GcMAF/Goleic. I've done a lot of research on immunotherapy. I believe it is what will cure most diseases; which I've believed for years, and I am convinced that it is the way of the future.

MASS MURDERING DOCTORS: THE TRUTH ABOUT ONCOLOGISTS, CHEMOTHERAPY AND CANCER

Immunotherapy is just starting to be "tested" because Big Pharma has to come up with a synthetic way or version that they can patent. Original GcMAF/Goleic is a natural human product that CANNOT BE PATENTED under FDA rules so they can't make any money from it until the scumbags find a way to patent it so they can rape the consumer. With any luck, Trump will win the election and put an end to the corruption in DC. I sure can dream, can't I? LOL I love America-and I owe her so much—but again—another story for another day.

My husband and I have a very emotional lunch, complete with beers and tears. This is his worst nightmare and I am responsible for it and I feel so bad. He's such a GOOD guy and he can't buy a break right now. He lost his dad, (my late father-in-law, who was a sure-by-God American hero) to small cell lung cancer in 2011 (11-11-11) and his mother's Alzheimer's disease presented shortly thereafter and I had to move to Baton Rouge in 2013 to look after her but now she is in Illinois with us while I battle this cancer.

We talk and he is nervous about the immunotherapy, since it's a human product and he has concerns he voices but we decide that those concerns don't enter into it now since I literally have nothing left to lose. If it doesn't work I won't have lost anything as I am essentially a dead woman walking. I had the GcMAF/Goleic at home in the refrigerator so we went back to Dr. Janet's office and spoke with her briefly about a treatment plan and she is on board and believes in immunotherapy and GOD LOVE HER she is willing to see that I get what I need prescription-wise to make this work.

We raced home from the doctor's office and pulled a bottle of GcMAF/Goleic out of the refrigerator, drew it up in a syringe and stuck it like a life-long junkie. I've just played my hand face up on the table. Now it's up to my nagalase-paralyzed immune system and macrophages to kill the cancer that came to kill me. If they do, I should make it all the way back, but the GcMAF/Goleic is not cheap, but what is your life worth? The people at the immunocentre will help you with a protocol and they have 4 clinics in Europe where you can get inpatient treatment for the cancer and they have a huge success rate and by all accounts I have a decent chance to live through this. I'm scared. Not of dying, we all die, but of the unknown. I can't bear to think about my beloved husband growing old all alone, or worse: getting Alzheimer's and I won't be there to look after him-or my dad having to bury yet another of his children in less than a year since he buried the younger daughter and had to bury a grandchild in

MASS MURDERING DOCTORS: THE TRUTH ABOUT ONCOLOGISTS, CHEMOTHERAPY AND CANCER

March of 2015 and a child 6 months later and possibly a second daughter in less than two years. He's 86 years old with a birthday in October and I don't want to put him through this but I have NO choice. In about 10 days or my next MRI I'll know if I have a chance to make it. If the immunotherapy thing I am doing works, I will be fine —and-it works FAST—according to the clinic people I should expect a 25% to 40% tumor shrinkage the first week and I am going to try to get another MRI within the next week – if Dr. Janet can't get my insurance to pay for it then I will go down to St Louis and pay cash at the "commercial" MRI place where they have a radiologist there and s/he will tell me right then and reads it right there at the time of the study and if there is the shrinking of the cancers that I hope and pray and sort of expect that there will be results either way as this is a very fast growing and aggressive cancer. My chances were never good, this cancer kills 98% in less than 5 years. I begged my sister to try this – as you know she died of this same cancer 90 days before I was diagnosed. I can't let my dad bury another daughter this year—it will kill him. He's 86 years old and Lori's death rocked him hard—harder than even the death of my nephew, his grandson in March of 2015. I don't know if he will survive this so I mobilize my friends and ask them to visit my dad and just talk to him and tell him I'm going to be fine. I need to go down to Florida and let him lay eyes on me so he can see I'm OK and hang out with him and talk for a few days so he will know I am not in any danger of dying soon and that the immunotherapy is working which I am fervently hoping it is—and I think it may be.

CHAPTER 19: YOU CAME TO KILL ME CANCER? REALLY?? LET'S ROCK!

It's game time. 2nd and 15 at the 35 yard line, down by 4 with less than a minute left on the clock. This crap just got extremely real. I have terminal cancer of the most aggressive most virulent and most deadly kind in high-grade serous carcinoma that has metastasized in my pelvis and this b*tch came to KILL me. It's f**king ON. I know what I got—let's see what that b*tch brought to this battle. I'm not done yet. I am following the treatment protocol to the letter. Paleo diet, no sugar, no wheat and no rice and a ten to twenty thousand IU dose of Vitamin D3 and I have to sit in the sun for 15-30 minutes a day. There are no side effects for the patient with immunotherapy, but it's devastating for cancer-and that is fine as frog hair with me!

MASS MURDERING DOCTORS: THE TRUTH ABOUT ONCOLOGISTS, CHEMOTHERAPY AND CANCER

I've just finished my first week on immunotherapy and I have 2 days till the next round starts. Good news: I FEEL GREAT!! I haven't felt this good in a year! I take that as a very good sign! I'm going to try to get to Chicago and finish things up with my clients (I'm a consultant) the week after next. I'm having another MRI next Saturday even if I have to pay for it out of pocket—there's an MRI in St Louis which is cash on the table, no Doctor's order needed, no bullcrap, no prescription. I can get one for $300-$500 cash if my insurance company balks at paying for it and if it shows the tumors shrinking, then I know I'm on the right track and if not, I will revisit the idea of chemo. The only way I might consider the chemo is for the possibility it offers that my Dad won't have had to bury a daughter in consecutive years—and he's just distraught. I'm the golden child to him—Lori was my mother's golden child, and while he loved her too, she wasn't the kid who spent years putting his dinner on the table every night and never had the bond with her that he does with me.

If chemotherapy buys me the time I need to bury my dad then I might do it. Mom is going to have to rely on my youngest sibling, my brother Keith.

I did the Rick Simpson protocol with the Cannabis oil that I started right after my surgery, and when my 3 month MRI was crystal clear, I was hopeful (as was my husband) that the surgery and RSO had done the trick and that we had caught the cancer in the nick of time. My treatment plan was close monitoring with an MRI every 3 months for 18 months since this very aggressive, virulent and highly malignant cancer recurs in 6 to 18 months with or without chemo so I didn't see the point in destroying my immune system with chemo since I thought I would need it down the road! I've been holding my breath and on Tuesday July 12th 2016 my worst fears materialized when the MRI came back with peritoneal tumors and the terminal diagnosis of peritoneal carcinomatosis which is essentially Stage III-B which is the midnight train to the Big Adios because while my tumors are very small, they are untouchable with any kind of conventional medicine. I am sure the immunotherapy is the way to go, and if it doesn't work then it's my time to die. I'm glad Dr. Janet is on board and is co-ordinating my care and making sure I get the tests and things I need that my insurance DOES pay for because they will not pay for the GcMAF/Goleic. I've got to have Dr. Janet to order up my MRIs and such and I need her to be my advocate and since she's not on my insurance; I pay her cash out of pocket as well. This is advantageous because the insurance company can't really say no to anything,

MASS MURDERING DOCTORS: THE TRUTH ABOUT ONCOLOGISTS, CHEMOTHERAPY AND CANCER

and they can't dispute her judgment or orders because they don't have the legal right to see her records since they aren't PAYING HER—I am. She works for me, not them. We talk, and I explain how GcMAF/Goleic works and she's good with it because she believes in immunotherapy as well so it wasn't a hard sell and I am very grateful for that! We all hug and leave and my husband is not convinced or sold on this immunotherapy but as he said, I've got NOTHING to lose, since I am on the midnight train to the big Adios and it's a one way ticket if this doesn't work. I'm scared. I draw a bath and cry in the bathroom so John doesn't see it, and I decide that if I have to cry again, then I will set a timer for 5 minutes and when it goes off I will have to stop. I have to be strong for John and Mama G. I have seen some changes in my body from the immunotherapy, or at least I think they are. First—I feel GREAT and I mean GREAT. I haven't felt this good in over a year, which, as close as I can figure is about when the cancer started. Second, my skin is noticeably smoother and softer rather that dry and itchy and a bit flaky. Third, an unhealed blister that I got two weeks ago and one I got the day before I started the shots are now both completely healed but the second one healed WAY faster—almost a week faster. My age-related gingivitis has cleared up as well. Another thing I noticed is that I've stopped losing weight—I didn't lose an ounce this week. I've dropped 30 pounds without any dieting or exercise and no matter how much I ate, I kept losing weight. I've dropped those 30 pounds since Memorial day weekend and today is July 17th 2016; so with my weight stabilizing I'm sure it's another good sign. I blew a vein with a bad IV stick and the horrible bruise I usually get was NOWHERE to be see. My appetite is back with a vengeance! Last and most interesting, the little basal cell Carcinoma on my upper lip I've been trying to get rid of for 5 years IS GONE—and I mean GONE. Individually these things don't mean much; but together they tell me something is going on and I believe in immunotherapy and I am so delighted that Dr. Janet also think it's the way of the future and is working with me. If it works I will make a 100% recovery and it will never come back—or if it does I just take some more shots and ramp up the macrophages. I'm scared but cautiously optimistic—and this stuff works FAST. In their clinics in Europe, they report that the tumors shrink an average of 25-40% a week—but that's with them injecting the GcMAF/Goleic directly into the tumor to get that kind of shrinkage—and when they are gone, you keep taking the shots for 8 more weeks after your nagalase level drops below .65 to seal the deal.

MASS MURDERING DOCTORS: THE TRUTH ABOUT ONCOLOGISTS, CHEMOTHERAPY AND CANCER

The more undifferentiated a cancer cell is, the easier it is for GcMAF/Goleic-activated macrophages to find it. High-grade serous-cell carcinoma is as undifferentiated as you can get, so I hope they kick some cancer ASS. I'm hopeful and I'm still feeling great which is excellent news since the cancer may also be in my spine according to the MRI. My whole life is in turmoil. I'm living with a death sentence in a few months because of a defective gene. February 12th 2016 I was living the dream. Six days later it became a nightmare I can't wake from. I'm scared—not of dying, but of the great unknown—what happens after the light? I've been in the light, but I didn't cross over to the other side, so all I know is the light. Will I find my sister and the rest of the family that has passed on? Will we know each other? Every religion has a difference of opinion on the subject, so I'm going with the Mormons on this one and assume I will find my family and be reunited with them, so I'm cool with that.

I'm following the immunotherapy protocol to the letter because I desperately want to live. My husband who watches me when I am writing this book said to me: "Please don't make me be the one to write the last chapter of your book" and I thought I would die right there with the poignancy of his request. I SO do NOT want to leave him alone in the world but I am unspeakably grateful that he supports my decision not to have chemotherapy. My poor sister's asshole ex wouldn't even consider anything but chemo and radiation because they are "medically proven" and "FDA approved" which is total bullcrap with the 2.1% cure rate. I've never met such an ignorant ass in my life and his crappy doctors killed my sister—however, my 18 year-old orphaned niece is going to be set for life after she sues the crap out of these doctors for malpractice and wrongful death. I'm waiting on approval for my next MRI and I am eager to see it since I am certain it will show progress. Dr. Janet ordered my study and now it is up to the insurance company to approve the MRI and as soon as I have it done, I will be able to see if I am going to survive this or not. If the tumors are shrinking, then in all likelihood I'll be OK and will be delighted to autograph your copy of this book!

CHAPTER 20: THE WAITING REALLY IS THE HARDEST PART

I've started my 3rd week on the GcMAF/Goleic and I still feel absolutely GREAT. My body feels like a fine tuned machine humming away, I swear my arthritis in my hands is not as painful as it was 2 weeks ago. John seems to think it's the placebo effect, but I know what I feel. I have the energy of a teenager—I got on the elliptical machine and did 15 minutes—and I didn't even pass out and I haven't used it since March. I wasn't winded and I feel even better now, so I think I might start using it again. It can't hurt and the immunocentre people said exercise is good for the immune-strengthening. GcMAF/Goleic wakes up 5 of the 6 components of your immune system in TEN MINUTES but it takes 3 weeks to get the 6th component to rev back up to full strength, so I should be there in 4 days. If this stuff is working, it is a miracle indeed. Everything I find and everything I've researched tells me that this cancer in my belly is going to kill me, but the way I feel and the things that are happening are giving me hope that I may just skate out of this and if I do, I am going to make sure the world knows that this is the cure! Perhaps this is my mission—to put an end to the suffering and death caused by cancer and perpetuated by **Big Pharma lies: "We're working on a cure every day" (but I have to toss the "bullcrap" flag on that one)** and oncologists marking up the poison the administer to desperate people by 5000% and pocketing the difference. I teased Dr. Janet and told her that if this worked we should start our own clinic! Stick everyone with GcMAF/Goleic on schedule and use the profits to defray the cost of treating those who can't afford it and blow the whistle on the American Cancer Society (Where's that TRILLION dollars we donated for the cure? Where's our cure??) and the Big Pharma lobbyists and the long list of politicians who took the bribes to control the FDA to let them market their POISON and tell us it was a cure—I'm going to blow the lid off of Cancer, Incorporated. I have no doubt they will come after me—I'd be taking 200 billion a year—EVERY YEAR—of their profits. The Merchants of Death won't like it, and there's a lot of evidence this will cure many things other than cancer. The list is long but it proves what I have believed ALL MY LIFE: Immunology is the key to ending all diseases known to man. I want the next MRI as soon as I can get it because this is a fast-growing very aggressive cancer and if the tumors are shrinking then I know we are on the right track and that I'm going to be OK and not die at 57. I just do NOT believe I can feel this good and die.

CHAPTER 21: WILL I LIVE OR WILL I DIE? ONLY THE MRI KNOWS...

MASS MURDERING DOCTORS: THE TRUTH ABOUT ONCOLOGISTS, CHEMOTHERAPY AND CANCER

I've been on the immunotherapy juice (GcMAF/Goleic) for 3 weeks and I feel better all the time. It's a pretty easy protocol actually, you take your injection of GcMAF/Goleic in the morning, 10-20,000 IUs of Vitamin D3 and 15-20 minutes of sunlight every day and some exercise along with a sugar-free and carbohydrate free diet which is fine with me as I rarely eat carbohydrate-laden foods anyway. When I am cured, there will be more chocolate cake in the world for me to eat, not like there's a flour and cocoa shortage!

I am eager to see the results of the MRI because I am sure the will be good; so the sooner the better as far as I am concerned—but at the same time I am afraid to look at the report in case it's bad and I really AM going to die. However, the little signs I've been seeing are very common among the immunocentre patients and they tell me it is a sign that the GcMAF/Goleic is working. Once again, I need a cleaner MRI so that I can breathe, and so that John can sleep.

My doc got my MRI approved so I will have it sometime this week hopefully and if the tumors are shrinking then I am going to beat this and from what the people at the immunotherapy place tell me, I will never have a recurrence because my immune system will be "trained" to fight this cancer, so that would be awesome. I would also be a survivor of peritoneal carcinomatosis with High-Grade Serous Carcinoma which is a 100% fatal which would certainly give both my book and the people who make the immunotherapy juice a ton of credibility.

The name ovarian cancer is a misnomer. There are 4 different kinds of cancer that start in the ovaries and three of them ARE survivable but not this one because it is so very virulent and aggressive. It's actually more correctly identified as High-Grade Serous Cell Carcinoma of the Pelvis. I had the cancer in both ovaries and in my uterus. In the uterus it's call Serous Cell Papillary Carcinoma, and when you have hysterectomy, as well as salpingo/oophorectomy, commonly referred to as an RRSO or Risk Reducing salpingo/oophorectomy, since they take EVERYTHING-tubes, ovaries, uterus, cervix-everything goes. Now, after you have this preventative surgery, you can still get High-Grade Serous Cell Carcinoma of the Pelvis which is then called Primary Peritoneal Carcinoma—but it's the same cancer. I know it's confusing but hang with me! Now, the TERMINAL condition of **all of these** when it metastasizes or

MASS MURDERING DOCTORS: THE TRUTH ABOUT ONCOLOGISTS, CHEMOTHERAPY AND CANCER

RECURS (my case) is called Peritoneal Carcinomatosis and it is invariably fatal/terminal and fast because this is a highly malignant, aggressive and deadly cancer, the Genghis Khan of cancers. The REASON I am terminal is because there's NO way to treat Peritoneal Carcinomatosis. You can't get it with IV chemo, and you cannot surgically remove the peritoneum. Radiation is not possible because the damage to the intestines would be unsurvivable. So, while my tumors are small or were 4 weeks age, they double in size every 6 weeks; which means they grow exponentially and fast so any recurrence of the high-grade serous cell carcinoma is untreatable and kills you within about 6 months. Clear Cell Carcinoma is a survivable ovarian cancer, so is Low-grade Serous carcinoma and stromal cell carcinoma, but HGSC is the BRCA1/2 as 71% of the cases are BRCA1/2because this the cancer that kills us—every time. There are no known survivors of peritoneal carcinomatosis, it is invariably fatal. This is my current reality—unless the immunotherapy GcMAF/Goleic works, I will die somewhere around December 2016—although I want to live to see Trump inaugurated.

I am still waiting for the insurance company to approve my pelvic MRI that was incorrectly ordered so I got approval for the abdominal MRI but not the pelvic MRI which is where my cancer (hopefully now smaller) is trying to kill me. GcMAF/Goleic and how it can eradicate the cancer and save your life. The science behind it it rock solid and you can research it on the internet but try not to be distressed by the BigPharma lies and smears! My insurance is a disaster thanks to that incompetent usurper Obama and his "reforms" that halved my care and DOUBLED my premiums and tripled my deductibles. It stops being a mere nagging expensive annoyance when your life is hanging in the balance.

Big MRI tomorrow. I am alternating between freaked out, batcrap crazy and scared to death. This is not a game any more—I think it must be what waiting to be sentenced is like—in a death penalty case. John is freaked out and my mother-in-law has been in the hospital for 9 days with the doctors refusing to listen to me until I insisted on all of them meeting with me and told them what I thought would be the best course of action for what is essentially MY patient, and that they needed to listen to me because what they were doing was going to kill her and soon! She was in severe pain so we rushed her to the ER where a CT scan revealed a perforated ulcer and severe peritonitis and she went from ER to OR (once again!) and then they medicated her on what they thought was the cat's posterior and ISN'T and she was babbling and screaming incoherently all the time so they tossed in ATIVAN to chill her out and she was even more incoherent and yesterday I told them flat out NO MORE Ativan and NO MORE Dilaudid (which works like SPEED on me) and to leave her fentanyl patch ON and if she needed a rescue dose, then a fentanyl push but NOTHING else. They thought that because she has Alzheimer's that she babbled incoherently all day at home. I told them NO!! She is continent, self bathes, self toilets, makes her own toast for breakfast every day, walks out to the end of the driveway every day for her newspaper and watches the critters in my private zoo wander through my yard-in and out of the woods and the wide variety of birds that eat at the feeders we have and never misses Jeopardy or Wheel of Fortune and they looked shocked! She hasn't known me or John since last Monday-and last night she still didn't. This morning when I went to the hospital she called me by name-and I just broke down and cried. Then I called John and told him Mom was going to make it-we had been talking about hospice last night trying to figure what to do if she didn't snap out of it-we thought she might have had a CVA we didn't know about. It's been a bad 10 days and tomorrow's MRI tells the story. I'm a head case right now.

CHAPTER 22 THE FIGHT FOR THE MRI AND THE AMAZING DR. JANET

It has been a nightmare getting this MRI approved. My insurance company, dumber than DIRT, but massively more expensive (Thanks Obama—you lying sack of crap) decided that I had no medical need for a pelvic MRI for a pelvis documented to be full of cancer, but approved an abdominal MRI which is pretty much the same place, but has no cancer. I can't wait to get another approval because if I need surgery to take out the big tumor I have to do it soon. I decide to go to the hospital where I am known and have friends. I brought a copy of the MRI report from the other hospital and quietly explained to the tech (who is a doll!) what I need and why and she's on board and she has a word with the radiologist who doesn't care, he gets paid by the hospital. They billed for an abdominal MRI that we pushed down to my pelvis. I am relieved that it wasn't a big hassle to fudge the insurance billing because in a worst case, we can always say it was the "Lower Abdomen". Anyway, I eat a handful of

MASS MURDERING DOCTORS: THE TRUTH ABOUT ONCOLOGISTS, CHEMOTHERAPY AND CANCER

Vicodin so that I can lay on that hard board for the next two hours without moving, and blindfolded with earplugs and headphones, she rolls me into the tube. It's with and without contrast so she started an IV as well to inject the dye later. The banging and whirring of the magnets starts and I try to relax and let the nice narcotic painkillers help me to drift off and lightly doze. I am rolled out for my dye injection and rolled back in for another half hour and focus on not moving. I listen to a few songs on the radio (through the headphones) and a news broadcast and the MRI ends. Then when I ask for some information they tell me they want my films from the last MRI so I set a new land speed record blazing to get the films and hand deliver them to the radiology department and tell him all I want to know is bigger, smaller or the same. The rest can wait—but that's what I desperately need to know. They tell me he will be there until 5 so I tell them I will be back and I go up to see my mother-in-law in her room and do some things for her. Frantic and stressed I do my best to focus on Mama G and try not to watch the clock. Finally at 4:40 pm I give up on waiting for the call and go back down to Radiology and am told the miserable bastard left at 430 when he was supposed to be there until 5 and they don't have the report but it looks like it's been done and has to go to my doctor's office. I could just scream I'm so frustrated and upset at having to wait another day so I go to dinner with my husband and drink 3 beers to settle my nerves—the first drink I've had since I found out I was terminal on July 12th when we had lunch and drank a few beers. I was so stressed and distraught but I did feel a lot better after the beers—no wonder people become alcoholics when life overwhelms them. John has to go to Louisiana tomorrow to do some things for mom so I tell him I'll call him and he says he'll stay if I need him but the hard day was finding out I was going to die soon, not the day I might find out I will be OK. Dr. Janet's office calls me to tell me they don't have the report so I drive over to the hospital and find out the radiologist won't be in until tomorrow which is Friday and if he doesn't get the report done then it will be a long and stressful weekend. My sister Sarah is furious that he did this and God help him she's a terror and one of the few people in the world that I would NOT want to have angry at me. She's brilliant and will not take crap from anyone—or let anyone she loves be abused and she is enraged because she knows how stressed I am. Several more close friends and family call to express support and concern, but there's nothing to do but wait. I will go back tomorrow and try and get the report again. I'm stressed and shattered but there's nothing to do but wait. I will deal with the radiologist down the road with a crappy review on the rate-your-doc websites and on Yelp but he works for the hospital so I can't really affect his practice—his paycheck depends on the hospital, not private patients, so he may be beyond my reach professionally. I'm upset and stressed but not particularly worried so I go upstairs to my mother-in-law's room to hang with her for a while to try and keep the hospital from killing her.

CHAPTER 23: A FUNNY THING HAPPENED ON THE WAY TO MY CURE

Finally I get the report late Friday afternoon and it is TERRIBLE news. My original tumor has markedly increased in size and I now have a SECOND one and the big one is now seeding my peritoneal cavity with cancer cells so I am in BIG f**king trouble. I discover to my horror that the pain medication I MUST have to live (for 21 years) is interfering with my GcMAF/Goleic and I have to change medications to what they recommend or I will die—and very soon. It made for a miserable pain-filled weekend as it's difficult to titrate a dosage from 2 different painkillers that work in distinctly separate ways. Dr. Janet prescribes the highest med dosage buprenorphine patches that come 4 to a box and are supposed to last for seven days. I had ripped off my Duragesic patches the second I read the report, and put on one of Butrans patches and six hours later I'm in too much pain to breathe. I add a second patch and swallow a handful of Vicodin (also forbidden) just so I can get to sleep and Sunday morning I am suffering but hesitant to add a third patch but I have to do it and so I am wearing 3 patches for a 60 mcg an hour dose of buprenorphine that isn't NEARLY as good as the 125 mcg and hour of Duragesic (fentanyl) and I can't take anything but aspirin as a rescue dose, so I'm going to have to suck up the pain for the duration of the immunotherapy because at least pain reminds me I'm alive and fighting to stay that way and I'm going to get my back fixed when this is over—assuming I do not die from the cancer than kills everyone. I have to get these 2 big tumors sliced out ASAP and since I am so desperate I call the lowdown scumbag Xynos' office and they inform me that their first available appointment is in OCTOBER. I will be DEAD by then so I called Dr. Katruna Murray at the women's oncology center www.womensonc.com and they got me in on Monday the 22nd of August and I am certain I will have surgery

MASS MURDERING DOCTORS: THE TRUTH ABOUT ONCOLOGISTS, CHEMOTHERAPY AND CANCER

within a week of seeing her. Interestingly, the smaller scattered tumors did not progress AT ALL and there are NO NEW ONES and my doctors are baffled that there aren't since the biggest tumor has been spraying cancer cells for five weeks. Dr. Xynos' office called me back 2 days later, but by then I already had the appointment with Dr. Murray so I blew them off—if they couldn't get back to a terminally ill woman on the same day, then God forbid I should have a problem after surgery—plus I loathe the SLU medical mill system. This is considered to be the MOST aggressive cancer known—high-grade serous cell carcinoma. There are NO known survivors of this kind of cancer so I have passed scared and I'm now terrified but I believe in GcMAF/Goleic because the science is solid. I am certain that chemotherapy will kill me and I would rather die than let them pump me full of POISON! Buprenorphine is not the painkiller that fentanyl is by a long shot! I've also discovered the fentanyl was masking, to a large degree, the severity of some of my other orthopedic issues. My love of horses and being an equestrienne in my youth means I've been thrown countless times, bitten, kicked, slammed into solid objects and having a horse fall twice with me aboard which could have been fatal—and I thought it was fun. If I knew then what I know now, I'd have gotten another hamster instead. After 5 back surgeries, I had kind of resigned myself to just living with it. **Last year I found out my surgeon (Paul B. Mitchell, MD Norfolk, VA) lied to me and covered up that he put an implant filled with bone growth paste in my spine (totally contraindicated for me) which is what caused my fusion to overgrow so horribly.** He never asked/told me he was going to do this because I would have told him not to and when it started overgrowing he told me it was forming a false joint but still never told me TO THIS DAY that he put bone growth crap in there. However, I know now why it over grew and that means it's fixable and I am going to look into it, assuming the cancer doesn't kill me—then I get the joy of narcotic withdrawal after 20+ years which ought to be at LEAST as much fun as chemo. The way things are going, I'm not sure how this is going to end and I'm pretty scared all the time—like a mild panic attack that never goes away. You KNOW if I'm gladly complying with very strict dietary rules AND giving up my highly effective yummy Fentanyl painkiller patches for the crap that is Buprenorphine and being in way more MAJOR pain, then you KNOW someone put the fear of GOD into me!! I had to buy a pair of jeans in a

MASS MURDERING DOCTORS: THE TRUTH ABOUT ONCOLOGISTS, CHEMOTHERAPY AND CANCER

size SIX, I was wearing 10s in July. My 10s and 8s are getting looser and I SWEAR I do nothing but eat!! Every time you look at me I'm chewing. Normally I would be under the impression that if I were constantly eating and LOSING 3-4 POUNDS A WEEK, that I would have ALREADY died and gone to heaven. However, the first-hand certain knowledge that 60 mcg/hr of Buprenorphine isn't jack crap compared to 125 mcg/hr of fentanyl which is 100 x stronger than morphine, tells me I have not left this mortal coil as of yet. I hear from the First Immune people and they tell me medical marijuana is OK to take as it doesn't interfere with the GcMAF/Goleic so between the buprenophine and the medical Mary Jane I don't care that my insurance company, (Blue Cross/Anthem and ExpressScripts on the FEDERAL EMPLOYEES GROUP PLAN) DENIED ME—A DOCUMENTED TERMINAL CANCER PATIENT—medicine to control cancer pain. I'm seriously considering tweeting out the denial and putting it on Facebook to let the insurance company have a taste of social media wrath—how does an insurance company DENY pain medication to a documented dying woman? How do they sleep at night? I finally decide to pay $89 for 14 pills because I am in such pain. I hate Anthem Blue Cross of Missouri for being dicks NOW when they've been good with me for years. Of course I am seeing a doctor whom they swore was on my plan and isn't and so I pay cash to see Dr. Janet but it also means she doesn't report to Blue Cross because they don't pay her—I do. She's been more than generous with her time with me and I try not to drive her crazy. I do not understand why they would make a pill for sublingual administration that is so horribly bitter and nasty tasting?? I tried to use it SubL and it was so NASTY that after 5 minutes I washed it down with tea and it gagged me and I had to swallow it mixed with the vomit that came up with it. I know, gross. I'm sorry to be disgusting but I can't have any other kind of pain killer and I will probably be having surgery next week, so I will need it. I'd be delighted to let the makers taste the horrible bitter pills that they expect me to hold under my tongue for 20 minutes. I start to gag in about 1 minute from them. I am SHOCKED that they would make a sublingual med that tastes this bad—but of course the real use is for junkies so I guess they make it taste bad to punish them just a little bit more. I am fully cognizant that after 20 years PLUS on fentanyl that I have a huge physical dependence but I am NOT an addict. I never take more than I need or more often that prescribed and I've never had to ask Dr. Janet to refill a prescription early in 10 years. I just want to make medical history by not dying!!!

Every doctor I've been to in the last 25 years, **other than Dr. Janet**, treats me like a scumbag street junkie. I can't tell you how humiliating that is—and because I usually need to see them for medical reasons unrelated to my severe pain issues I have to put up with their BS and the terrible way they treat me—like I'm a scumbag because I'm in pain. I've had them call me a junkie, a drug whore, doctor-shopper, addict and worse. I can't even really get John to understand the difference between addiction and physical dependence, as much as he loves me and as smart as he is. Addiction is a state of mind when you panic and freak out and are willing to do anything to get your fix. Physical dependence is what the drug has done to my body after all these years-and if I didn't have pain like this I would NEVER even take an aspirin. Chronic pain sufferers are the 21st century lepers and the patients no one wants. Now let's add an incurable cancer into the mix and see how that shakes out. The Fentanyl patches have allowed me to have a fairly comfortable life with no addictive behavior, as there is no way to abuse them for a quick buzz but they give me good round-the-clock pain management and I never get a high—just peel one off and put another one on and keep right on going. I asked Dr. Trejo to give me the patches back in 1990-something because I was having to take pills all the time and I'd get a wicked whack of narcotic and then it would wear off leaving me searching for my pills in a panic because I was in such pain. He started me on a high dose of oxycontin which was better that the Percodan because it was a 12 hour pill but I hate pills anyway so when the patch came out I asked for it. The change was remarkable. I never panic any more. NO med spike ever—no "buzz" to learn to LOVE and NO addictive behavior like panicking when I couldn't find my pills or the stress of being in pain for a period of time because it was too soon for another pill. I would force myself to wait until it was time for the next dose even if I was crying in pain because I knew-I KNOW-that the first step on the slippery slope of addiction is to take more of a med than I am prescribed and I have a terrible fear of being addicted which is why I am so very very careful to take meds EXACTLY as directed by my doctors. I use one doctor and one pharmacy so that I keep everything above board.

MASS MURDERING DOCTORS: THE TRUTH ABOUT ONCOLOGISTS, CHEMOTHERAPY AND CANCER

CHAPTER 24: MEETING DR. MURRAY AND POTENTIAL SURGERY #3

Dr. Karuna Murray is a first-rate money grubbing Big Pharma whore. She coerced me into signing financial responsibility by saying that she wouldn't see me unless I did. I am pulling a complaint with Blue Cross Anthem Missouri about that. With a definite diagnosed HGSC she still felt it would be necessary to do a biopsy and that I would have to have chemo as well and a PET scan that my insurance won't pay for. I thanked her for her time and John and I got up and left. The problem is that the standard of care is chemo, surgery, more chemo and then death while the oncologist (and let us not forget the HUGE profits they get on the drugs they buy and RE-SELL to the patient at a huge markup) gets rich by poisoning me. No thanks Dr. Murray—but if you want to die, she's the doctor for you. Chemo is her thing and she didn't even want to hear about the immunotherapy so she's a bad doctor in addition to being a bad person. I don't know if I am going to be able to get a doctor to remove these two tumors, as it will apparently violate the current idea of standard of care to NOT kill me with poison, which then may leave them open to a charge of medical malpractice and in these litigious times she isn't going to deviate from what she learned in medical school and is pushing the 39-year old chemo treatment with the 2.1% success rate and the $50,000.00 in her pocket for each unsuccessful treatment as she turns me from healthy and vibrant to bald, vomiting and dying. f**k her and her cisplatin and carboplatin taxane flavored POISON. I'll stick with GcMAF/Goleic and if I die, then it is my time to go. If I make it, then I am going to devote my life to ending the routine poisoning of cancer patients by the doctors who are trying to kill them for large amounts of money and the thirty THOUSAND dollar markup on the chemo drugs they buy and re-sell to desperate dying people. The Big Pharma whores and supporters are unable to synthesize GcMAF/Goleic so they want to keep it off of the market because they want to keep selling and administering poison to the patients who don't know how to stop them from doing this, or don't know they have a choice for a REAL cure. However, Dr. Murray violated the standard of care in a lot of ways with her greed and I tried filing a medical malpractice action against her since she insisted upon a treatment that is held by virtually all oncologists as useless in the treatment of peritoneal carcinomatosis. Sadly, she got away with attempting to kill me under the myth that useless chemo is the ONLY (and most profitable by far) is the only mantra

MASS MURDERING DOCTORS: THE TRUTH ABOUT ONCOLOGISTS, CHEMOTHERAPY AND CANCER

of big Pharma. For her to insist on a useless therapy that puts hundreds of thousands of dollars in her pocket is nothing but unmitigated greed. Wanting a biopsy (to make sure it's cancer when she's already telling me I have to have chemo) is nothing but bill padding. I handed her an MRI that's 10 days old and she wants another one ($1000 out of pocket) and a PET scan that my insurance won't pay for is, again, just bill padding and I am sure that the treatment center (conveniently next door) is going to be the place I would be sent and she forced me to sign for financial responsibility which she is not allowed to do under the contract with Blue Cross. I am looking for a lawyer for this since she tried to force me to have chemo that is contraindicated for my cancer since it can't help me but is a million-dollar bill for my insurance company. Additionally, it would keep me out of ANY drug trials for immunotherapy because it would destroy my immune system and won't help me, so the f**king greedy whore signed my death warrant if the GcMAF/Goleic can't overcome the tumors DOCTOR Murray wouldn't remover without my agreeing to chemo. If the b*tch didn't have an M.D. after her name, injecting me with POISON like what is in chemotherapy would be considered ATTEMPTED MURDER and she'd be arrested. The best I could do was file a complaint with the Missouri state medical board and leave factual reviews on every doctor rating site I could find—and her ratings are abysmal. She's a terrible doctor and a worse human being and she's pushing 40 year old poison because she's so totally out of touch that she has no clue about cutting edge oncology. Go somewhere else—unless you're in the mood to die suffering horribly. She's only interested in selling you ancient poison at a 100 grand a pop—90K or more of which goes right in her pocket on drug markups. Her survival rate for cancer has to be abysmal, it wouldn't surprise me to find out she also owns a funeral home—it would be a natural accouterment to her non-existent medical prowess and what must certainly be an abysmally low survival rate. If you want to die, she's definitely the doctor you need to see—dying a little bit every day while being poisoned by this miserable b*tch while she pretends what she's doing isn't legalized murder. I heard back from the Medical Board of Missouri. Apparently they will take up to a year to investigate my complaint, but I will according to the doctors, be dead in six months, so I am going to tweet out a picture of their idiotic reply about taking a year with a reason they should expedite the investigation on my complaint. Thanks Missouri State Board of Medicine—

apparently it doesn't occur to you that someone with a deadly cancer probably won't be around in a year—thank God my husband was in the room as a witness and that I taped the entire appointment—I tape ALL my doctor appointments and if you have a serious disease you should too. I use and recommend an app called "Voice Record Pro" it's free and it's GREAT. It's absurd that it takes THAT LONG to investigate a doctor and I find myself questioning if the delay is because there are SO MANY complaints about Missouri doctors (oh dear GOD!!) or because they just don't give a crap about complaining patients. Neither answer gives me any reassurance and it's unlikely I will find out what happens.

CHAPTER 25: OK GcMAF/Goleic/GOLEIC SHOW ME WHAT YOU'VE GOT!

I am following the GcMAF/Goleic protocol to the letter for the past 12 days. First Immune had some shipping issues so my order is a week late and I'm OUT of the immunojuice (GcMAF/Goleic) and I'm panicking because my order is being held in customs and I end up being told I have to pay $32 in taxes and duties and my GcMAF/Goleic that is supposed to be kept cool has been in the hot warehouse all week so I am worried sick that it won't work—and I've gone a week without it. I'm going to see if I can get a little bit put back in case of shipping issues in the future. Hopefully I will get it tomorrow and UPS is the worst international shipper there is— they are TERRIBLE. A 4 am Monday call to UPS does nothing and I am still without my desperately needed GcMAF/Goleic and I am still in a stressed out tiz over all of this. The biotech company is not responsible for this, it's an FDA/government bullcrap delay but the GcMAF/Goleic must be kept cold and has now been in a hot warehouse for over a week. I've been out of it over a week, so I am totally flipping out since it's the only thing standing between me and the midnight train to the Big Adios, and my piece of crap Obamacare-compliant insurance company Blue Cross/Anthem federal employees HMO servicer called Express Scripts has STILL not approved my pain meds —but it's only been two weeks since my doctor prescribed it so what's the rush? Let the dying cancer patient suffer—we have our rules and regulations. Thanks Obama— you lying sack of crap! I have an appointment with the doctor in the clinical trial for immunotherapy at the University of Miami Sylvester Cancer Center, Dr. Brian Slomowitz. They made a special spot for me because I pointed out to the doctor that

MASS MURDERING DOCTORS: THE TRUTH ABOUT ONCOLOGISTS, CHEMOTHERAPY AND CANCER

if his immunotherapy cured me-and it would have a MUCH BETTER chance of doing so because my immune system hasn't been demolished by chemo—that his project would conceivably become a FIRST-LINE treatment replacing chemo rather than the final resort that it is now—because Big Pharma doesn't want to give up chemo profits which are 200 to 300 billion a year—EVERY year!! If immunotherapy patients live longer but have a recurrence—they keep them alive with MORE $$$$$ Chemo and more profit. HOWEVER with me, a cure (or LONG remission) makes his treatment very attractive first-line options—and immunotherapy has none of the miserable side effects of chemo which would make it WAY more popular than chemo. I'll go to Florida to see Dr. Slomowitz with the Miami University cancer center immunotherapy trial and that's the one I WANT to get into and I WILL. He's smart and he wants me in his trial BADLY because he and I have had a meeting of the minds—here's how bad he wants me in his trial: 8 minutes after I emailed him an inquiry about getting into his trial, HE CALLED ME ON THE PHONE at 6:30 am to talk to me. SOP is the patient is sent on a records hunt and has to fill out a bunch of forms. They CALLED ME and took all my information over the PHONE-unheard of-and they let me email them DIRECTLY with the PDF of my records which is MORE than adequate for them to document I am a BRCA1+ and I do have peritoneal carcinomatosis and that my sister was the same and died from the same high-grade serous carcinoma I had. I am super stoked about this immunotherapy trial but as it turns out, it wasn't what I thought it would be. The trial in Houston and Chicago told me I'd have to have had chemo to qualify. I got out in front of this by pointing out to Dr. Slomowitz that because I have NOT been chemo-ed my immune system was fully operational which in theory AND REALISTICALLY gives his trial a much better chance of success which could turn it into a FRONT-LINE medication/procedure rather than the last resort. The profit difference would be staggering-which I also pointed out to him. Doctors are crapty businessmen, but a hard science gal like me with an understanding of how he can profit massively by saving my life to show him the way to Jesus and the promised land of great wealth. I build BEAUTIFUL castles in the sky and people cannot wait to move into them. Also, I don't know that the Euro-juice isn't working although the issues with getting it have caused a very stressful week. They ship in a metal thermos-which can look like a pipe bomb to Customs-and it comes from FRANCE where they have had so many terror issues lately so I told them the foil pack was a better idea-it came right to me-and so did last month in the metal Thermos but it is STILL in a warehouse in Philly under review and has been for a week, so they MUST think it's dangerous or I would have it by now.

Unfortunately, they have NOW decided that they cannot ship to the USA at this time and there's no telling when/if they will ever be able to ship again to the USA so we had to have it shipped to a UPS depot in Windsor, Canada and John (who has a valid passport, mine expired in 2008 and I didn't bother to get another one) is going to have to go across the border to pick it up and disguise it as insulin so that he can smuggle it into the USA. I'm trapped in a Dallas Buyer's Club scenario when all I really want to do is cure my cancer—and that totally corrupt piece of crap Barack Obama has put so many stops along the way for what should be MY choice that it's just unbelievable. I'm so stressed and scared over all of this, but I am desperately trying to pull it together. I am also starting the RSO oil again, I packed 30 capsules with 90% THC containing Crown Royal cannabis that I have from earlier in the year. I bought a lot of it figuring it would go up in price as I've seen it bringing $100 a gram on dispensary websites so I stocked up since I didn't know about GcMAF/Goleic at the time and since I can't GET my GcMAF/Goleic, and I may not get into the trial if I am upfront about not doing chemo, I may have to pretend that I am willing to do chemo when there are NO circumstances under which I would ever consider chemo. I'm doing a rice-grain size dose of RSO 4 times a day—every 6 hours to build up my tolerance. The First Immune people said that a lot of their patients used medical marijuana, so maybe it helps the GcMAF/Goleic to work? I see no reason not to use it as well at this point. I have NOTHING to lose, I am going to die soon if it doesn't work. I am flat out in a total panic, my husband is going to have to drive 1000 plus miles and risk getting arrested to try and help me and I'm laying on a heating pad in my bed, more freaked out than I have EVER been since this whole thing started. I'm doing a decent job with getting my head around that I'm going to die young but I am not looking forward to it—and my husband and family are frantic that I should not die because of the family trust situation that is terrifying them as my death leaves my brother as the sole heir which cuts them out of the money forever as they think Keith isn't going to take care of anyone but Keith. I'm freaked out that there is not a problem with the UPS delivery in Canada since they now are waiting for a POWER OF ATTORNEY which I am hoping and praying will be handled by the time John has to leave for Canada and I am so terrified I can barely breathe. I'm going to die without the immuno-juice so I am going to have to round up all of my marriage licenses again and get my passport renewed in case I have to go to France to get the vials that are the only thing that I think may help me. I'm beyond frightened at this point. My husband is willing to risk his job and freedom to try and save my life and I don't know If I can handle it if something goes wrong. I am so freaked out that the idiots at the FDA are interfering in something that is none of their business and now I'm about to have issues in Canada! The BEST part of this is that it came right through Louisville which is a 3 hour drive which would have been way more convenient. I'll be picking up 2 marriage licenses copies in GA and one in Martin county and another in Palm Beach country to get my passport renewed in case I need to go to Europe. I'll have to borrow some money from my dad as I hate to ask my husband and I've spent through my retirement and he will need his to live out his lifespan and if he develops Alzheimer's he will need every penny he has and then some in all likelihood. What a mess—but I am hoping that if they can slice out these tumors soon in Miami then I will buy some time to get to France for more immuno-juice and my stepmother has relatives in Germany so I could rent a room from them for a month or six to give the immuno-juice time to work. However, I have received word that the GcMAF/Goleic is safe at the UPS depot in Canada, and John will be going there tomorrow to get it and I am wound up beyond words—and Sarah is going with him—so I have 2 of the 3 most important people in the world to me risking a lot to save my life—on a treatment that hasn't worked yet and I am scared—really scared. If it wasn't for the RSO I'd be in a screaming little ball all day and all night. My hands are shaking, it's hard to type when I am this stressed out and worried. I'm going to get my passport renewed so that if there's another trip to be made to Canada, I can do it, not John! He left this morning with Sarah to smuggle my "unapproved" GcMAF/Goleic into the USA since the FDA can't stop protecting Big Pharma's profits as their leash holders demand since they are bought and paid for by the bribes—uh—CAMPAIGN DONATIONS to Congress and the Senate. Our government is beyond corrupt and Trump is our only hope— although I may be dead before that happens as conventional doctors have written me off as terminal. John calls and tells me he is back in the USA with my GcMAF/Goleic and I get an email from Immuno-Biotech that they think they have their shipping issues resolved and hopefully another trip to Canada won't be needed. I'm back on schedule with my GcMAF/Goleic and I am vaping and eating RSO as well to try and manage the tremendous back pain that changing medications has caused and since it doesn't interfere with the GcMAF/Goleic I am getting some pain relief although I am pretty bashed from my husband hitting an idiot who pulled out in front of us in a truck last night and then taking off—and my husband CHASED HIM DOWN and CAUGHT HIM in the bashed Prius! The headaches of dealing with a possibly totaled car and body shop and rental car and cancer and Mama Gloria with Alzheimer's and my own parents in their 80s and other family drama is an absolute NIGHTMARE. I'm on my way to Miami to talk to Dr. Slomowitz about his immunotherapy trial. I'm not opposed to double dipping—this is my LIFE!

CHAPTER 26: WELCOME TO MIAMI UNIVERSITY CANCER LIES CENTER

I'm here in Miami at the UM Sylvester cancer center explaining to idiots why their immunotherapy is not successful and showing them how to triple their funding and then get rich with a slightly different protocol. I'm a VERY valuable lab rat, they may NEVER get another one like me. I am BRCA1+ I have an EXTREMELY rare cancer and the kicker: I have NOT had any form of chemotherapy. This means (as I explained to the doctors—I'm the owner of a MENSA card and a hard science education) that they are doing their protocol INCORRECTLY. They are trying an immunotherapy protocol on women who have had their ENTIRE IMMUNE SYSTEM DESTROYED BY CHEMO and wonder WHY it's not a roaring success. Here's a clue idiots: You don't do immunotherapy AFTER chemo destroys the immune system—you do it BEFORE chemo! Immunotherapy should be a front-line treatment and it isn't BECAUSE THE PROFIT CANCER, Inc. generates is 200 billion A YEAR—EVERY YEAR—and they can kiss it goodbye with a cure they are determined to suppress. Also, don't forget that our friendly oncologists are allowed to sell patients the drugs directly for the chemo "cocktail" and they pay 5K and resell it for 100K and pocket the difference. THINK about that one: **Oncologists are allowed to sell patients the drugs directly for the chemo "cocktail" and they pay 5K and resell it for 100K and pocket the**

MASS MURDERING DOCTORS: THE TRUTH ABOUT ONCOLOGISTS, CHEMOTHERAPY AND CANCER

difference. Why else would they push a 40-year-old "treatment" with a 2.1% "cure" rate? Every "round" of chemo puts 75-100K in the oncologist's pocket—why else would they tell you the bullcrap about how they have to 'shrink' the tumors before removing them. How could it POSSIBLY matter WHAT size the tumor is? It's CANCER so you cut all of it out—no matter what the size. You don't see them trying to shrink NON-CANCEROUS tumors now do you? No. They just slice them out—even when they weigh 20-plus POUNDS. If the tumor shrinkage is so important, why is it ONLY the MALIGNANT tumors that are deemed important to "shrink" before removal and ENORMOUS benign tumors are removed as is? I'll tell you why: YOU CAN'T SELL A MILLION DOLLARS WORTH OF POISON CHEMO TO SOMEONE WHO ISN'T TERRIFIED OF DYING OF CANCER!! How does it matter if it's bigger? It's not like shrinking it by POISONING the poor victim for a hundred grand in their pocket changes the tissue to NON-CANCEROUS and they LEAVE IT BEHIND—it's just to make money. That's why that miserable b*tch Dr. Murray tried to force me to have chemo to "shrink" the tumors—which is bullcrap—all it does is poison me so she can drop 100-500K in her pocket. Greedy Big Pharma whore in love with chemo—as evidenced by all the scrawny, pale, bald, puking and dying women in her office both of them—but at 50K or more per infusion, you don't need more that 5 patients a month to make a bunch of money. What kind of SCUM of the Earth DOES THIS and still has the BALLS to pretend to be a healer? However, Dr. Murray is definitely the role model for window wenches worldwide because in addition to being a greedy piece of crap, she's a miserable b*tch. She learned HER bedside manner from Josef Mengele School of Medicine and was without a doubt a STAR pupil and honors graduate!

SIDEBAR: MY REFUSAL OF CHEMO AT MIAMI UNIVERSITY CANCER CENTER

Here is the letter I wrote to Brian Slomowitz who lied to me to lure me to Florida with the promise of an immunotherapy trial and tried to rope-a-dope me into NINE ROUNDS of chemo—when the limit is supposed to be six rounds. He said it would be low dose to of course "shrink the tumor". I have the entire appointment on tape naturally, I tape all my appointments.

Dear Dr. Slomowitz:

I like you, so I'm going to be straight up and direct with you.

MASS MURDERING DOCTORS: THE TRUTH ABOUT ONCOLOGISTS, CHEMOTHERAPY AND CANCER

I have a couple of questions:

Please tell me what you know about high-grade serous carcinoma that over 100,000 of your colleagues do not know?

Could you explain how it is that the exact same carboplatin/cisplatin with taxanes cures your patients when EVERYONE else's HGSC patients—on the entire planet—die from it?

I am writing a book about BRCA1 and HGSC **(the one you are reading)** and have done extensive research—and have written nearly 200 pages of sourced information about it. I've studied HGSC 5-8 hours a day 6-7 days a week since February 19, 2016 and have read over 1000 clinical studies of HGSC and over 100 studies of the efficacy of platinum-based chemo on HGSC and ALL of them died with the progression-free survival (PFS) averaging less than a year. None lived more than 22 months after initial diagnosis at stage III-IV. I never worked in oncology and this is one of two cancers I have studied, but I know a LOT about it—way more than 5 of the 6 oncologists I have seen. I have been to 17 physicians and 6 oncologists. Each and every one of non-oncologists has told me that IV chemotherapy cannot and will not help me, but every oncologist has tried to force me to have it with two of them asking me to leave their office when I asked them what was their markup on the resale of the chemo drugs that they buy for 5K and ALL of them giving me the "shrink first" lies. Additionally, I have read over 100 studies that tell me that IV chemotherapy cannot help me. It is not because I am some big holistic medicine fan that I am refusing chemo. I am not. I am a firm believer in better living through pharmaceuticals and always have been. I personally believe that holistic medicine is bullcrap. However chemo does nothing for me except make me suffer, puts $50-$100,000 for each resale of the chemo cocktail drugs in your pocket, and I still die in January-ish 2017. I'm not interested in "time" for the sake of time—I am interested in a CURE which will ONLY come through immunotherapy. There are European immunotherapy trials as well and I can afford to go there and will seek an immunotherapy trial overseas if it comes down to it, and I am renewing my passport in Miami on Monday. I went back and re-read the parameters of the immunotherapy trial. They clearly state that I cannot participate in the trial if my current tumors have been treated with chemotherapy. I can see no

MASS MURDERING DOCTORS: THE TRUTH ABOUT ONCOLOGISTS, CHEMOTHERAPY AND CANCER

medical reason to chemo them before removal, reaping the profit on the markup of the chemo drugs isn't a medical justification. Benign tumors weighing POUNDS are removed without "shrinking them" which I am sure is due to the fact that people without cancer can't be terrorized into allowing themselves to be voluntarily poisoned. The FDA may have been bribed into approving any drug that shrinks a tumor for 28 days to be an effective cancer treatment, but you and I both know that doesn't mean JACK toward a cure. I'm not signing up for ANCIENT 39-year old chemotherapy. Where's the TRILLION dollars of research money that joke of a charity ACS conned out of the public? Why is an almost 40 year old treatment the BEST you've got? Especially since the survival rate is 2.1% overall and ZERO percent for HGSC? There are NO KNOWN SURVIVORS of what I have. NONE. There are four kinds of ovarian cancer—three of them are survivable—but HGSC which is 74% of all OVCA cases (of which 48% are BRCA1/2+) is not survivable when there's a recurrence, and peritoneal carcinomatosis is "always fatal complication of ovarian and all other abdominal cancers" in which EVERY SINGLE PAPER AND STUDY I HAVE READ concurs that I am going to die and that IV chemo cannot help me. When the tumors progress to where they are problematic, I'm sure that going to some ER far from home screaming in pain will result in an a CT and then immediate trip to the OR where they will nip out the tumors causing the bowel obstruction because they won't know what they are until they are biopsied (and I'll be long discharged and out the door by the time that happens) as my records are not on the electronic portal and they never will be, I have refused to use it or to allow my records to go on it, and I'll deny any cancer history and tell them I had a hysterectomy a few years ago—they have no way of knowing it's not true. In the urgency of the moment, they will operate and then try to send me for chemo yet again. I can game the system just as well as a welfare scumbag if I have to do so, but I didn't want it to come to that. If you don't want the surgery money, then I'll go back to Illinois and wait until it's bothersome and let some ER surgeons handle it down the road, makes no difference to me who slices me open. After over 30 surgeries in my life, I view surgery like most people view having their teeth cleaned at the dentist's office—not fun, but no big deal.

If you'd like the fee for removing the tumors and you can get my insurance to approve it, I'm fine with you doing the surgery and banging BCBS/Anthem for the fee, but there's NOT going to be any chemo. I think they paid the original gyno $6500. It was about 45 minutes on the table and I'm sure they will pay about the same to you for nipping out the tumors. Your call. I know you pretended you wanted to help me and it's not a holistic medicine love/belief that stops me from accepting your help. It is the certain knowledge that you cannot do anything for me except cause my hair to fall out, damage my kidneys, heart, lungs, liver and make me puke until my teeth fall out. That is not how I want to spend the potential last few months of my life. I'm not having chemo. EVER. I'd rather die. My family and I have discussed this and they are totally supportive. If you are not interested in nipping out the tumors I'll seek care elsewhere, and all the best to you. I'm not afraid to die—and I've already been given the Last Rites 3 times so I've been on borrowed time for a LONG time. We all die—it's just a question of the state of your health up to the end. 9 weeks is potentially the rest of my life and I'm not spending them bald, puking, sick and miserable with a totally demolished immune system WANTING to die—that's just not going to happen. I want a cure, not a remission. I want my LIFE at 100 mph with my hair on fire which is the way I've lived my entire life—not some miserable sick existence. Nothing else is acceptable. If I die, so be it—but I'm dying on MY terms, and the only platinum ANYTHING that is getting near me is shiny metal set with E-F VVS diamonds, not injected into my veins by a Haz-Mat gowned nurse.

Very Truly Yours,

Nothing from nothing, If the nurse has to be specially protected from this crap, then there's NO WAY IN HELL I will allow anyone to inject it into my veins. NO WAY!!

CHAPTER 27 IT'S NOW JUST UP TO ME, GcMAF/Goleic AND GOD

Since I am in Florida and will not be getting chemo from the scumbag con artists at Miami University Hospital, I am spending the week with my family. I'm staying at my Dad's house and seeing the friends and family I haven't seen in almost a year since my sister died and her dear friend Geri, who is also very dear to me, took her death very hard and I have been terribly worried about her so I have spent time with her while I was here. She was also kind enough to give me my GcMAF/Goleic injections intravenously which means they are even MORE potent than when I give them subcutaneously. I tried to stick it IV myself but I blew the vein twice because the fine

MASS MURDERING DOCTORS: THE TRUTH ABOUT ONCOLOGISTS, CHEMOTHERAPY AND CANCER

motor skills in my hands are gone. However, the very best way to take this is intravenously as it passes through the spleen and activates more macrophages and getting my immuno-juice 3 days in a row (she's going to stick me tomorrow before I leave) is going to be a big boost to killing off these pesky tumors!

I have given up on doctors other than Dr. Janet who I will be seeing next week. I could have another MRI but I'm going to wait for a while. I don't think John would be able to take another study without seeing any improvements, I think it would kill him. He's under tremendous stress with his mother's Alzheimer's and my terminal cancer and I don't want him to stress any further. I have no symptoms whatsoever. No bloating, no swollen lymph nodes and no weight loss. I feel fine—great in fact—other than my insurance company keeps refusing to approve my pain medications and I am in terrible pain with my back. I find it ironic that they paid for my 30 fentanyl patches and 90 Vicoprofen every month but won't pay for 12 buprenophine patches and 90 buprenophine tablets which are HALF THE COST OF WHAT THEY USED TO PAY FOR!! Unbelievable!! I am banging them hard on social media and when I get back to Illinois I am going to sodomize them in the media for this—I put the refusal of medication up on Twitter with the caption "what kind of insurance company denies pain medicine to a dying cancer patient?" Blue Cross Blue Shield Anthem Federal Employees HMO denies pain medication to me EVERY TIME I HAVE A NEW PRESCRIPTION FOR IT. Thanks Obama—you lying sack of crap.

However, it's now just me and God with the GcMAF/Goleic being the only thing standing between me and the midnight train to the big Adios. The "doctors" that refused to surgically remove my tumors and tried to force me to have chemotherapy THAT CANNOT HELP ME are:

Dr. Brian Slomowitz, MD University of Miami Sylvester Cancer Center, Miami, Florida. He tried to force me to have 9 rounds of chemo and then lied to me about getting me in an immunotherapy trial. He tried to make me do what he called "low dose chemo" which makes absolutely no sense at all, why would you bother with a lower dose of poison that wouldn't do anything but kill healthy cells? He promised me the immunotherapy to get me to come to Florida from Illinois when I told him on the phone that there was NO WAY I would ever do chemo before I drove 1500 miles to

MASS MURDERING DOCTORS: THE TRUTH ABOUT ONCOLOGISTS, CHEMOTHERAPY AND CANCER

see the lying sack of crap. He's just another greedy scumbag oncologist that wants to make a few hundred grand by poisoning me with something that has NO chance of helping. He also wanted to prescribe oral chemo (Oleparib) which I'm not going to take either. I have the entire appointment on tape as Florida is a single consent to recording state, and he clearly coerces me to do chemo.

Dr. Karuna Murray, MD Women's Oncology Center, St. Louis Missouri. This miserable b*tch is in a class ALL BY HERSELF. I have never met such a C**T in my entire life. She was the only doctor who was able to see me in a few days—which tells you she's a terrible doctor, there was a 2 month wait to see a GOOD oncologist like Dr. Xynos and 3 days to see her. Her ratings on WebMD and the other doctor rating sites are terrible. I taped the entire appointment again (Missouri also being a single consent state) and she is the most miserable b*tch on the planet. She not only wanted to chemo me for profit, she wanted a BIOPSY of an already-documented cancer, insisted on a PET scan at the facility conveniently located in the same building (and possibly owned by her as well—illegal in Florida but maybe not in Missouri) and is so incompetent she couldn't even feel the tumors during the pelvic—however they still needed to be "shrunk down" before surgical removal. I filed an official complaint with the Missouri State Board of Medicine for this first class Big Pharma whore. She doesn't deserve to have a license to practice medicine—she's not a healer, she's a greedy quack poisoning people for fun and profit without regard to anything but how much money she can make. She's the first doctor I have ever filed a formal complaint about in my life, but at the rate this is going, she may not be the last. I don't like her and I don't trust her.

Dr. Francisco Xynos, M.D. St. Louis University Oncology St.Louis, Missouri

Dr. Xynos tried to force me to have chemo after telling me I had a 100% removal of the cancer. When I refused, he told me (on a taped recording as well) that I would die "vomiting feces". Charming. When I had the recurrence in August and called to set up surgery, his office told me his first appointment was in October. I told them I was a patient with a recurrence and they said they'd call me back that day. They never called until two days later when I already had the appointment with Dr. Murray. I liked Dr. Xynos but he's 71 years old and while he's an excellent surgeon, he's in

MASS MURDERING DOCTORS: THE TRUTH ABOUT ONCOLOGISTS, CHEMOTHERAPY AND CANCER

love with chemo and has the WORST BREATH of anyone I've ever met. Get your teeth cleaned and buy some mouthwash or STAND BACK about 3 feet!! I've already described the horrible medical mill that he works in and for that reason alone I wouldn't go back to him, so just as well his office staff sucks.

It's not just physician greed nor Big Pharma profiteering, it's something much more ghastly that keeps cancer from being cured. Health systems worldwide are underfunded. Health systems can't afford a cancer cure. For the good of insolvent retirement and health trust funds and life insurance companies the elderly must die on time. That is the hidden determinant that blocks adoption of any cancer cure, and the reason is because they have been robbing all of us BLIND and if we don't die on time, they are in deep crap because they DO NOT HAVE THE MONEY TO PAY ALL THEIR OBLIGATIONS to pensions, insurance and Social Security. In an article entitled "Chemotherapy: Snake-Oil Remedy?" that appeared in The Los Angeles Times of January 9, 1987, Dr. Martin F. Shapiro explained that while "some oncologists inform their patients of the lack of evidence that treatments work...others may well be misled by scientific papers that express unwarranted optimism about chemotherapy. Still others respond to an economic incentive. Physicians can earn much more money running active chemotherapy practices than they can providing solace and relief...to dying patients and their families."

The failure of chemotherapy to control cancer has become apparent even to the oncology establishment. Scientific American featured a recent cover story entitled: "The War on Cancer — It's Being Lost." In it, eminent epidemiologist John C. Bailar III, MD, PhD, Chairman of the Department of Epidemiology and Biostatistics at McGill University cited the relentless increase in cancer deaths in the face of growing use of toxic chemotherapy. He concluded that scientists must look in new directions if they are ever to make progress against this unremitting killer.

Adding its voice, the prestigious British medical journal The Lancet, decrying the failure of conventional therapy to stop the rise in breast cancer deaths, noted the discrepancy between public perception and reality. "If one were to believe all the media hype, the triumphalism of the [medical] profession in published research, and the almost weekly miracle breakthroughs trumpeted by the cancer charities, one might be surprised that women are dying at all from this cancer" it observed. Noting that conventional therapies—chemotherapy, radiation and surgery—had been pushed to their limits with dismal results, the editorial called on researchers to "challenge dogma and redirect research efforts along more fruitful lines."

John Cairns, professor of microbiology at Harvard University, published a devastating 1985 critique in Scientific American. "Aside from certain rare cancers, it is not possible to detect any sudden changes in the death rates for any of the major cancers that could be credited to chemotherapy. Whether any of the common cancers can be cured by chemotherapy has yet to be established."

In fact, chemotherapy is curative in very few cancers — testicular, Hodgkin's, choriocarcinoma, childhood leukemia. In most common solid tumors — lung, colon, breast, etc. — chemotherapy is NOT curative.

SIDEBAR: WHY HAS GcMAF/Goleic NOT BECOME THE MAINSTREAM CURE?

Why has GcMAF/Goleic gone unnoticed? ----- Dr. Tim Smith

"It's kind of a language problem: if someone shouts "Cancer Cure!!! Cancer Cure!!! Cancer Cure!!!" in Swahili, it is quite possible that earth-shattering-ness of it all won't get through, and everyone will go on about their business as if nothing happened." To a stodgy medical community that's resistant to change, GcMAF/Goleic is just another "unproved therapy." And an "alternative" one at that. Unproved therapies are not to be trusted. (Even if they're harmless and bio-identical.) "Proving" this discovery the conventional way would involve developing and promoting a lucrative drug. Doing that takes about a decade and costs over 100 million dollars. Beyond time and money, it requires a lot of biochemical know-how and some sophisticated equipment. Brewing it up in your basement lab with a chemistry set and a bunch of buddies is not an option. However, a motivated pharmaceutical company could do it overnight! (Note: They did: First Immune Biotech and you can visit it at: GcMAF/Goleic.se which is their website and they have the cure available for purchase and 4 clinics to visit.) Big Pharma isn't interested because there's no cash cow at the end of this rainbow. GcMAF/Goleic—like all chemicals our body is programmed to make—can't be patented because it fits the FDA's definition of "natural" (translation: can't get a patent). We are thus confronted with the supreme pickle: is it possible to conduct open-minded, nonprofit driven research in an era of corporate and politicized medical science? I yearn for the olden days when science was done for the sake of science. It wasn't that long ago. **The cancer industry does not really want cancer to go away. This may seem harsh, but it's true.** Many incomes would be interrupted if cancer and HIV suddenly ceased to exist. Government agencies would have to be closed, oncologists would have to be retrained, researchers redirected, cancer treatment centers shut down or converted to screening and prevention facilities—and that's just the tip of the iceberg. We're talking profound social upheaval here. Cancer is entrenched, profitable and institutionalized, and vanquishing it would cause major fireworks. These fears are largely unfounded, however. For optimum effectiveness, GcMAF/Goleic and Nagalase testing will need to be integrated into the existing cancer care system, so we need the system.

To understand GcMAF/Goleic and Nagalase we must embrace an entirely new model— a completely different approach to cancer and chronic viral infections. There is no super drug, no magic bullet. Our bodies already know how to cure cancer and viral infections; we simply need to enhance these systems using natural medicines. That's how GcMAF/Goleic works. The scientific community, however, is deeply resistant to the idea of natural medicines bolstering the immune system.

If we are going to commit to stopping these epidemics our new direction must be annual screening (with Nagalase or AMAS testing) for early detection, then nipping cancer in the bud with GcMAF/Goleic. The old "wait until its gotten so big we can see it on imaging and then slash, poison and burn" approach has got to go".------Dr. Tim Smith.

CHAPTER 27: THE WAITING IS THE HARDEST PART...

I am continuing with the GcMAF/Goleic injections as there is nothing else I can do. I'm going to have to smuggle it back in from Canada again as the goddam FDA grabbed it again even with a different shipper. It's a thousand mile round trip every 4 weeks but since we are talking about my LIFE and not seeing any other alternative I'm sticking with the program and have a brand new passport so I can go to Canada. I've also named my cancer—I've named it Obama so I can REALLY hate it. I am still completely asymptomatic—no belly pain, no bloating, no ascites, no swollen lymph

MASS MURDERING DOCTORS: THE TRUTH ABOUT ONCOLOGISTS, CHEMOTHERAPY AND CANCER

nodes. ALL of these are good things, and I should be presenting symptoms by now—particularly considering how aggressive this cancer is. That I am not; means the immuno-juice (GcMAF/Goleic) is working. I'm in a lot of pain from my botched back surgery—which is another book all by itself. Buprenorphine STILL isn't the pain med fentanyl is but I'm getting by. My amazing husband got me an awesome chair cushion/pad with firm memory foam and it sure helps pad my now-bony rump. I'm not losing weight from the cachexia, but I am on a super low-carb diet that I am practically religious about maintaining (and recommended by First Immune) to give the immuno-juice the best possible chance of success since I can't get any of these greedy bastard oncologists to remove my cancer because they want to make a quick half million by poisoning me first—and I can't seem to get a general surgeon to do it, so I guess if it comes down to it I'll go with my ER plan for removal. ER surgeons like to cut and get paid to cut and in an emergency they will do it because they will NOT know they are malignant which precludes any of the greedy gyno-oncologists from deigning to remove them. John has mastered giving me my GcMAF/Goleic IV and I am feeling great! Since it's a naturally produced substance in your body, there are NO side effects. No hair loss, nausea, anemia, liver, kidney, heart or brain damage either! I feel better than I have in years and everyone in Florida told me I look great and can't even believe I have cancer. I tell them—it's not the CANCER that makes you sick, it's the chemotherapy that kills you!

SIDEBAR: FOR OBAMACARE FANS WHO WANT SINGLE PAYER:

By the way, for those of you who are fans of single-payer, here is the situation in England: In the UK the National Health Service is billions of dollars in debt. Hospitals there have resorted to withdrawing drinking water from bedridden patients, which is the perfect way to cull this patient population, as it leaves no fingerprints. According to one news report, 12,000 are "killed" annually in British hospitals due to dehydration. Elderly patients report they have averted dehydration by drinking water from flower vases. A more horrific report delivered to the Royal Society of Medicine in London by a leading professor of medicine claims 130,000 patients annually in the National Health Service system have been placed on a "death pathway" instead of a "care pathway." [Daily Mail UK] No one gives a crap about the cancer patient other

MASS MURDERING DOCTORS: THE TRUTH ABOUT ONCOLOGISTS, CHEMOTHERAPY AND CANCER

than the oncologists who are only interested in poisoning for profit since their chemo poison has such an abysmally low success rate. We are expendable and represent a dollar profit UNMATCHED in any other kind of medicine—after all, it's hard to get people to agree to pay a million bucks to be poisoned unless they are told they'll die without it—but they conveniently forget to mention that 50% of patients DIE from the chemo poison LONG BEFORE the cancer would have killed them had they done nothing.

The FDA dickheads grabbed my GcMAF/Goleic because it's "unapproved" and therefore much too dangerous (total bullcrap) BECAUSE the corrupt FDA doesn't do anything that might affect the profits of BigPharma. A harmless substance that cures cancer isn't allowed, but highly INEFFECTIVE POISON chemotherapy is just fine and dandy and come on down! We all have to die on time because the totally corrupt governments worldwide have robbed us BLIND and stolen our money and borrowed ANOTHER 20 TRILLION for us to PAY BACK for their thievery. Trump is the ONLY chance America has and by the time you are reading this, hopefully he will have been elected. If Hillary Clinton is elected, America is finished. She needs to go to jail for what she did, not the Oval Office. Just my two cents. I'm in a "Dallas Buyers Club" situation, so perhaps you can figure out from here the issues of GETTING the GcMAF/Goleic. I have to go to Canada with my husband every month to pick up my monthly supply of GcMAF/Goleic because of the FDA morons. No wonder people hate government.

CHAPTER 28: DR. JANET VISIT OCTOBER 12, 2016

I had an appointment with Dr. Janet who is a phenomenal doctor and the ONLY doctor I will EVER trust. We discussed my care plan and will be doing a MRI in a month or so and if it looks like the GcMAF/Goleic isn't working then I will stop taking it and put my Duragesic patches back on and finish putting my affairs in order. I've started to do a little of that as only a fool would not be doing this in my situation—and I am no fool. I believe the GcMAF/Goleic will work but since I have no definitive PROOF that it is working (YET) I am nervous and unfortunately I do not have the luxury of not being able to put off doing this. The GOOD news is that Dr. Janet did an exam of my belly, mashing firmly, and there's no fluid and there's no pain, so she was

MASS MURDERING DOCTORS: THE TRUTH ABOUT ONCOLOGISTS, CHEMOTHERAPY AND CANCER

surprised that I am not presenting symptoms but pleasantly so although she has to write something on my chart to justify the pain meds we have had to fight Blue Cross Anthem Federal Employees Insurance HMO tooth and nail (actually ExpressScrips—the WORST SERVICE EVER) just to get PAIN MEDS that are HALF the cost of the Duragesic patches and 90 Vicoprofen that they paid for every month like clockwork. Assholes all of them—what kind of insurance company denies pain medication to a woman that is officially listed as dying for an agonizingly painful cancer? Anyway, Dr. Janet must be pretty confident that I'm doing OK because she told me I didn't have to come back for 3 months so I must be doing pretty OK. I feel GREAT and if I didn't know I had cancer, I would NEVER know I had cancer. The RSO (Rick Simpson Oil/Medical Marijuana) in a vaporizer does a very good job helping the pain that the buprenophine doesn't touch and I sleep on a heating pad; so between the medical marijuana and the heating pad, chair pad, hot baths and just in general sucking it up and living with the back pain, I'm getting by. I hope it's worth it—although I did point out to my husband that no matter how much my back hurts it can't be as bad as chemotherapy. Nothing is as bad as chemotherapy—a slow miserable death being slowly poisoned by your DOCTOR. Keep in mind that if anyone other than your doctor injected you with the SAME CHEMO poison, it would be attempted murder—something to think about when you are signing up to be voluntarily poisoned. Anyway, I'm doing fine for the moment and I don't think I'm going to die in January—at least not THIS January. The November MRI tells the story though—if the tumors have not reduced then I will die in March or so and this book will have been a pointless effort to spread the word of a cure that didn't work for me!

CHAPTER 29: CANADA AYE? ROAD TRIP AND INTERNATIONAL SMUGGLING

At 2 am John and I leave for Canada and we get to the border about 1130 am. Since the FDA snatched 2 of my GcMAF/Goleic shipments, John is worried I might be on a watch list and be stopped and searched. We agree we cannot take the risk and he ditches me at a Cracker Barrel about 20 miles from the border. I go in and sit down and decide to try and eat something. My server, Lea, was super nice and I tipped her massively for taking up a table for her entire lunch service, but they weren't really that busy, so I sipped my iced tea and ate my bacon and eggs and tried not to have a

MASS MURDERING DOCTORS: THE TRUTH ABOUT ONCOLOGISTS, CHEMOTHERAPY AND CANCER

nervous breakdown while my amazing husband risked his career, future, income and possibly arrest with future imprisonment to smuggle the GcMAF/Goleic over the border to try and save my life. I pray to God he will just get back safely. After what seems like an eternity, he calls and tells me he's safely over the bridge and the UPS store manager was good enough to put the GcMAF/Goleic in the refrigerator which means that we don't have to RACE to get there before it goes bad because it must be kept cool, so next time we can go on a Saturday and John won't have to take the day off from work and we can spend the night and come home on Sunday which means we won't have to do 1000 miles in the car in a day. It's a grueling trip and we start for home. We get home at 8:30 pm, exhausted but having to make sure Mom is OK and get her night medications and get her put to bed. Her Alzheimer's has progressed markedly in the last 3 years and it's wearing on John. I have to get her out of here and back to Baton Rouge to give John a break but I don't want to leave him. He's coming unglued from the stress at home and we had an argument—so rare in our long and happy marriage and he revealed his biggest fear that he will end up like Mom with Alzheimer's and have no one to look after him—which is MY biggest fear as well. I cannot bear the thought of John with no one who loves him to care for him and it gives me the will to keep fighting this cancer and sticking to the protocol and dietary restrictions to the letter. I'm so tired that I went to lay down for just a second and pass out immediately. We celebrated our 9th wedding anniversary the next day and it was nice but also bittersweet as neither of us know whether or not it will be our last. I misbehaved and had 2 bites of a potato side dish and 3 bites of the big cheesecake slice they gave us for our anniversary. I also had 2 glasses of sparkling chardonnay wine which is the first alcohol I've had since August. I've had 4 beers, 1 glass of red wine and 3 glasses of white wine counting my anniversary splurge. The alcohol doesn't affect the GcMAF/Goleic but the sugar gives the cancer cells a boost of a meal. It was wonderful and since we go to this place regularly, they were so kind to us, they are aware of our situation. It was nice but the next day we are back on the protocol and John hits the IV push perfectly with the new longer needles and I get the nice energy rush of the GcMAF/Goleic and hope and pray for the best. I am also cautiously optimistic as I'm is no pain and thanks to Miralax I am pooping on a fairly regular basis for the first time in my life but I have to keep the bowel moving because my normal habits would hide issues. There are two kinds of people in the world: crapters and Camels. My husband is a crapter, he goes 3 times a DAY—I am a camel —I go 3 times a month—maybe, but at the moment my back pain is too severe to strain and push so I suck down the Miralax every 3rd day as a precaution and to make it less painful. I know, it's gross—but this cancer kills you by blocking the bowel—so I have to keep pooping no matter what. Still, so far so good, I'm OK and have sufficient pain meds at the moment so I am getting along well. I'll have another trip to Canada coming up in about 2 weeks, but right now I'm feeling good and going to Louisiana for two weeks to take my Mother in law to her doctor appointments before another smuggling trip in November.

CHAPTER 30: SO, WHAT IS GcMAF/Goleic AND HOW DOES IT WORK?

Discovery and basic study of GcMAF/Goleic GcMAF/Goleic, discovered by Dr Nobuto Yamamoto in 1991, is derived from the group specific component (Gc) protein (vitamin D binding protein), a member of the albumin superfamily. GcMAF/Goleic is an interesting serum glycoprotein with various biological activities. It is reported that during an inflammatory response, β-galactosidase of an activated B-cell and sialidase of a T-cell hydrolyze the terminal galactose and sialic acid saccharides of Gc protein to produce GcMAF/Goleic which has interesting biological activity; it activates macrophages via super oxide radical generation and phagocytic activation 4, and has been demonstrated to have anti-angiogenic and anti-tumor activity in vivo. GcMAF/Goleic also directly inhibits proliferation and migration of human prostate cancer cells or human breast cancer cells independent of its macrophage activation ability. Clinical study of first-generation GcMAF/Goleic for cancer and HIV treatment Clinical trials using GcMAF/Goleic in patients with metastatic breast cancer, prostate cancer, and metastatic colorectal cancer have been conducted. Cancer did not recur over a four to seven year period in all subjects administrated weekly doses of 100 ng of GcMAF/Goleic for 7 to 19 weeks; a result that took everyone by surprise. However, there are some problems with these clinical trials: there were no clear classifications of patients' histo-pathological types, grades, and stages, and the curative judgment was based solely on a patient's Nacetylgalactosaminidase (Nagalase) activity, and neither tumor markers or cytokine levels were measured, and there was no control group.

MASS MURDERING DOCTORS: THE TRUTH ABOUT ONCOLOGISTS, CHEMOTHERAPY AND CANCER

There is also an interesting clinical report of HIV treatment using GcMAF/Goleic. The weekly administration of 100 ng of GcMAF/Goleic to 15 non-anemic HIV-infected patients showed that the number of CD4+ cells increased to normal levels within 6 weeks, and were maintained for the entire 7 years after GcMAF/Goleic therapy, while the number of CD8+ cells decreased to normal levels, and the amount of HIV-1 RNA and p24 as well.

Serum Gc protein (known as vitamin D3-binding protein) is the precursor for the principal macrophage-activating factor (MAF). The MAF precursor activity of serum Gc protein of prostate cancer patients was lost or reduced because Gc protein was deglycosylated by serum α-N-acetylgalactosaminidase (Nagalase) secreted from cancerous cells. Therefore, macrophages of prostate cancer patients having deglycosylated Gc protein cannot be activated, leading to immuno-suppression. Stepwise treatment of purified Gc protein with immobilized β-galactosidase and sialidase generated the most potent MAF (termed GcMAF/Goleic) ever discovered, which produces no adverse effect in humans. Macrophages activated by GcMAF/Goleic develop a considerable variation of receptors that recognize the abnormality in malignant cell surface and are highly tumoricidal. Sixteen non-anemic prostate cancer patients received weekly administration of 100 ng of GcMAF/Goleic. As the MAF precursor activity increased, their serum Nagalase activity decreased. Because serum Nagalase activity is proportional to tumor burden, the entire time course analysis for GcMAF/Goleic therapy was monitored by measuring the serum Nagalase activity. After 14 to 25 weekly administrations of GcMAF/Goleic (100 ng/week), all 16 patients had very low serum Nagalase levels equivalent to those of healthy control values, indicating that these patients are tumor-free. No recurrence occurred for 7 years at the time of this writing.

What is MAF—Macrophage-Activating Factor?
MAF is a protein that activates our macrophages, the microscopic white cells that kill invading microbes and cancer cells. MAF is made from a precursor protein called the Gc protein.
Cancer is Clever—It Inactivates Our Immune System

MASS MURDERING DOCTORS: THE TRUTH ABOUT ONCOLOGISTS, CHEMOTHERAPY AND CANCER

In a way, cancer cells are clever little devils because they disable our immune system in order to enhance their own survival. Dr. Yamamoto discovered that cancer cells do this by secreting an enzyme called Nagalase, which prevents the precursor protein Gc from being converted to MAF. This Nagalase-enzyme activity can actually be measured in cancer patients, and greater tumor burden corresponds with higher Nagalase enzyme activity (as one would expect). Elimination of the tumor results in reduction of Nagalase activity to lower, more normal values.

Dr. Yamamoto devised a technique for restoring Gc-protein activity, which creates the most potent macrophage-activating factor ever discovered, having no adverse effects. He called it **GcMAF/Goleic.** Macrophages treated in vitro with GcMAF/Goleic (100 pg/ml) are highly effective at killing breast-cancer cells. (A picogram is 1 TRILLIONTH of a gram).

GcMAF/Goleic for Metastatic Breast Cancer—Human Trial

Dr. Yamamoto then studied his GcMAF/Goleic in human metastatic breast-cancer patients with weekly injections of 100 ng of GcMAF/Goleic. Dr. Yamamoto found that over time, as treatment with GcMAF/Goleic progresses, the MAF-precursor activity of patient Gc protein increased, and the serum Nagalase decreased. After 5 months of weekly GcMAF/Goleic injections, the cancer patients' elevated Nagalase activity had returned to normal levels, same as healthy controls. Over the next four years, these sixteen treated metastatic breast-cancer patients remained cancer free with no recurrence. In 2008, Dr. Yamamoto published his landmark study on human breast cancer.

GcMAF/Goleic for Metastatic Colorectal Cancer—Human Trial In 2008, Yammamoto published his study on 8 patients with metastatic colorectal cancer. They all had significant metastatic disease after primary resection. Nagalase activity fell to normal levels with GcMAF/Goleic injections, and remained low with no cancer recurrence over 7 years of observation. This was supported by serial CAT scans that remained negative.

MASS MURDERING DOCTORS: THE TRUTH ABOUT ONCOLOGISTS, CHEMOTHERAPY AND CANCER

GcMAF/Goleic FOR THE TREATMENT OF CANCER, AUTISM, INFLAMMATION, VIRAL AND BACTERIAL DISEASE

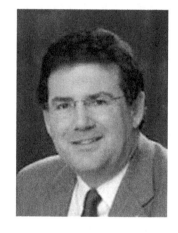

by David Noakes (**I owe this man my life**)

Human GcMAF/Goleic, otherwise known as Vitamin D binding protein macrophage activating factor, holds great promise in the treatment of various illnesses including cancer, autism, chronic fatigue and possibly Parkinson's. Since 1990, 59 research papers have been published on GcMAF/Goleic, 20 of these pertaining to the treatment of cancer. 46 of these papers can be accessed through the GcMAF/Goleic web site.

GcMAF/Goleic is a vital part of our immune system which does not work without it; and is part of our blood. GcMAF/Goleic stimulates the macrophage element of the immune system to destroy cancer cells. It also blocks the supply of nutrients to cancer cells by stopping blood vessel development to the site (anti-angiogenesis). Cancer cells are weakened and starved, making them more vulnerable to attack by the GcMAF/Goleic stimulated macrophage system. Research has shown macrophage activation and stopping diseased blood vessel development can also help in various neurological diseases such as Parkinson's, Alzheimer's, rheumatoid arthritis, inflammatory conditions, and diabetic retinopathy.

David Noakes might just be the person to bring GcMAF into the mainstream. He's the CEO of Immuno Biotech Ltd. and spokesperson for First Immune GcMAF, a project he describes as, "PhD and BSC biochemists and biomedical scientists with external doctors, oncologists and scientists who kindly provide advice, committed to bringing some of the increasing number of published but relatively unused medical cures to as many people as we can." At the moment, Noakes and his colleagues are supplying GcMAF/Goleic to 30 countries where it is legal, via a network of "around 300" doctors. Their GcMAF/Goleic is made to extremely high standards, and is being used in ongoing clinical research by Noakes' collaborators and others. Their ultimate goal is to, "Build the case that GcMAF/Goleic is effective for various illnesses, which will help to make it

MASS MURDERING DOCTORS: THE TRUTH ABOUT ONCOLOGISTS, CHEMOTHERAPY AND CANCER

available to the public". I got my GcMAF/Goleic from First Immune, the company he owns and I owe him my life as this works—no doubt about it!

OTHER USES FOR GcMAF/Goleic

In the case of autism, Dr. James Bradstreet had treated 1,100 patients with GcMAF/Goleic with an 85% response rate before he was MURDERED. His results show a bell curve response with 15% of the patients showing total eradication of symptoms and 15% showing no response. In addition, experimental and clinical evidence confirms that GcMAF/Goleic shows multiple powerful anti-cancer effects that have significant therapeutical impact on most tumors including breast, prostate, and kidney. GcMAF/Goleic is created in the body by the release of two sugar molecules from a GcProtein molecule.

HOW DOES NAGALASE INTERFERE WITH THE IMMUNE SYSTEM?

Tumors release an enzyme known as Nagalase. Nagalase degrades GcProtein to the point it is unable to become GcMAF/Goleic. Since GcMAF/Goleic only lives for about a week in the body, without continuous conversion of GcProtein the stores of GcMAF/Goleic are depleted rapidly in the presence of Nagalase. However, Nagalase can only destroy GcProtein and not GcMAF/Goleic. Thus the introduction of external GcMAF/Goleic through injection into the body has been shown to be effective. GcMAF/Goleic has no side effects of its own, but in under 10% of cases the immune system, which will be rebuilt in just three weeks, can produce considerable side effects in autistic children. The treatment consists of an injection with a tiny diabetic sized syringe once a week. The duration depends on the severity of the disease. Research also reveals that in cancer cases that are stage I and II, the success rate approaches 90% inside 6 months. Nagalase and immune system levels can be measured in the blood and thus offer a marker for cancer and other diseases.

In conclusion, GcMAF/Goleic restores the energetic balance in the cell. Cancer cells driven by sugar metabolism become healthy oxygen driven cells, so tumor cells no longer behave as parasitic organisms. GcMAF/Goleic stimulates macrophages to consume the cancer cells and cells invaded by viruses. This stimulation of the immune system and the anti-angiogenetic effect surrounding the tumor is beneficial in cancer and several neurological disorders like autism, chronic fatigue, Parkinson's, and Alzheimer's, and it is available to the general public.

MASS MURDERING DOCTORS: THE TRUTH ABOUT ONCOLOGISTS, CHEMOTHERAPY AND CANCER

WHAT IS NAGALASE?

Nagalase is a protein made by all cancer cells and viruses (HIV, hepatitis B, hepatitis C, influenza, herpes, Epstein-Barr virus, and others). Its formal, official chemical name is alpha-N-acetylgalactosaminidase, but this is such a tongue-twisting mouthful of a moniker that we usually just call it "Nagalase."

Why is Nagalase important?

Nagalase causes immunodeficiency. Nagalase blocks production of GcMAF/Goleic, thus preventing the immune system from doing its job. Without an active immune system, cancer and viral infections can grow unchecked.

As an extremely sensitive marker for all cancers, Nagalase provides a powerful system for early detection. Serial Nagalase testing provides a reliable and accurate method for tracking the results of any therapeutic regimen for cancer, AIDS, or other chronic viral infection and many diseases not thought to be viral are also cured with GcMAF/Goleic too!

NAGALASE PROVES THAT CANCER CELLS BREAK ALL THE RULES

Normal healthy cells cooperate with one another in a concerted effort to further the good of all. Cancer cells refuse to play ball. Their disdainful attitude toward the rest of our cellular community is appalling. For example, these cellular scofflaws ignore clear messages to stop growing and spreading and encroaching on their neighbor's space. How would you like it if your neighbor moved his fence over into your backyard?

Of all the rules cancer cells break, none is more alarming than the production of Nagalase, the evil enzyme that completely hog-ties the immune system army's ability to stop cancer cells. Virus particles also make Nagalase. Their goal is the same as that of the cancer cells: survival by incapacitating their number one enemy: the immune system the most powerful defense system known to science and not understood well. Like a stealth bomber, the Nagalase enzyme synthesized in and released from a cancer cell or a virus particle pinpoints the GcMAF/Goleic production facilities on the surface of your T and B lymphocytes and then wipes them out with an incredibly precise bomb. How precise? Let me put it this way: Nagalase locates and attacks one specific two-electron bond located at, and only at, the 420th amino acid position on a huge protein molecule (DBP), one of tens of thousands of proteins, each containing millions of electrons. This is like selectively taking out a park bench in a major city from six thousand miles away. More astonishing, if that is possible, Nagalase never misses its target. There is no collateral damage.

As you already know, GcMAF/Goleic is a cell-signaling glycoprotein that talks to macrophages, enabling them to rapidly find, attack, and kill viruses and cancer cells. By activating macrophages, GcMAF/Goleic triggers a cascade that activates the entire immune system. Blockage of GcMAF/Goleic production by Nagalase brings all this wonderful anti-cancer and anti-viral immune activity to a screeching halt, allowing cancer and infections to spread in their silent killing spree while you are unaware of the cancer until too late.

What does Nagalase actually do? How does it destroy immune functioning and deactivate macrophages? Once synthesized and released into nearby tissue or into the bloodstream, Nagalase, like that drill sergeant at boot camp, shouts harsh commands at the vitamin D binding protein (DBP) that is about to be turned into GcMAF/Goleic. Nagalase demands that DBP not, under any circumstances, attach itself to a specific sugar molecule (galactosamine). If DBP has already grabbed (i.e., connected to, using a two-electron, "covalent" bond) a galactosamine sugar molecule, it is commanded to immediately let go. "Leave galactosamine alone, or you'll be in big trouble!" is the Nagalase sergeant's command. We'll probably never know whether or not, on some deeper level, DBP knows that Nagalase's motives are dastardly—but it doesn't really matter: DBP will definitely always obey. Like the army private, the DBP literally has no choice. Because of the way hierarchies work in cellular biology, proteins must do the bidding of their enzymes. The enzymes, like Nagalase, are the drill sergeant and the proteins, like DBP, are the privates. That's just the way it is. Obeying the drill sergeant's command means DBP can't do its assigned task, that of becoming GcMAF/Goleic. It is rendered useless. For DBP, on a molecular level, life no longer has meaning.

Unfortunately for cancer and viral patients, DBP had been on its way to becoming GcMAF/Goleic until the Nagalase drill sergeant so rudely interrupted. Now GcMAF/Goleic—the one protein our bodies need in order to activate our immune systems—can't be made. Immune activity screeches to a halt. The defense system protecting us from cancers and viruses has been snuffed out.

MASS MURDERING DOCTORS: THE TRUTH ABOUT ONCOLOGISTS, CHEMOTHERAPY AND CANCER

Nagalase, using this astonishingly simple yet cunningly subversive technique, emasculates the GcMAF/Goleic precursor protein (DBP) by knocking off its three sugar molecules. One quick whack by Nagalase and the DBP protein that would have become a GcMAF/Goleic molecule now limps off into the sunset, permanently disfigured and disabled. With one simple, swift maneuver, Nagalase has brought the entire immune system to its knees.

Here's how Dr. Yamamoto put it (for clarity, I've replaced some of the technical words): "Serum vitamin D3-binding protein (DBP) is the precursor for the principal macrophage activating factor (GcMAF/Goleic). The precursor activity of serum DBP was reduced. These patient sera contained alpha-N-acetylgalactosaminidase (Nagalase) that deglycosylates (removes the sugars from) DBP. Deglycosylated DBP cannot be converted to GcMAF/Goleic, thus it loses the GcMAF/Goleic precursor activity, leading to immunosuppression." (Microbes Infect. 2005 Apr;7(4):674-81. Epub 2005 Mar 22. Pathogenic significance of alpha-N-acetylgalactosaminidase activity found in the hemagglutinin of influenza virus. Yamamoto N, Urade M.)

Nagalase testing: former mass murderer now works for the good guys

It's easy to be a little bipolar about Nagalase. On the one hand, this nasty protein's behavior toward us has been reprehensible and disastrous. Working in cahoots with cancer and HIV—not shy about getting into bed with our mortal enemies—Nagalase can rightfully claim direct responsibility for billions of human deaths. Nagalase would just as soon add you to the list, so we don't have to be shy about placing Nagalase in the "genocidal murderer" column. With the advent of Nagalase testing, however, this bad actor now will be harnessed to a useful purpose. By providing us with precise and reliable advance information about enemy operations, Nagalase blood level testing becomes a "Deep Throat" double agent for cancer. He helps us by giving us an early warning sign. Early detection (using AMAS or Nagalase) saves lives. You don't want a cancer to have gotten out of control by the time you find and start treating it. When cancers are still young and small, gentle natural therapies are the most effective. Alternative treatments work best on early small cancers by enhancing immune functioning and removing the source of the inflammation that is causing the cancer in the first place. Cancers that have become large enough to see on imaging pose a much more significant threat, and the big guns now become necessary.

MASS MURDERING DOCTORS: THE TRUTH ABOUT ONCOLOGISTS, CHEMOTHERAPY AND CANCER

The current method for diagnosing most cancers requires us to wait until a mass shows up on imaging (e.g., a mammogram, chest X-ray, or colonoscopy). This approach wastes valuable time and causes needless deaths. But long before imaging can find it, a positive Nagalase (or AMAS test) can tell us that early stage cancer exists somewhere in the body. By enabling earlier and therefore less invasive treatment options, this information provides a huge head-start. Normally present at only trace levels, Nagalase shows up in the blood when a cancer or virus appears The malignant and viral entities that make Nagalase are not normally present, so its appearance is a big deal from a diagnostic perspective. When Nagalase shows up, even in very small amounts, we have the earliest glimpse of a new cancer or viral infection. The old adage, "Where there's smoke, there's fire" applies here. A positive Nagalase test notifies us that a cancer (or a nasty virus) lurks within. Nagalase appears in the blood stream when a nascent cancer is just a minute cluster of abnormal cells, long before conventional diagnostic methods can detect it. Through blood testing, we can find this red flag, even when present at exceedingly low levels. Providing us with this early warning sign might not quite qualify Nagalase for the "Good Samaritan" award, but I could go with "extremely useful." Like a rehabilitated criminal on parole, the potential for harm is still there. For now, however, he's staying out of trouble and doing community service. Turn your back and he's a mass murderer again. Rising Nagalase levels indicate a cancer or virus is growing and spreading. Conversely, Nagalase levels will decrease if the cancer or infection is being effectively destroyed. Any treatment that lowers cancer cell (or viral numbers) will lower Nagalase levels. Nagalase will, for example, always drop after surgery (whether or not the entire tumor was removed). Chemotherapy and radiation also reduce Nagalase levels. So does GcMAF/Goleic. If, after these treatments, the depressed level begins to rise again, this is the warning sign that the cancer was not completely removed, and/or that metastatic disease is hiding out somewhere. With viral infections, increasing Nagalase levels indicate return of the infection. Consecutive rising Nagalase levels are therefore a red flag, warning us it may be time to entertain new treatment options. Conversely, if levels are going down, stay the course: the cancer or virus is going away. Many medical professionals don't feel comfortable with "nonspecific" tests like Nagalase. It drives them nuts to discover that a cancer is

MASS MURDERING DOCTORS: THE TRUTH ABOUT ONCOLOGISTS, CHEMOTHERAPY AND CANCER

lurking somewhere inside without knowing exactly where it is located. "How," they ask, "do you expect me to treat a cancer I can't see? Why, I'm not going to tilt at windmills!" This may be a signal that you need to find a different doctor, perhaps one who works in an alternative cancer clinic. Here you will find highly-trained professionals who understand the concept that cancer is a molecular biological change long before it presents visually (by this I mean becomes viewable on imaging). When GcMAF/Goleic becomes available (available at First Immune Biotech, www.GcMAF.se) the answer will be easier: a six month course of weekly 100 ng GcMAF/Goleic intramuscular injections with monthly Nagalase level tests to follow the Nagalase level as it goes back down to baseline. The cancer can be declared cured, even though it never reached life-threatening proportions.

Nagalase, arguably our most immuno-suppressive protein molecule, poses an enormous threat in terms of cancer perpetuation and viruses' ability to continually defeat us. Yet cancer researchers have not shown any interest in it. (Maybe I'm being a little too generous here; perhaps "clueless" would be more a more accurate depiction.) Why don't they get it that blasting cancer cells into oblivion with chemo and radiation is usually not sufficient to stop advanced disease and does nothing to address the cause: immunosuppression. **CANCER IS AN IMMUNO-SUPPRESSIVE DISEASE.** Even if we ignore for the moment the excessive collateral damage caused by chemo drugs and radiation, the patient also needs—requires—a healthy immune system to finish the job. **If we don't revive immune function by disabling Nagalase, the cancers and viruses will just keep roaring back.** When the immune system is destroyed by chemo, there's nothing to fight back with and the cancer will recurs since this process makes cancer cells immortal. Restoring immuno-competence by negating the stultifying effect of Nagalase should therefore become a primary research goal. Cancer secretes nagalase that deglycosolates 3 molecules that prevent the body's immune system from making the GcMAF/Goleic needed to kill the cancer cells. Cancer is an immune system deficiency, nothing more and nothing less. Replacing the GcMAF/Goleic will kill tumor based cancer in 6-12 months of twice weekly injections and it never recurs. Yammamoto was 100% correct and I am going to tell him so if he is still alive when this is over (he's in his early 90s at this writing), assuming I don't die. I will owe him my life and I want him to know it.

MASS MURDERING DOCTORS: THE TRUTH ABOUT ONCOLOGISTS, CHEMOTHERAPY AND CANCER

As of the 3rd of August, 2017 I am still not presenting any cancer symptoms. I'm scared to death every second of every day. I made a huge gamble on a long held belief of mine, but if I'm wrong, I'll pay for it with my life. I don't feel the least bit brave—but I knew chemo couldn't help me and I didn't want to go through the last 6 months of my life sick, puking and wanting to die—or worse—surviving to a miserable sick existence dependent on my husband to take care of me. I didn't live that way and I won't die that way either. I put up a brave front for John but believe me when I tell you I am f**king SCARED. It's the chemotherapy that causes the new cancers. Immunotherapy is what cures cancer, NOT chemotherapy. Chemotherapy is the biggest bullcrap lie in medicine. My sister and I had/have the same cancer. She died—not from the cancer—from a ruptured esophagus from vomiting from the chemo and BLED TO DEATH IN FRONT OF MY PARENTS WHO ARE ELDERLY as she was 55 and I am 57. I have not had ANY chemo and I have already lived longer than she did with all the chemo poison they could pump into her and I feel perfectly fine and normal. If I didn't KNOW I have cancer, I would never believe I do. Here's a new article about how people who have survived cancer get new cancers from the chemotherapy 5 years down the road—and the 40 year old platinum poison they tried to give me causes LEUKEMIA (among others) down the road. It's all about profit and money and corruption. Read this happy bullcrap put out by Cancer Treatment Centers of America (CTCA) who built a medical empire on poisoning people for profit—and calling it medical treatment—and financed by—you guessed it; Big Pharma.

CHAPTER 31: CHEMOTHERAPY CAUSES FUTURE CANCERS IF YOU SURVIVE

Metachronous cancer: A growing concern for cancer survivors

CTCA May 02, 2016

For many survivors, beating cancer brings a welcome sigh of relief. But for some, even those **VERY FEW (author-added**) whose cancer never regrows or spreads, it won't be their last battle with the disease. Research suggests that a growing percentage of cancer survivors are being diagnosed with "metachronous" cancers—new primary tumors unrelated to the patients' previous cancers. As troubling as repeat bouts of cancer may be, rising rates of metachronous cancer may actually underscore how

MASS MURDERING DOCTORS: THE TRUTH ABOUT ONCOLOGISTS, CHEMOTHERAPY AND CANCER

much progress is being made in survival rates, doctors say. **The longer cancer patients live, the more likely they are to develop new diseases,** since cancer risk grows with age, says Dr. Sagun Shrestha, Medical Oncologist at the (CTCA) hospital in Tulsa. The five-year survival rate for breast cancer patients, for example, has more than doubled over the past 50 years, from 40 percent to nearly 90 percent. Of the 14.5 million cancer survivors in the United States, two-thirds have survived for more than five years, according to the American Cancer Society. **"As patients get older, we do see second or even third primary cancers,"** Dr. Shrestha says.

A 2013 study by researchers with the Rhode Island Cancer Council and Brown University analyzed more than two decades' worth of cancer data, taken from the Rhode Island Cancer Registry. The results suggested that about 20 percent of new cancers were metachronous. In the late 1980s, that figure was about 12 percent. **The study found the average interval between first and second cancers was 6.5 years for men and 4.8 years for women. Four cancer types accounted for a majority of the new primary cancers: lung, colon, breast and prostate.** Those statistics underscore the need for continued cancer screening for survivors, particularly for the four cancer types, the authors noted. Besides avoiding tobacco, the focus on cancer prevention should emphasize a variety of healthy habits, including frequent exercise, good nutrition, stress reduction and adequate rest, doctors say. Choosing carbohydrates that have a lower glycemic index, meaning they are metabolized more slowly, may be one strategy. That means avoiding refined white bread, white rice and sweets, and instead choosing whole grains, fresh fruits and a variety of colorful vegetables. When a new cancer erupts, some patients are relieved to hear that their previous cancer hasn't regrown or spread, even if it means fighting another cancer, says Dr. Maurie Markman, President of Medicine & Science at Cancer Treatment Centers of America (CTCA). The new primary cancers are often caught in the early stages, before they have spread to other areas of the body and when they tend to be easier to treat. "The new primary cancer may be dealt with in a manner quite different from metastatic cancer," Dr. Markman says. "Sometimes, the news that a patient is dealing with a new primary is not bad." **Author's note: Of course not Dr. Markham—it puts more money in your pocket when the cancers come**

back because you are treating them incorrectly. Cancer is an immunodeficiency disease. Period.

Courtesy of Natural News: One of the side effects of chemotherapy is, ironically, cancer. The cancer doctors don't say much about it, but it's printed right on the chemo drug warning labels (in small print, of course). If you go into a cancer treatment clinic with one type of cancer, and you allow yourself to be injected with chemotherapy chemicals, you will often develop a second type of cancer as a result. Your oncologist will often claim to have successfully treated your first cancer even while you develop a second or third cancer directly caused by the chemo used to treat the original cancer. There's nothing like cancer-causing chemotherapy to boost repeat business, huh?

It may surprise most people to find out that one of the most common treatments for a variety of cancers is chemotherapy and that it actually has its origins in World Wars I and II. Given that most people consider the treatment of cancer to be a war, then it shouldn't come as much of a surprise. The fantastic science of chemotherapy began because it was noticed that Mustard Gas caused the destruction of fast growing cells. In the average human body, the fastest growing cells are hair follicles, stomach lining, immune system, intestinal lining and bone marrow. This serves to explain why Mustard Gas was an effective agent of warfare damage to such major systems of the body would cause obvious illness and death. After World War II, a number of other chemotherapy agents were developed, all of which operate in basically the same way: attacking and killing growing cells.

As an analogy, suppose you were to tell an exterminator that you have a termite infestation in your home. The exterminator, a profession whom you are entrusting, tells you that the best course of action will be to use a chemical which is known to eat away at both the wood and the foundation of homes, as well as causing irreparable damage to furniture and windows. Unfortunately, after all, you really do want to get rid of those termites, right? Basically, the use of chemotherapy is the same type of treatment. Another way to look at it would be using a sledgehammer to open a peanut. Chemotherapy is, admittedly, effective at reducing tumors because it's a highly effective and very toxic poison. It's designed to kill cells and it does its job very

MASS MURDERING DOCTORS: THE TRUTH ABOUT ONCOLOGISTS, CHEMOTHERAPY AND CANCER

well. It's also very effective at hampering the immune system, damaging the gastrointestinal system and, effectively, causing a great deal of damage to the human body. Chemotherapy treatments are effective at many things, especially at diminishing the quality of life for cancer patients. Chemotherapy treatments also happen to be carcinogenic. Yes, a carcinogenic. Remember, a carcinogen is something that has been shown to increase the chances of developing cancer. During all this, the pharmacists are peddling these toxic chemotherapy chemicals to their customers as if they were medicine (which they aren't). While preparing these toxic chemical prescriptions, it turns out that pharmacists are exposing themselves to cancer-causing chemotherapy agents in the process. And because of that, pharmacists are giving themselves cancer and they're dying from it. People who live in glass houses should never throw stones, they say. You might similarly say that pharmacists who deal in poison shouldn't be surprised to one day discover they are killing themselves with it. Chemotherapy drugs are extremely toxic to the human body, and they are readily absorbed through the skin. The very idea that they are even used in modern medicine is almost laughable if it weren't so downright disturbing and sad that hundreds of thousands of people are killed each year around the world by chemotherapy drugs. Now you can add pharmacists to that statistic. For decades, they simply looked the other way, pretending they were playing a valuable role in our system of "modern" medicine, not admitting they were actually doling out chemicals that killed people. Now, the sobering truth has struck them hard: They are in the business of death, and it is killing them off, one by one. The Seattle Times now reports the story of Sue Crump, a veteran pharmacist of two decades who spent much of her time dispensing chemotherapy drugs. Sue died last September of pancreatic cancer, and one of her dying wishes was that the truth would be told about how her on-the-job exposure to chemotherapy chemicals contributed to her own cancer.

The Occupational Safety and Health Association (OSHA), it turns out, does not regulate workplace exposure to toxic, cancer-causing chemotherapy chemicals. At first glance, that seems surprising, since OSHA regulates workplace exposure to far less harmful chemicals. Why not chemo? The answer is because the toxicity of chemotherapy has long been ignored by virtually everyone in medicine and the federal government. It has always been assumed harmless or even "safe" just because it's

MASS MURDERING DOCTORS: THE TRUTH ABOUT ONCOLOGISTS, CHEMOTHERAPY AND CANCER

used as a kind of far-fetched "medicine" to treat cancer. This, despite the fact that chemotherapy is a derivative of the mustard gas used against enemy soldiers in World War I. Truthfully, chemotherapy has more in common with chemicals weapons than any legitimate medicine. So today, while workers are protected from secondhand smoke in offices across the country, pharmacists are still being exposed every single day to toxic, cancer-causing chemicals that OSHA seems to just ignore. The agency has only issued one citation in the last decade to a hospital for inadequate safety handling of toxic chemotherapy drugs.

As the Seattle Times reports, "A just-completed study from the U.S. Centers for Disease Control (CDC) -- 10 years in the making and the largest to date -- confirms that chemo continues to contaminate the work spaces where it's used and in some cases is still being found in the urine of those who handle it..." That same article goes on to report more pharmacists, veterinarians and nurses who are dead or dying from chemotherapy exposure:

• Bruce Harrison of St. Louis (cancer in his 50's, now dead)

• Karen Lewis of Baltimore (cancer in her 50's, still living)

• Brett Cordes of Scottsdale, Arizona (cancer at age 35, still living)

• Sally Giles of Vancouver, B.C. (cancer in her 40's, now dead)

The great contradiction in cancer treatments As the Seattle Times reports:

"Danish epidemiologists used cancer-registry data from the 1940s through the late 1980s to first report a significantly increased risk of leukemia among oncology nurses and, later, physicians. Last year, another Danish study of more than 92,000 nurses found an elevated risk for breast, thyroid, nervous-system and brain cancers." The story goes on to report how new safety rules are being put in place across the industry to protect pharmacists, veterinarians, nurses and doctors from toxic chemotherapy chemicals. But even the Seattle Times, which deserves credit for running this story, misses the bigger point: If these chemicals are so dangerous to the doctors, nurses and pharmacists dispensing them, how can they be considered "safe enough" to inject into patients who are already dying from cancer? It's a serious

MASS MURDERING DOCTORS: THE TRUTH ABOUT ONCOLOGISTS, CHEMOTHERAPY AND CANCER

question. After all, if nurses can become violently ill after merely spilling chemotherapy chemicals on themselves (it's true), then what effect do you suppose these chemicals have when injected into patients? The cancer industry, though, has never stopped injecting patients long enough to ask the commonsense question: Why are we in the business of dispensing poison in the first place? Poison, after all, isn't medicine. Not when dispensed in its full potency, anyway. The whole idea of "safety" in the cancer industry is to find new ways to protect the health care workers from the extremely dangerous chemicals they're still injecting into the bodies of patients. Something is clearly wrong with this picture... if health care workers need to be protected from this stuff, why not protect the patients from it, too?

It makes no sense that we would use a drug to treat a cancer patient that causes cancer in the person administering it. Nobody ever died from handling herbs. In contrast to all this, consider the truthful observation that no naturopath ever died from handling medicinal herb, homeopathy remedies or nutritional supplements. These natural therapies are good for patients, and as a bonus, you don't have to wear a chemical suit to handle them. Furthermore, medicinal herbs, supplements and natural remedies don't cause cancer. They support and protect the immune system rather than destroying it. So they make patients healthier and more resilient rather than weaker and fragile. However, herbs, supplements and natural remedies don't earn much money for the cancer industry; only the highly-toxic patented chemotherapy drugs bring in the big bucks. So that's what they deal in poison for the patients. And when you deal in poison, some of it always splashes back onto you. Chemotherapy doesn't work either. Beyond this whole issue of pharmacists and health care workers dying from exposure to secondhand chemotherapy, there's the issue of whether chemotherapy actually works in the first place. Scientifically speaking, if you take a good, hard look at what the published studies actually say, chemotherapy is only effective at treating less than two percent of the cancers that exist. And that two percent does not include breast cancer or prostate cancer. Yet chemotherapy is routinely used to "treat" breast cancer even though it offers no benefit to breast cancer patients. In effect, the cancer industry is engaged in a criminal treatment hoax that promises to make you healthier but actually gives you even more cancer which is great for repeat business, but terrible for the cancer patients who suffer under it. The

MASS MURDERING DOCTORS: THE TRUTH ABOUT ONCOLOGISTS, CHEMOTHERAPY AND CANCER

level of quackery at work right now in the cancer industry is simply astonishing. You would think that if doctors and pharmacists were dishing out these chemicals to patients, they would make sure there was some sort of legitimate science to back them up. But they haven't. The science doesn't exist. Chemotherapy doesn't work at anything other than causing cancer and it accomplishes that indiscriminately, damaging any person it comes into contact with. Merely touching chemotherapy chemicals is dangerous for your health.

The so called "war on cancer" is a dismal failure after squandering upwards of a trillion dollars over the past 50 or so years, but the cancer doctors can't even tell us what cancer is let alone how to cure and prevent it in the human body. Obviously they don't know what they are doing and don't want to know what they are doing. Cancer is not hundreds of different diseases as they falsely claim, one for every organ, but one disease: immune deficiency. As Warburg showed, all cancer cells metabolize via anerobic glycolysis or the wasting disease which dumps lactic acid into the body instead of CO_2 out the lungs as normal oxygen based respiration does. This disease, observed in all advanced cancer patients has been given the disease name: CACHEXIA. The cancer doctors are guilty of scientific misconduct, fraud, medical quackery and crimes against humanity and must all be fired and jailed. Are bacterial infections different for different organs of the body? Why would cancer be a different disease for every organ? **All approved cancer treatments are life threatening. Therefore when a patient under treatment dies, they could have died either from cancer or treatment or both, but usually falsely reported as from cancer instead of treatment. This is a gift to the doctors who are becoming rich off this biggest medical scam of our time. The only way to prove the cause of death is via an autopsy by a top pathological laboratory which is never done. Those involved in this scam, doctors and pharmaceutical companies, love this so they can never be charged with murder.** What is really bothering me about the immuno-therapy is that if it works I don't know how my family is going to feel about it because I so wanted my sister to skip chemo and do this as well and she wouldn't hear of it. I BEGGED HER to let me help her and she would NOT DO IT so if the cure is the immuno-juice, then I don't know how I will live with not FORCING her to listen to me. Both my parents are still alive and watched her

MASS MURDERING DOCTORS: THE TRUTH ABOUT ONCOLOGISTS, CHEMOTHERAPY AND CANCER

die—from the chemo by the way, NOT the cancer—although they wrote "cancer" on her death certificate. She bled to death in front of BOTH of my parents from a ruptured esophagus caused by chemo-induced vomiting. All I have to say about this is that I am SURE I made the right decision to refuse chemo—it gives you cancer again in a few years. This is because they are not treating the cancer correctly from the beginning. CHEMO IS NOT THE RIGHT CHOICE, EVER!

A team of researchers looking into why cancer cells are so resilient accidentally stumbled upon a far more important discovery. While conducting their research, the team discovered that chemotherapy actually heavily damages healthy cells and subsequently triggers them to release a protein that sustains and fuels tumor growth. Beyond that, it even makes the tumor highly resistant to future treatment.

Reporting their findings in the journal Nature Medicine, the scientists report that the findings were 'completely unexpected'. Finding evidence of significant DNA damage when examining the effects of chemotherapy on tissue derived from men with prostate cancer, the writings are a big slap in the face to mainstream medical organizations who have been pushing chemotherapy as the only option to cancer patients for years. The news comes after it was previously ousted by similarly-breaking research that expensive cancer drugs not only fail to treat tumors, but actually make them far worse. The cancer drugs were found to make tumors 'metasize' and grow massively in size after consumption. As a result, the drugs killed the patients more quickly.

Known as WNT16B, scientists who performed the research say that this protein created from chemo treatment boosts cancer cell survival and is the reason that chemotherapy actually ends lives more quickly. Co-author Peter Nelson of the Fred Hutchinson Cancer Research Center in Seattle explains: WNT16B, when secreted, would interact with nearby tumor cells and cause them to grow, invade, and importantly, resist subsequent therapy." The team then complimented the statement with a word of their own: "Our results indicate that damage responses in benign cells... may directly contribute to enhanced tumor growth kinetics." Ever since chemotherapy was introduced into the practice of western medicine, doctors and oncologists have been trying to answer this nagging question: Why does

MASS MURDERING DOCTORS: THE TRUTH ABOUT ONCOLOGISTS, CHEMOTHERAPY AND CANCER

chemotherapy seem to work at first, but then cancer tumors cells grow back even more aggressively while the body becomes resistant to chemotherapy?

It turns out that chemotherapy damages healthy cells, causing them to secrete a protein that accelerates the growth of cancer tumors.

This protein, dubbed "WNT16B," is taken up by nearby cancer cells, causing them to "grow, invade, and importantly, resist subsequent therapy," said Peter Nelson of the Fred Hutchinson Cancer Research Center in Seattle. He's the co-author of the study that documented this phenomenon, published in Nature Medicine. This protein, it turns out, explains why cancer tumors grow more aggressively following chemotherapy treatments. In essence, chemotherapy turns healthy cells into WNT16B factories which churn out this "activator" chemical that accelerates cancer tumor growth. The findings of the study were confirmed with prostate cancer, breast cancer and **ovarian cancer tumor**s. This discovery that chemotherapy backfires by accelerating cancer tumor growth is being characterized as "completely unexpected" by scientists. The chemotherapy fraud exposed As Natural News has explained over the last decade, chemotherapy is medical fraud. Rather than boosting the immune response of patients, it harms the immune system, causing tumors to grow back. This latest researching further confirms what we've known for years in the holistic health community: That chemotherapy is, flatly stated, poison. It's not "treatment," it's not medicine, and it's not prevention or a cure. It's poison with virtually no medicinal value except in perhaps one to two percent of cancer cases. The No. 1 side effect of chemotherapy is, by the way, cancer. Cancer centers should technically be renamed "poison centers" because they are in the business of poisoning patients with a toxic cocktail of chemicals that modern science reveals to be a cancer tumor growth accelerant! Meanwhile, dirt cheap substances like turmeric and ginger have consistently been found to effectively shrink tumors and combat the spread of cancer. In a review of 11 studies, it was found that turmeric use reduced brain tumor size by a shocking 81%. Further research has also shown that turmeric is capable of halting cancer cell growth altogether. One woman recently hit the mainstream headlines by revealing her victory against cancer with the principal spice used being turmeric. This

MASS MURDERING DOCTORS: THE TRUTH ABOUT ONCOLOGISTS, CHEMOTHERAPY AND CANCER

accidental finding reached by scientists further shows the lack of real science behind many 'old paradigm' treatments, despite what many health officials would like you to believe. The truth of the matter is that natural alternatives do not even receive nearly as much funding as pharmaceutical drugs and medical interventions because there's simply no room for profit.

"Cancer is the biggest medical failure of our time and the biggest medical scam of our time. I have been studying the failed war on cancer for over 15 years since my wife was nearly killed from the treatment rather than from breast cancer." —Winfield J. Abbe, Ph.D., Physics

The kindness of people I've met during this battle has been amazing, but the prayers mean the most of all. I will be having an MRI soon—but I am so terrified of what it might say. I've been allowing myself the luxury of engaging in denial and pretending to myself it's all going to be OK. It might be, but I won't know until the next MRI. I have been doing an immunotherapy drug I got in Europe. My education is all hard science and the science is solid. They've had tremendous success, enough that they are on the hit list of the FDA (so I am in a Dallas Buyer's Club situation) and Europe's version of Big Pharma is trying to discredit them—but they have a huge success rate. It's not cheap but it's 1/10th the cost of chemo but of course my insurance doesn't pay for it—but they would shell out a million bucks for chemo in a heartbeat. I'm seriously considering trading a signed waiver for any and all future chemotherapy in return for a check for 50K to defray the cost of the GcMAF/Goleic shots but I doubt they will go for it. They'd rather pay for a ton of poison for a million bucks than to pay for 25 grand worth of GcMAF/Goleic!

My pain issues are from having to switch to a highly ineffective painkiller from a very effective one that interferes with the immuno-juice so I had to change it and to add to THAT my idiot insurance company THAT I HAVE NEVER HAD AN ISSUE WITH TILL NOW decides that paying HALF of what my meds USED to cost them and they keep denying it. My doctor (Dr. Janet—you'll read all about her) is ready to kill them, and if the immuno-juice works, I will owe her my life as well since she has made sure that I get anything I need to facilitate this even though she was skeptical although she is now "cautiously optimistic" since I have no current cancer symptoms. My dad (86 and he had to watch his youngest daughter bleed to death a year ago on the 18th of November 2015) said he thought I was "incredibly brave" because I flatly refused chemo and found what I hope is a cure. We'll see soon enough. I DON'T feel very brave though—I'm scared to death about all of this most of the time.

CHAPTER 32: THE NOVEMBER MRI—WHERE THE RUBBER MEETS THE ROAD

It's time to call Dr. Janet for the next MRI. This one tells the story of life or death for me. If the GcMAF/Goleic is working, then I am going to see smaller and/or disappearing tumors, and if it's not, I've got maybe 6 months to live. I'm so scared I can't even BREATHE—so very much is riding on this MRI—like my whole life. We are going to Canada tomorrow to get next month's supply of immuno-juice (GcMAF/Goleic) and once again my husband will risk his job, career, security clearance and freedom to save my life. I am grateful that President Trump was elected yesterday as I hope to be able to break the stranglehold that BigPharma has on the "approved" permitted medicine for those of us forced to buy Obamacare—also soon to be a bad memory. My insurance that is willing to pay an oncologist hundreds of thousands of dollars to poison me with chemotherapy to the tune of 900 thousand dollars; will not give me a penny toward paying for the GcMAF/Goleic even though I estimate the cost of my cure will be about $75,000.00 but I would think that the cost will go down when it is made by a major drug company, proven effective and approved under a Trump administration and it would be covered by insurance and administered by oncologists.

SIDEBAR: INTERNATIONAL DRUG SMUGGLING PART DEUX

I'm sitting in a hotel room in Detroit shaking with nerves as my beloved husband once again risks EVERYTHING to smuggle a Vitamin-D binding protein into the USA from Canada. My life literally hangs in the balance as he goes to Canada for the THIRD time in as many months to sneak the vials of GcMAF/Goleic back into the country so that I can continue my fight against the killer cancer in my pelvis. The stakes are as high for him as they are for me. He holds a Top Secret security clearance which is required for his job and if he gets caught doing this, his clearance, job and career are GONE along with our health insurance, income and way of life—and **HE DOES NOT CARE.** He is the bravest and toughest guy in the world and I am a basket case of

MASS MURDERING DOCTORS: THE TRUTH ABOUT ONCOLOGISTS, CHEMOTHERAPY AND CANCER

nerves waiting for the call to tell me he's safely over the border with my "unapproved" medication. I hope President Trump (Yaaaaayyy!!! by the way) will clean up the corruption in DC and get rid of the unholy alliance of BigPharma, the bought-and-paid-for FDA and the scumbags in Congress who take their money to keep us sick and dying when the cure is out there for everyone—but since these same scumbags have looted our pension funds, Social Security and Medicare and because we have to die without taking out the money we put in—which they've STOLEN and are content to let us die of cancer and other diseases that are cured with GcMAF/Goleic. Is this so they can conceal the theft of our money? I don't have ANY problem believing that even though it makes me sound like a crazy conspiracy theorist which I'm not. However, look at the pension fund shortages in many states. Look at how they've robbed Social Security. If millions of people stopped dying of cancer, how much MORE would they cost? Quite a bit. Let's also think about all the money spent on these "Cancer Center" hospitals. Those have to be paid for, if people stop dying of cancer, they go broke. You think Cancer, Inc. doesn't have friends in Congress they are paying off? Think again! Finally my cell rings and John is safe on the US side of the border with my GcMAF/Goleic tucked into it's chilled case for transport back to Illinois. I am so relieved I want to cry but I don't since it upsets John to see that. He's worried when he gets back and tells me they asked a lot more questions this time and different ones than usual. Passports have a bar code now so they KNOW he's been there 3 months in a row about a month apart so it looks like he's making regular trips—which he is, so I am going to have to make the pickup by myself next month. I hope and pray I have the kind of steely nerves and ice-water blood to casually smuggle unapproved GcMAF/Goleic back into America in order to save my life. I'll go alone next time—no need to drag poor John and Mom along. Last month we did the trip in one day, leaving at 2 am and getting back to Illinois 1100 miles later at 9 pm, stopping only to use the rest room and get gas. Meals came through a window and we hauled ass because Mom was alone at home. We decided to take her with us on this trip and we spent the night in a hotel and it was a lot easier for everyone. I'm waiting on approval for my pelvic MRI to see if the tumors are shrinking; as I feel they must be given my total lack of symptoms although I have some symptoms of a cold—which can also happen if your cancer is almost gone and your intake of GcMAF/Goleic stays

MASS MURDERING DOCTORS: THE TRUTH ABOUT ONCOLOGISTS, CHEMOTHERAPY AND CANCER

at a high level. It kicks your immune system into high gear with nothing to fight so you get symptoms of a cold—which I have now had for 8 days so if it's not an allergy then it has to be because my cancer is on the verge of being killed—I HOPE and PRAY but this MRI I am trying to schedule is the one that will tell me if I am going to live out my projected life span or die sometime in the summer of 2017. It's scary and stressful and everything—including my life—riding on the results. No wonder I'm flipped out scared right now—I have NO idea what the MRI will tell me—it will definitely let me know if I'm going to die in a few weeks OR it will tell me I have a chance to beat the incurable unbeatable cancer and make medical history. I have been allowing myself the luxury of denial for the past few weeks since I feel fine. If I didn't KNOW I am supposed to be dying, I would never have a clue that anything is wrong. There's a reason they call this cancer the silent killer, there are NO symptoms or warning signs. As I write this diary of a fear-crazed terminal cancer patient, I STILL have no idea how it will end. Will John—after all he has been through with me on this journey—will he have to write the last few pages of this book to say how I died bravely fighting the killer cancer? Or will I be on a book tour blowing the whistle on the corruption of BigPharma and their bought-and-paid-for politicians? Will people with cancer listen to me and get cured using GcMAF/Goleic? Will it become the accepted treatment for all cancers and put Cancer, Inc. out of business who will probably have me killed for spite; and of course, the 200-300 billion plus in LOST annual profits? I would give anything for a tiny peek into a crystal ball, it is the not knowing that is the hardest thing. Hope for the best and prepare for the worst is the most chickencrap motto ever but it's what I have to do right now. I pray the same prayer every day—several times. It goes like this:

Please God don't take me away from John, he needs me! If it is your will, let me survive this cancer to show the way to the world; so that your gift of a cure through the miracle of GcMAF/Goleic and your Grace in providing it to Dr. Yammamoto, can end the terrible suffering of all your children struck down by this horrible disease and perpetuated by Satan's demon doctors. Amen.

I hope He is listening and that the answer is yes and that I will be delivered into grace. The MRI will tell me the answer, but I am so scared that my hands are shaking

MASS MURDERING DOCTORS: THE TRUTH ABOUT ONCOLOGISTS, CHEMOTHERAPY AND CANCER

when I call Dr. Janet's office to start the process of getting the insurance approvals for the MRI that will tell me if I will live to see my 59th birthday in December 2017.

It's been three days since I called about getting an MRI and I still haven't heard when it would be, so with Thanksgiving next week, I will probably end up making the December Canada drug-smuggling run for my immuno-juice by myself before we go back to Baton Rouge—all of which will be contingent on what the MRI says. I feel fine, no symptoms and John gives me my immuno-juice IV every day which has become the new normal to me. Today is a sad day though, it was a year ago today, on November 18th 2015 that my sister—about whose battle with cancer this book was originally about—until I was drafted into the same desperate battle for my life with a cancer than has a zero percent survival rate—died. I call her sons, my nephews and chat briefly with them and they sound OK, just sad like me. I try to call my beloved Carleigh and there's no answer so I text her after dinner as she is a lot like me and I know she doesn't want to TALK about it. We exchange texts, she says she's OK, but I am worried so I tell her I will call her in a few days and I tell the kids that I will let them know how the MRI turns out. I always feel so positive and confident that I will be OK until I remember the survival rate. I want to get this over with so that I can know something—I've allowed myself to have hope. Not good. It's the worst feeling in the world to want to know the answer to something while being totally terrified of what that answer might be. I'm sick with fear knots and I have NO idea how in God's green earth I am going to be able to lay in the claustrophobia-inducing MRI tube with all of this terror crashing around in my head. It's going to require medication I'm NOT ALLOWED TO TAKE but I will suck it up and get it done as I have no other option. It's like the Paleo diet I am supposed to follow: salmon, chicken livers, butter, cream and the ever-popular canned pig's brains. I hate salmon but you wouldn't know it watching me eat it. I choke the nasty salmon down. Chicken livers are also on my menu and I eat them 2-3 times a week and force down salmon the rest of the time. I have stuck to the diet like glue other than my anniversary, and if I had been sure it wouldn't be the LAST ONE I would have choked down salmon and not had the glass of wine rather than the tasty steak, glass of wine and 2 bites of the cheesecake dessert that came with the meal on the Prix fixe menu.

MASS MURDERING DOCTORS: THE TRUTH ABOUT ONCOLOGISTS, CHEMOTHERAPY AND CANCER

OK. It's on for Tuesday, November 22, 2016 at 12:30 pm at St Joseph's Hospital, or as we like to call it: The Hospital in the Corn Fields. They are singularly unsurpassed in the number of times they have incorrectly filed my insurance and I keep telling them the correct information but they keep filing the insurance claim with the WRONG insurance company—no matter WHAT I do! I would normally let them twist in the wind for their utter incompetence and stupidity, but their total lack of comprehension of these words: "I'm on Blue Cross MISSOURI, NOT ILLINOIS so you need to bill MISSOURI" creates work for my poor husband. I am so not looking forward to this because, while it might potentially tell me that I am going to live, it can just as easily tell me that I am toast and going to die in a few months. I didn't even want to have the MRI because I feel fine, but I have to know because John wants to take a fancy trip somewhere—the "Teri's Going To Die Tour" or fun, fun, fun—till Daddy takes the T-bird away. He wanted to go to New Zealand but if I'm going to die, I want to go to Germany and die drunk on good beer, sausages and pastries! If the radiologist gets the report done I MIGHT find out tomorrow. Either way I think I'm going to have to break training and have a drink or three depending on the news. I'm a trembling basket case at the moment. John has threatened to put me outside in the cold until I'm too tired, cold and hungry to keep doing the caged lioness pacing thing. The radio was playing "The Waiting is the Hardest Part" as I'm leaving the hospital after the MRI. God has a sense of humor and he drinks. Oh yeah—and his last name is Murphy. As there are no known survivors of this, I am prepared for the worst. However, I have to believe it must be doing SOMETHING because the general consensus is that I should be a LOT sicker and a lot easier to coerce into chemo but my oncologists are baffled. I gave every one of my oncologists a paper on GcMAF/Goleic and told them what I was doing and EVERY ONE of them glanced at it and pooh-poohed it without reading it. Now they are baffled and scratching their collective ignorant heads and wishing they'd kept the paper because I won't give it to them now. I don't want them interfering. They've literally done EVERYTHING short of holding a GUN to my head to try to force me to do chemo—they are utter scum. I am certain that if I had been a minor they would have tried, and probably succeeded in Obama's America, to get a court order to force me to be chemo-ed. I call the hospital and Vernie tells me that my report is ready and she left it with Judy at the reception desk so I throw on jeans and a t-shirt and race to the hospital in the cornfield and get the envelope containing the report. I'm crying by the time I reach the car and my hands are shaking like an alcoholic needing their first drink of the morning. From what I have learned about this cancer; it is extremely aggressive and doubles in size every 6 weeks or so in addition to seeding the peritoneum. I race home knowing John is on his way and as I park the car in the driveway, I tell myself that I've already resigned myself to dying from this and that there's no reason not to know. With shaking hands, I tear the envelope open and start to read the report that possibly tells me how much longer I will have to live and begin to read the report.

CHAPTER 33: I'VE A LOT TO BE THANKFUL FOR ON THANKSGIVING 2016

I read the report hyperventilating and shaking. The print is blurry through my shaking and tears and I have to read it 3 times for it to sink in. The largest tumor has NOT grown at all and appears to be more solid, but the smaller tumor HAS SHRUNK BY almost ¾ of a centimeter!! There's no mention of the small scattered milliary tumors so I am assuming they are gone. The bigger one has not increased in size and the smaller one is 0.7 cm smaller—and this cancer doesn't GET smaller so....the only possible conclusion is that the GcMAF/Goleic is working—it HAS to be or I'd be dead by now. While I am not out of the woods by a long shot, I've found the breadcrumb trail and hopefully it leads me to a cure. I have hope where before I had none. I go into the house and sit at the kitchen counter and read the report again looking over every word and I am still crying now—but it's relief and joy. I had been steeling myself for enormous tumors that would mean my death in February or maybe March —as the oncologists had told me would happen—but the GcMAF/Goleic is working!! IT'S WORKING!!! I might not die after all from the cancer that is 100% fatal—I might survive it and bring the news that there really IS a cure to all the cancer patients in America. I think of my sister who died a year and 4 days ago when this would have saved her life had she only listened to me when I BEGGED her to stop the chemo that eventually killed her and let me help her with the GcMAF/Goleic. She just would NOT listen to me—or maybe it was her dickhead ex-husband—she listened to him instead of me and paid for it with her life. I hear from the grapevine that HE has cancer now too, but I'll be damned if I want to tell him about GcMAF/Goleic—he deserves to die

MASS MURDERING DOCTORS: THE TRUTH ABOUT ONCOLOGISTS, CHEMOTHERAPY AND CANCER

the same horrible death that Lori died from the chemotherapy he was so sure was the only answer. However, I am sure that my mother will tell him since they are all buddy-buddy these days—after she loathed him with the fire of 1000 suns on steroids for a DECADE—NOW, after he killed the golden child by taking her to the Moffit Cancer Center with the most incompetent doctors in the state, she loves him. They pumped her full of their million-dollar 40-year-old chemo poison and told her she would be fine—which they HAD to know was a f**king LIE because this cancer is 100% fatal when it goes to peritoneal carcinomatosis which it did for her and for me. It's how BRCA1+ women die—this cancer kills a lot of us.

I have been given official confirmation that the GcMAF/Goleic has the ability and TIME to save my life even though the scumbag oncologists refused to remove the tumors without poisoning me with chemo first. I just have to figure out how to keep getting the GcMAF/Goleic over the border from Canada so that I can save my own life and bring the miracle cure of GcMAF/Goleic to every cancer patient in the world. If it cures my cancer with it's 100% mortality rate, it will cure ANY cancer, and I will become the ONLY known survivor of the deadliest cancer known. That should give me some credibility if nothing else! John walks in the door and sees me crying with the report in my hand and I tell him the good news—and we are both crying now. It's a snotfest of epic proportions and I'm going to have to buy stock in Kleenex soon with all the crying we've been doing since February 18th when I found out I had cancer. John has been giving me my GcMAF/Goleic injections intravenously and has gotten very good at it, and I am hoping my veins will continue to hold up since John isn't comfortable with anything but hand veins as they are easier to hit. We decide that a celebration dinner is in order and we will have to make some reservations for Saturday. I text the good news to my friends and family and they are all happy. I'm relieved for a lot of reasons, but the biggest one is that I now KNOW that if anything happens and my beloved nieces or nephews are struck with this terrible cancer that they WILL NOT DIE from it. That's what I am the most thankful for on this cold Thanksgiving Day in 2016. At the tender age of 57-almost-58 I have gotten a chance to live out my projected life span instead of dying 6 months after diagnosed with the killer cancer. I am giving thanks to God, First Immune, Dr. Yamamoto for discovering GcMAF/Goleic and Dr. Dan O'Connell for telling me about it. It HAS to be working and since it seems to be shrinking and killing the tumors, I am certain that my next MRI will show further shrinkage of this silent killer that steals so many lives—with the help of the corrupt medical establishment. My sister Lori lived 13 months from diagnosis to grave with every kind of chemo poison they could pump into her while lying to her about how she was going to get well. I know they knew she was going to die from the get-go, but the lousy bastards sold her false hope which is unforgivable in my view. It wasn't ENOUGH that the lying sacks of crap were banging her insurance for 100 grand a pop for their poisoned promises of a cure, they were lying to her every step of the way. I have lived LONGER with NO chemotherapy than she did with all they could give her; until she vomited from it SO VIOLENTLY that it ruptured her esophagus and she bled to death with my elderly parents watching it happen. It's monstrous and unforgivable and I curse them and will continue to curse them from heaven's door if it comes to that. BASTARDS!

I am reading the MRI reports more carefully, and it mentions that the largest tumor becomes "indistinct" with the bowel loops which is unusual and I also think it becomes indistinct because it's being eaten up by the macrophages—or at least I HOPE that's why. It also says that there are more solid components of the tumor which means that it is imploding as this cancer is not a dense highly undifferentiated cancer. Either way, I am certain that the immuno-juice has taken hold and if we stay the course, we might just pull this off. I think it took longer because I have a LOT of cancer and it's the MOST aggressive, malignant and deadly of ALL they gynecological cancers and I had a high tumor load. I am also certain that John giving me the shots IV is making a difference as well and while I feel bad that mom wants to go home, I feel that it is critical to my ultimate survival to keep doing the IV injections. I can run her to Louisiana if she needs to go which she doesn't as I have a year's worth of Rx refills for her diabetic meds and her AD meds are good through mid-January. I think that after the next MRI in 90 days the cancer should be much better and if the tumors are smaller then I can go to subcutaneous or intramuscular injections without compromising anything, but my life is hanging in the balance here and I am literally at the tipping point where we win or we go past the point of no return—which I am pretty sure I was close to and even though we have progress on this MRI, I'm not even close to out of the woods yet, this can still go south and very easily. Mom is going to have to suck it up a little longer—and she's not suffering NEARLY as much as she thinks (and wants US to think) nor is any doctor going to increase her pain meds as she's at the max that I would give her because of the danger of OD. She does the exact same thing here she does at home—reads the paper and watches the news, so her life is exactly the same but I can STILL—and very easily—die from this cancer. I can't get carried away because I am making progress because if I don't stay the course and backslide to the point of no return then I can still die from this wretched cancer. When I watch John do the IV push of the immuno-juice I mentally curse the tumors—and mentally scream at them: "DIE MotherFUCKERS!!!!!!

I'm still scared to death, but I know I have a CHANCE to beat this cancer for a real CURE and survive the unsurvivable cancer. I just have to stay the course with lousy painkillers and strict diet for another 3 to 9 months as this cure could take up to a year. I feel that since the tumors are starting to shrink that the GcMAF/Goleic activated macrophages now have the upper hand and are eating up the tumors and that the progress will pick up from this point—or at least I hope this is the case because I am still betting my life on this immuno-juice. It's definitely the acid test of putting my money where my mouth is, so to speak. I've bet my life on this—literally. There was nothing chemo or anything else could do, so if this didn't work, I was going to have to start making decisions and putting my affairs in order so that it wouldn't be a huge pain in the butt for my poor grieving husband, and to make sure that the transfer of my assets to him go smoothly. That I actually have a CHANCE to survive is just mind boggling. I had the results in an envelope and I could barely bring myself to open it as my hands were shaking so badly and I was crying so hard because I knew it could be bad—and since no one survives this, it was VERY likely to be bad news. I had to read it three times because I just couldn't believe it and I'm still scared —but now it's because I am terrified I'll screw this up. I have so many doubts and fears but the MRI went a long way to calming down my husband and settling my nerves but I'm more determined than ever to stay the course and hopefully win this battle for me and for all the cancer victims killed by oncologist and Big Pharma's greed, for all the cancer patients suffering through the bullcrap LIE that is chemotherapy and for the people in the future who will GET cancer and will NOT have to suffer through chemo because they will be able to call First Immune and get their

MASS MURDERING DOCTORS: THE TRUTH ABOUT ONCOLOGISTS, CHEMOTHERAPY AND CANCER

cancer CURED with the miracle that is GcMAF/Goleic because if it cures my cancer, it will cure ANY cancer. I'm rededicating myself to following this protocol as closely as possible, and the only thing left to worry about is whether or not I'll be able to continue to GET the GcMAF/Goleic from Canada and smuggle it over the border. I am making trip #4 next week and I'm scared—my LIFE is now literally going to depend on being able to smuggle the immuno-juice into the USA. How I loathe and despise the scumbags on the FDA who are willing to let me and every other cancer victim in the country DIE to protect the profits of Big Pharma. They like to tell you they need to charge all this money for research but it's nothing but bullcrap since the standard chemotherapy they use on EVERYONE is this chickencrap 40 year old protocol with the pathetic cure rate. The ones who really want it left alone are the oncologists who are marking this poison up 10,000% and reselling it to dying, desperate cancer victims who are scared out of their minds and willing to pay to be voluntarily poisoned by the most evil, greedy pieces of crap in the universe: their doctors. I do not understand how these oncologists live knowing what utter scum they are. How do they SLEEP at night??

CHAPTER 34: CANADA AYE? TRIP NUMBER 4, SOLO AND SCARED

Getting ready to go to Canada for the 4th time. I hope and pray that I've got what it takes to smuggle the GcMAF/Goleic into the country. I am going to need the steely nerves that John has so admirably demonstrated that HE has, I am going to have to rise to the occasion and suck up that my LIFE literally DEPENDS upon my being able to get this stuff back to the USA to keep attacking this terrible cancer. I have a grudging respect for the SOB cancer—it's tough as nails and doesn't want to lose. It's determined to kill me and it's about 10,000,000–0 and has NEVER lost at this stage of the game and it's NOT going to go gently into being dissolved into amino acids at the cellular level without a fight. It has taken 3 months to beat it back to where it starts to shrink and to kill off the milliary tumors, but we are on the track to a cure and as long I can keep using the GcMAF/Goleic—which means smuggling it back to the USA— I don't die. Not like there's any PRESSURE or my life hanging in the balance or anything like that. I am going to drive up, go pick up my GcMAF/Goleic and spend the night in Detroit, assuming I am not in JAIL and then head home the next morning.

MASS MURDERING DOCTORS: THE TRUTH ABOUT ONCOLOGISTS, CHEMOTHERAPY AND CANCER

I've decided to get the hotel room and drop off my gun and medical marijuana and all the other things I can't take into Canada. I'll drive over the border in a rental car—as they don't need to get my tag number and it's not unusual to have a rental car on a business trip which is my cover story. Also, I've been using medical marijuana which may have left traces of it in my car—not enough to be visible to the naked eye but what I really need is to get rid of the scent because if the dogs hit on the scent, they will tear my car apart to find medical marijuana that isn't even in the CAR which is why I'm renting a car. There won't BE any in the car, but they will still screw up my car and find the GcMAF/Goleic. It's simpler to rent a car for 2 days and just drive the rental to Canada. I want to go across the border while I'm tired from the long drive so that I won't be as jittery and nervous over my LIFE depending on my ability to smuggle unapproved medication over the border. I don't even know what they will do to me if I get caught. Will I go to jail? Prison? If I do, I'll die because I won't be able to get the GcMAF/Goleic if I'm locked up and I'll die from the cancer without it. I can't keep thinking this way or I will go NUTS long before I get to Canada. I am also worried about going in the winter as well since I'm a 5th generation Florida native and snow driving isn't something I have a lot of experience with or knowledge about doing. I usually stay home when it snows!

I'm still so very overwhelmed by the news in the MRI. I've had 5 months of getting my head around that I was going to die soon and the possibility that I might NOT die and have a CHANCE to survive has just been so earth-shaking that I'm having a really hard time getting my head around it. No one has ever survived this cancer. EVER. That's why my doctors are STUNNED that the immuno-juice is working. I'm sure the prayers had a lot to do with it as well. I didn't pray for a cure, I just prayed for God to SHOW me the way to a cure if it was His will, and I would do the rest. I'm just still in shock over it all—but I'm not out of the woods yet—not by a long shot.

I have to go to Canada on Tuesday morning to get December's immuno-juice as they questioned John rather extensively since he's been there 3 times in the last 3 months so it looks like he's making a regular trip to pick up something—which he is—so I'm going this time. John says I'm a terrible criminal with no ability to lie and he's worried sick. I'll be OK though. I'm doing the 500 mile drive and going over the border as soon as I get there so I should be tired enough not to be shaking with nerves. One of my friends who moved here from Detroit says they won't search an empty rental car or a purse/backpack since they are looking for CARLOADS of stuff so with a little luck (and a couple of pain meds to chill me if needed) I'll be all right. John also pointed out that a rental car won't have had time to be customized with a hidden compartment for smuggling, so it gives me a better chance of not being searched. I'm spending the night there so I'm dumping my bag with all my contraband and gun at the hotel and I'm also using a rental car to keep them from tagging my plate if I'm on a watch list. Luckily I don't fit the profile but I'm still scared to death—I'm such a chicken and my husband is SO brave I can't stand it! I go with John to pick up the rental car and we get a little bonus. The econo-box I rented for cheap isn't available (never is at this place) and they give me a big Toyota Highlander SUV for the trip. It's a great car, and it also fits what a woman like me would drive in the profile I am trying to fit: Affluent middle-aged woman with no criminal intent and no plans to do anything illegal other than smuggle lifesaving unapproved cancer drugs into America. It's not like my life hangs in the balance or anything like that....oh...wait..it DOES!

I've decided that I am going to channel my best CIA-agent inner self and that I am going to DO this. I'm going to GET OVER on the Customs agents at BOTH borders and bring my immuno-juice back home and laugh about how stupid they are when I get home. When this book comes out, they are going to be pretty hacked off about it but I do NOT care. They would let me die because corrupt elected officials have passed laws to prevent desperate, dying cancer patients from having ANY chance of being cured, and put them in jail for bringing a Vitamin-D binding protein into America. I don't have a choice and I can't fail—or I will die. No pressure there, aye?

Tuesday morning at 4 am I am up loading the car and hitting the interstate to the city where I will cross the border into Canada, go to the UPS depot and grab my immuno-juice, strip the labels and put them in the chilled case a GET them BACK over the border into America. I drive the 500 miles and stop at my hotel just long enough to check in and drop off things I can't take into Canada. I leave my big purse and grab a small handbag and put my passport, wallet and a few other things in it. I chew up a rescue med pain pill to further chill me out and get back on the road. I get to the

MASS MURDERING DOCTORS: THE TRUTH ABOUT ONCOLOGISTS, CHEMOTHERAPY AND CANCER

checkpoint on the Canada side where they ask me why I'm going to Canada and I tell them I'm doing some Christmas shopping and he waves me through and I follow my directions to the UPS depot and pick up the package and head for the Wal-mart where I rip open the package, take out the vials of GcMAF/Goleic and put them in the chilled case and pop it in the cooler. I throw away the shipping materials and customs forms in the Wal-mart trash can. I buy some things in the Wal-mart for John—he loves the Nestlé Aero bars and the Breton crackers so I buy several packages of each and leave the store. Now I just have to get over on the US Customs guy and I am home free for another month. I drive over the border and the Customs agent asks me what I bought and I show him the candy and crackers and he asks if I bought any alcohol and I tell him no and he waves me through the checkpoint and I am home free. I am almost collapsing with relief as I head back to the hotel—and the continuation of being able to treat my cancer for another month. I am exhausted from the drive and the stress of smuggling the GcMAF/Goleic back to the USA. I go into my hotel and lay down on the bed and take a few deep breaths and let the reality that I got the job done sink in. I also realize that I am starving so I look up some places to eat on Yelp and choose one. As I head out the door of the hotel, I see the Wendy's across the parking lot and realize that I can be eating in 5 minutes if I go there. I walk across the parking lot and get a couple of Junior cheeseburgers off the Dollar Menu and a large chili and head back to my room. I toss the burger buns and hash up the meat and stir it into the chili and pop it into the microwave to get it boiling hot to kill anything bad in it, since it was about room temperature when I bought it—another epic fail in food safety standards. I wolf it down, it's flavorless but I don't care and finish it and fall asleep checking my email. I woke up a couple of hours later and went and got another round of chili and cheeseburger patties and eat that as well. I go back to sleep and wake up around 5 am, get dressed and grab my stuff and head for home. I get back about 1 pm Central time and John and I return the Toyota to Enterprise and we grab some McDonald's for dinner and head for home. He gives me my shot IM since he couldn't hit the vein, a rare miss for him, and I drop like a rock and sleep the sleep of the righteous. I'm exhausted from the long (1000 mile round trip) drive and the poor sleep from the uncomfortable bed at the hotel. I would have expected to sleep from pure exhaustion, but it was not to be, so it's good to be home safe and not in jail in Canada for smuggling life-saving medication.

CHAPTER 35: STAYING THE COURSE AND SPREADING THE WORD

I now have definitive proof that the GcMAF/Goleic works. It is killing off the incurable cancer than came to kill me about 14 months ago. I have already survived LONGER with NO chemo than my poor sister who was 13 months from diagnosis to grave. She didn't have to die and the chemo killed her, not the cancer. If she had listened to me, she would have had a CHANCE to make medical history with me. I am going to survive this cancer as long as I keep doing what I'm doing and don't lose sight of the goal, and I feel guilty for being tired of being sick when I'm being spared the horrors of chemotherapy. I'm really tired of eating salmon that I hate. I've been eating zero sugar and carbs for a three quarters of a year now (and I've gone from a size 12 jeans to size 6s and may end up a size 4 before all this is over) so the diet isn't difficult for me to stick with since it's pretty close to my previous eating habits. I'd love some chocolate and a potato or some pasta or some rice. A couple of beers would also be awesome—but there's a whole world of carbs and beer out there for me when I beat this killer cancer. I'm surprised at how much I would like to have a beer and can't because of the sugar (maltose in beer is a 105 on the glycemic index so there's NO way I can have it, and since I rarely drink, I don't understand why I miss it so much. With this latest MRI showing that the GcMAF/Goleic is starting to kill off the tumors—that I believe I have at least a fighting chance to beat this. If I do, I am going to blow the whistle on Big Pharma. They killed my sister just like they've killed so many people's sisters and Moms. Dads. Wives. Husbands. Grandparents. Cousins. Brothers. Uncles. Children. Aunts. It's time to end the scourge that is cancer and the scumbags that profit from the suffering and death of their fellow human being.

That's the half of me that thinks we can beat this cancer and then spread the word and shout it from the mountaintops wanting to save people from this horrible suffering for profit racket these oncologists seem to have going on. The other half of me is telling me to be cautiously optimistic and lay low and not attract attention. Good advice considering I still have to smuggle the GcMAF/Goleic into the country for another year maybe—so I need to be discreet until I am CURED of this killer cancer.

MASS MURDERING DOCTORS: THE TRUTH ABOUT ONCOLOGISTS, CHEMOTHERAPY AND CANCER

I'm also surprised by how emotionally fragile and needy I am right now. Everyone is telling me how brave and courageous I am because I literally bet my life on this immune-strengthening drug but I'm not brave, I'm scared to death. I prayed for God to show me the way and if I survived this, I'd do my very best to spread the message and deliver his children from the suffering of cancer, and I will. Right now, I'm in no condition to do that; I'm an emotional cripple at the moment with everything that has happened but I am going to regroup and soldier on. I believe that God has allowed me to find this cure and has allowed it to work so that I can spread the word to ALL of the cancer victims in the world. I believe that Big Pharma will have me killed or silenced in some way, but if that happens, this book will serve as my legacy and will carry hope to cancer victims like myself that there is a cure and that they do not have to be poisoned with useless chemotherapy that does not worth to enrich BigPharma and the oncologists of the world who pretend to care but don't. GcMAF/Goleic is the CURE. If it cures my cancer, it will cure ANY cancer. I have put my story on a website that tells you how to order GcMAF/Goleic and to contact me or First Immune for help with cancer. They are terrific people and they have the CURE: info@help.vg and my website which has info and a synopsis of my story is here at the website I built to share my story. www.GcMAFCancerCure.com Go there if you want to live. I am hoping to prevent an assassination attempt by BigPharma by the public knowledge that there is a cure and that if something happens (or has happened) to me, that it was NO ACCIDENT and that I was murdered in order to protect the hundreds of billions of dollars in chemotherapy PROFITS for the scumbag oncologists and BigPharma worldwide. These people that are being murdered by chemo and "doctors" are the real victims of the bribery of the FDA and the greed of our elected officials for their thinly disguised as "campaign donations" bribes. My life means NOTHING compared to the huge amounts of MONEY they will lose with the cure. It's another h.Pylori scandal in the making and they cannot have that—or their lickspittle lackeys the oncologists who push their 40-year old POISON losing the 80% of their income that is generated by FAILED chemotherapies. The supreme irony here is that if there were oncologists CURING CANCER with GcMAF/Goleic they could probably charge ANYTHING they wanted and people would pay it. What's your life worth? However, they either don't know—or don't care which is worse. I could understand them

MASS MURDERING DOCTORS: THE TRUTH ABOUT ONCOLOGISTS, CHEMOTHERAPY AND CANCER

pushing their poison if they sincerely believed it worked, but that they MUST KNOW how useless it is and are poisoning people for PROFIT makes it that much more insidious and evil and means they are essentially mass murderers. I'm angry that they murdered my beautiful baby sister who kept ME beautiful with her professional skills. I didn't just lose my sister, I also lost my hairdresser of over 30 years! My hair is never going to look right again and my niece and two nephews are orphans because of the LIES of Big Pharma and I'm pissed off about it. I'm further enraged by the fact that they tried to kill me as well with their million-dollar USELESS CHEMOTHERAPY POISON and I have dedicated the rest of my life to spreading the word and bringing them down. GcMAF/Goleic is saving my life and can save the life of ANY cancer patient. The lies of Big Pharma killed my sister and I'm going to bring them to task for it. I can't bring Lori back—I wish to GOD I could—but I can't. I can, however, try to prevent them from continuing upon their campaign of mass murder and torture of cancer victims. The truth will set you free—but first it will **PISS YOU OFF!!**

CHAPTER 36: THE WAITING IS THE HARDEST PART, PART DEUX

I'm back to the waiting. I'm seriously considering going back to work full time but I am also very emotionally fragile at the moment and get panicky when John isn't around. I find his presence comforting and reassuring—as if nothing bad can ever happen to me while he's looking after me and I don't have to be afraid. I've got a lot of motivation to beat this cancer but there's another factor as well. Big Pharma murdered my sister with their lies and false hope to convince her to keep letting them bill her insurance for the USELESS chemo that had ZERO chance of helping her. I begged her to listen to me—on my KNEES but she believed the lies they told her about the "next chemo should be the one" that killed all her tumors that were like mushrooms. She didn't die from the cancer. She bled to DEATH in front of my elderly PARENTS from a ruptured esophagus brought on by chemo-induced vomiting. The doctors murdered her for my parents to watch—as if losing a child just wasn't ENOUGH. I'm mad about it—and if I survive this cancer, I am going to make it my life's work to make them pay for it. I want GcMAF/Goleic to be the only medicine people even consider using for so many things—because it works!

MASS MURDERING DOCTORS: THE TRUTH ABOUT ONCOLOGISTS, CHEMOTHERAPY AND CANCER

I'm finding it very difficult to get my head around that I might live. When I had no hope, I had resigned myself to the fact that I was going to die from this cancer as the tumors blossomed and grew like mushrooms in my pelvis until they crowded out and compressed the visceral organs and prevent them from functioning and I die. I was OK with it after I got my head around it, I am a woman of faith and I've had some close brushes with death already in my life. I'm not afraid to die. I've had an amazing life and if I died tomorrow I would still think I was the luckiest SOB that ever drew breath. I have had some time to get used to the idea of dying and now I am looking at the possibility that I might not die. Maybe God has a plan and I was supposed to cure my sister and when that didn't work out God gave me the cancer so that I'd cure the incurable cancer and spread the word that there is a cure. I've put up a website, and I've taken steps to protect the truth because if I do become the only known survivor of this cancer and become a threat to Big Pharma's hundreds of billions of profits, they will have me killed. They are already murdering over a million people a year with their criminally overpriced poison and one more death means NOTHING to them. Oddly enough, in the last two years, 60 doctors who were using GcMAF/Goleic to cure their patients of cancer have been MURDERED and to date, no one has been arrested or charged with these murders. I have no doubt that they would try to silence me as well. I am a woman of faith and I believe strongly that God has shown me the cure and allowed me to find the way to survive the unsurvivable cancer so that I could try to stop the slaughter of his children for the greed of Big Pharma and their oncologist lickspittle lackeys who push their poison for profit. EVERY SINGLE ONE of them KNEW AND KNOW that the chemo treatment, to which they tried to make me submit, could NOT HELP ME and that the only reason to give me chemo was for PROFIT. The same platinum-based chemo that they tried to force on me—A FORTY YEAR OLD PROTOCOL—is the first-line treatment for virtually ALL tumor cancers. Chemo kills 50% of the patients, NOT the cancer.

SIDEBAR: HERE ARE SOME MORE TERRIFIC FACTS ABOUT CHEMOTHERAPY

Chemotherapy is a 100 year old poison that started life out as World War One mustard gas. In the Auschwitz concentration camp they experimented on inmates

MASS MURDERING DOCTORS: THE TRUTH ABOUT ONCOLOGISTS, CHEMOTHERAPY AND CANCER

and started using it as a medicine. Today globally 1.5 million people a year are murdered by chemotherapy for profit.

Every doctor who prescribes it breaks his Hippocratic oath to "administer no poison". It is a $200 billion dollar industry mostly based in the USA. The chemo lobby is possibly the most powerful in the world. They've changed the laws in most western countries so that only their product, the poison of chemotherapy, is allowed to be prescribed by doctors. And good, life saving treatments for cancer, of which there are many, are concealed from patients who are pressured into chemo, usually with ghastly results. The oncologists I have seen: Francisco Xynos MD, Karuna Murray MD and Brian Slomowitz MD all tried to FORCE me to have chemo as a pre-condition to them surgically removing my tumors that were the smaller than the first joint of my thumb. They **LIED TO ME** by telling me that they had to shrink the tumors before they could be removed. This is an absolute f**king lie—they routinely remove BENIGN (non-cancerous) tumors that weigh 20 POUNDS or more without "having to shrink them first" because it's impossible coerce someone who doesn't have cancer and is terrified of dying into allowing themselves to be voluntarily POISONED for profit. Also, it's illegal to poison people and chemo drugs are POISON, plain and simple. If someone gave you this poison who either wasn't a doctor or you didn't have cancer, they would be arrested for attempted MURDER if you live and Murder if you die. My sister didn't die from her cancer. She died from a ruptured esophagus brought on by chemotherapy-induced vomited so VIOLENT that she ruptured her esophagus and BLED TO DEATH IN FRONT OF MY PARENTS in November of 2015. Her death certificate reads "CANCER" but it's a lie. The scumbag oncologist(s) sold her false hope and robbed her of three-quarters of a million dollars to treat a cancer that DOES NOT RESPOND TO IV CHEMOTHERAPY ACCORDING TO EVERY RESEARCH PAPER ON THE SUBJECT. The side effects of chemo are nothing short of horrific – your organs shut down, you may lose the sight of one or both eyes, you get "chemo brain" where your brain is often permanently damaged and you can't function, you may become unable to walk due to painful neuropathy in your feet and hands, severe vomiting, anemia from red blood cells being killed, your immune system is totally destroyed meaning any kind of infection can kill you AND you get cancer AGAIN in a few years (guaranteeing FUTURE PROFITS for Big Pharma) mouth sores that keep you from

MASS MURDERING DOCTORS: THE TRUTH ABOUT ONCOLOGISTS, CHEMOTHERAPY AND CANCER

eating along with ulcers in your intestines/bowel—losing all your hair is irrelevant by comparison! Many of these side effects are or can be PERMANENT.

Worse, chemo totally and absolutely destroys your immune system and blood counts, so particularly in stage 4, you are likely to to catch some infection you would normally have fought off and die from it. Many chemo drugs are listed as "a known carcinogen." The poison is so powerful that nurses who administer it have to be protected from it with gloves and monthly tests. Some chemos can't become safe even if they are heated to 1,800 degrees centigrade. John Cairns of Harvard University published in Scientific American that chemo drugs help, at most, one in 20 of people they are given to, my research shows the cure rate to be 2.1% with all of them happy to die to end the suffering. I've lived LONGER with NO chemo than my poor sister lived with every chemo (and all that false hope) the scumbag oncologists sold her.

CHEMO MAKES CANCER CELLS IMMORTAL

"When chemotherapy (is given) to kill the bulk of your cancer cells, a small remnant of these stem cells regenerate and renew the cancer, too" --------Siddhartha Mukherjee, MD "The Emperor of All Maladies" According to the Fred Hutchinson Cancer Research Center, Seattle, Washington, USA in their WNT16B paper, cancer cells become resistant to chemo, "chemotherapy resistance" which makes the disease worse. Yes, chemo may shrink a tumor, but it makes the cancer come back stronger, and with your immune system totally gone, your body has NOTHING LEFT TO FIGHT WITH— NO IMMUNE SYSTEM to fight off what I am certain is an immunotherapy disease. In particular it usually creates the secondaries that kill you 2 years later. The FDA considers ANY treatment that shrinks a tumor by 50% for 28 days to be an effective cancer treatment. Shrinking a tumor doesn't do JACK crap toward curing cancer but the bought and paid for Big Pharma whores on the FDA don't care how many people are suffering and dying from a curable disease as long as they protect their 200-300 BILLION a year—EVERY YEAR—in profits. They control organizations. The FDA in the USA has chemotherapy corporation directors on its board. They want $900 million spent over ten years before they will authorize a new drug. That way they ensure no inexpensive, effective treatment ever makes it to the public which protects their blood money profits, they are the scum of the EARTH. The FDA will license a chemo drug

MASS MURDERING DOCTORS: THE TRUTH ABOUT ONCOLOGISTS, CHEMOTHERAPY AND CANCER

provided it is below LD-50. That means a lethal dose, it ONLY kills 50% of lab animals that they test it on, so if it kills ONLY half of the rats, it will be approved. Think about that one: The FDA standard for drug safety is known as LD 50, LD stands for lethal dose, and **the 50 is the percentage threshold of lab animals poisoned to death by the drug tested**. As long as the percentage killed is under 50%, FDA will approve it! In the UK they fund the MHRA, which is the British FDA that licenses drugs in England. Their men (BigPharma) sit on the boards of licensing authorities so the drug companies license their own drugs. That's why they kill so many—around 2 million people a year including chemotherapy.

Cancer Research is still fraudulently raising money for cancer research when more than enough cures have already been found. It trashes and discredits these, to promote chemotherapy. All they care about is protecting the profits of oncologist and Big Pharma. The Big Pharma lobby is in government medical departments, making laws. They control charities with their directors on its board. American Cancer Society fraudulently raises money to find a cure for cancer, when a dozen cures have been found over the last 100 years. They use the money they raise to trash established cures—because if people know the cures have been found, there is no point in giving money to any "Cancer Research" charity since they spend 90% plus of their donations on salaries and "administrative expenses" which means they are not doing any kind of research, they are bloated, festering cash sucking cows, interested only in the survival and perpetuation of their false narrative. The charity should either concentrate on getting the cures out to the people, or close itself down and put its officers up for trial, arrest and imprisonment, because it has been killing people by concealing the truth. **Their real purpose is to push the poison of chemotherapy and increase the profits of the pharmaceutical corporations.**

Big Pharma uses these "charities" to attack university professors, PhD's and doctors who are researching or using excellent treatments that are a threat to chemotherapy and other drugs. They try to get scientifically excellent research papers that are published in prestigious journals retracted if they are a threat to their drugs. If you try to update Wikipedia pages they don't like, for example, by adding the names of scientific research papers, in minutes someone has deleted it. As an experiment I checked this out and my entry was erased in 2 minutes. Wiki enables you to have an email conversation with them, and they don't give a damn about the lies and destruction they perpetrate. Who funds them? It can only be chemo controlled charities. Whereas most doctors and nurses are doing their best. the people at the top of the medical and pharmaceutical industries are deeply involved with murder for profit. It's a BigPharma scam, a mafia, but they kill many millions more than the mafia's few hundred victims. There are many pharmaceutical company directors, medical government officials and hospital directors/managers who need to be arrested on criminal charges. They are murdering cancer patients—desperate, frightened and suffering people for MONEY. It's wrong—WAY wrong. I want to stop them and this book is part of the way I want to do it. Only by making the public aware of the cures that DO exist; will there be a chance to stop the death merchants from continuing to profit from the DEATHS of innocent, frightened cancer-stricken people who TRUST THEM to save their lives. They are treating them with 40 year old poisons that kills most of them and makes the doctors rich and BigPharma richer from the suffering and deaths of cancer victims. It's WRONG—no it's WAY f**king WRONG and if I survive this killer cancer, I am making it my life's work to STOP the slaughter of innocent people who BELIEVE that doctors are supposed to help them. My experience is that oncologists are the scum of the Earth, and to my dying breath I will try to stop them from their ongoing genocidal behavior toward cancer patients. Also, the **American Cancer Society is a fraud**. They are using your donations to trash REAL cures as **NINETY PERCENT of the money they weasel from the public is spent on salaries and expenses, NOT research**.

Ask yourself this: If they are doing all this research, then **why is the PRIMARY FRONT-LINE treatment for cancer STILL a 40-year old protocol?** They are using your donations to keep you sick and dying. Do NOT support the ACS, or the Susan G. Komen foundation, they are robbing you blind. They are liars and in bed with Big Pharma using donations to keep information from REAL cures from being spread online.

I bet MY OWN LIFE on the efficacy of GcMAF/Goleic—MY life. Not money, not a material item, but my OWN f**king LIFE that this would work for me and cure the

MASS MURDERING DOCTORS: THE TRUTH ABOUT ONCOLOGISTS, CHEMOTHERAPY AND CANCER

cancer that has **NO KNOWN SURVIVORS** for one reason: I believe the science and I am making the ultimate put up of shut up bet. I have never had ANY chemotherapy and I NEVER will. I believe in GcMAF/Goleic all the way. It's working far better than ANY chemo has EVER worked on any victim of high-grade serous-cell carcinoma and I know this because there are no survivors of HGSC when there has been a recurrence. NO SURVIVORS. If you don't think this is scary, think again. I went in for surgery to prevent a cancer I that I had NO idea that I already had. Then, I have a recurrence NINETY DAYS after two top surgeons tell me that they got 100% of my tumor and that I am cancer free, so I go from cancer free to terminal in 3 months! THEN I find out that I have the MOST deadly cancer there is—that there are no survivors and that chemo cannot help me. My only choice was to do the research and use my brain and education to find a scientifically solid CURE—because every oncologist I saw had nothing to say but "chemo, chemo, chemo!!" and was determined to poison me to the point that the greedy bastards turn down $6500 or so for a 45 minute surgery to remove 2 walnut size tumors to give the immunotherapies a better chance. Both of them insisted on the lie that they had to "shrink the tumors" before removal which as we already know is a bullcrap lie. If you have cancer, you better get proactive about saving YOUR OWN life because if you let the oncologists chemo you, then you WILL die. Not right away though—unless you die from the chemo which 50% of cancer patients do, you will have chemo and be sick and suffering for a year and when you start feeling better, your cancer will be back. Then the oncologists bang you for ANOTHER million bucks worth of poison because THEY CAN—you're desperate to live. If by chance you happen to be one of the 2.1% who are cured, then in ALL likelihood you will get ANOTHER cancer (metachronous cancer) in a few years FROM THE CHEMO so that you can start the poison, the MILLION-DOLLAR chemotherapy AGAIN until it finally kills you in 1-8 years of suffering and sickness and you're GLAD to die instead of facing chemotherapy again. THIS is your new reality. If you don't want that, then you better call First Immune because not only will you be CURED—not a stupid "remission" but CURED once and for all. **CANCER IS AN IMMUNO-DEFICIENCY disease, plain and simple and once your immune system is rebuilt and retrained your cancer is CURED and it will NEVER COME BACK.** No side effects either! It's a stupidly simple protocol to follow as well. Here's my treatment. While the NO-carb diet was boring and monotonous (not to mention how much I totally loathe and despise salmon) it's necessary and low-carb/no sugar kicks the crap out of the horrific "treatment" that is chemo. Here's what you have to do:

1. You MUST take injections of GcMAF/Goleic/Goleic as recommended by First Immune

2. You MUST adhere to a no-sugar and low-carb diet no matter how much you weigh

3. You MUST take 10-20,000 IUs per day of Vitamin-D3 (not regular vitamin D)

4. You MUST take 200 mcg of Vitamin K2 (again, not regular vitamin K)

5. It's best to eat: Salmon, Chicken livers, White meats, yogurt, pickles and other fermented foods. You WILL lose weight, but you won't be sick. Your weight will stabilize down the road and even though you might get skinny, you will be OK. Check with First Immune if you have any questions. They are not doctors but they know the protocols for successful cancer treatments and they know their product inside and out and are terrific about answering your questions. They are very good about replying to emails in a timely manner and you are always able to call them even if it is an international call. David Noakes is a great man and he is making history every DAY with the actual cure for cancer, and fighting BigPharma lies and corrupt politicians EVERY DAY to bring it to millions of cancer patients. Your oncologist has half a million reasons (and all of them are dollars) to poison you for fun and profit and only YOU can stop them. Say NO to the fake "cure" and YES to the real one! It's not easy to take a leap of faith when your doctor is trying to kill you, but if you want to live, you need to do it. I'm right now watching one of my dearest friends deal with her daughter being poisoned by chemo, another one I begged not to do it. However, when all your insurance will pay for is chemotherapy, the people who can't afford to pay for the GcMAF/Goleic/Goleic are stuck being poisoned and murdered by their "doctors" which is one MORE reason that immunotherapies MUST become the front-line treatment for all cancers and get rid of chemotherapy once and for all!

CHAPTER 37: MOTOWN HERE I COME AGAIN, SCARED AND DETERMINED!

On my way to Detroit and Windsor in January 2017 with a container of hot cocoa mix and a cake for Abdul and his family, as it turns out they liked the mix a lot. I pick up

MASS MURDERING DOCTORS: THE TRUTH ABOUT ONCOLOGISTS, CHEMOTHERAPY AND CANCER

my immuno-juice and do some shopping at Wal-Mart and slide back across the USA border without incident although I was sure the Customs agent could hear my heart pounding. Since I was in an Illinois-plated vehicle, they didn't realize it was a rental car—or maybe he did. They have that little screen that they look at and you can't see what they are reading and I'm sure they are waiting for me to start babbling so I focus on being pleasant and polite and not in a hurry and so far we've made 5 successful smuggling trips so I am not as terrified as I was on the first time, but I'm still scared crapless. If I lose a shipment, not only will I go on a list, but I may not be able to get into Canada again to get my immuno juice so I'd have to start enlisting friends to take a terrible risk for me—and I know they would—but I SO HATE to ask. It's scary creepy and so very hard to do and I wonder if they recognize me—and how long will my shopping story hold up? I bought $125.00 worth of stuff at Wal-mart no less and while I like what I bought, I'm going to go to Costco next time—I hear they have stuff you just can't get at the USA stores. I hate all the chemicals in the clothes in the USA, the ones in Canada don't have that—so much softer and nicer—and CHEAPER. Anyway, I make it back to the hotel, have another yummy Wendy's meal and pass out from exhaustion and slept until 8 am. I loaded up the rental Prius—a fricking GOLF CART car (my husband also has a Prius so he laughed his butt off when I ended up with a rental one) if there ever was one and headed back to IL and turned in the car. Another month of immunotherapy bringing me closer to the clean MRI I have to have in order to be cured. I have to take the shots for 8 weeks after I have a clean MRI and then I should never have a recurrence—I will be cancer-free for the rest of my life. I get back home without incident and pack up Mama G for the return to Louisiana since there's no reason for us to freeze in January in Illinois .

I get my mother in law packed up and the car loaded and we leave for Baton Rouge for some warmer weather until I have to go back to Canada in February. John wants to go, but I am worried about it. If I go to jail we have problems but he would still have his job and our health insurance so it is better if I take the risk. Then, my final nightmare comes true. Lori's two youngest children BOTH popped the test for BRCA1+ and my oldest nephew (with 2 kids of his own, my "grands" that I love) was recently tested after being mercilessly coerced by me. My oldest nephew has been waiting for the results of his genetic testing and finally he calls me and tells me he is

MASS MURDERING DOCTORS: THE TRUTH ABOUT ONCOLOGISTS, CHEMOTHERAPY AND CANCER

also BRCA1+ and when we stopped talking and he hung up, I cried for a solid hour. I had so hoped and PRAYED that this terrible genetic defect would pass him—even though it tagged his siblings, this was not to be and now my two grands are also at risk. I am just sick about this. On a 50-50 shot, Lori was 3 for 3; she passed the BRCA1+ genetic defect to EVERY one of her kids. It was all I could do to STOP crying I was so upset from the news. I can't believe that ALL of my beloveds share the BRCA1+ genetic killer and worse—Justin may have already passed it on to either or BOTH of his two children. It's better to KNOW though—and that means that ANY symptom that MIGHT be cancer WILL be thoroughly investigated instead of the kids being told "You're too young for cancer" because when you are BRCA1+ you are NEVER too young for cancer.

As heartbroken as I am that all the kids got the defect, it galvanizes my resolve to continue the battle against cancer and chemo. It's now it is more important than EVER that I make this CURE the front-line mainstream treatment for cancer. I have to survive this unsurvivable cancer and I have to take on BigPharma who will not doubt try to silence me one way or the other. The easiest way to silence me would be the keep me from getting the immuno-juice (GcMAF/Goleic) and let the cancer do their dirty work for them which is why this book can't come out until I am cancer-free which I am hoping will be in the summer. First Immune says it takes six to eighteen months to become cancer-free so I hope that my March MRI will show that the tumors are still shrinking and then I can breathe a little bit. I was literally holding my breath for the results of the November MRI which were good enough to let us all take a breath. I was supposed to be dead by now, but I still don't have as much as a swollen lymph node so while I might die in January, it's NOT going to be in January 2017 since it's the 14th of January as I type this, symptom free.

My mother sent me a text that said she was very proud of me and compared me to Jonas Salk (as mothers will do) and said that I was always the tenacious one willing to fight for what I believed in. What I'm fighting for now is to stop the slaughter of over a million people worldwide who are murdered by BigPharma's poison chemotherapy every year. They profit 200-300 BILLION a year, EVERY YEAR, from pushing their poison with it's 2.1% cure rate—that causes future cancer down the road and results in—wait for it: MORE CHEMO which equals MORE PROFITS. With GcMAF/Goleic the cure is permanent and there is never a recurrence of the cancer. First Immune is the only place in the world that is making this product right now and while it is saving lives, Big Pharma and the rest of the worldwide conspiracy to push chemo are desperate to keep it quiet and off of the market. They don't care how many people suffer and die as long as their profits are protected. Do you have a loved one who went through chemo? Remember what that was like? 2 million people go through chemo every year. HALF OF THEM DIE FROM THE CHEMO yet they will not consider an alternative because the message of the media is that chemo is the ONLY way. It's not and they are only looking to protect their profits. It is my most fervent hope that President Trump brings them to heel and allows Americans to have the CURE for cancer than isn't the poison chemo that doesn't work. It's the only chance for the cure that so many cancer victims are desperate to have—who would submit to chemo unless they were in fear of dying? NO ONE would and that's what the scumbag oncologists and Big Pharma is counting on—fear of dying make the nightmare of being slowly poisoned to death with chemo seem like a viable alternative. It has to stop!

CHAPTER 38: ANOTHER MONTH, ANOTHER TRIP AND ANOTHER MRI

I am getting ready for another trip to Canada to pick up my immuno-juice and I am faced with a dilemma. First Immune has asked me to courier some GcMAF/Goleic to people who desperately need it and can't get to Canada to pick it up. I am terrified but I don't see how I can say no. I can explain away 10 vials of GcMAF/Goleic as insulin for my diabetic husband but I can't explain a crapload of vials, I don't think I can take the risk of more than 25-30 bottles unless I did it in 2 or 3 trips—but again with the bar codes on the passports these days, they'll know I've made several trips over the border in a short amount of time. I don't know the details yet, but I am compelled to help other people who are in need of this medicine but the risk is much bigger than I am comfortable with and if I get caught, I will also die from the cancer. My survival literally depends upon continuing to get the immuno-juice and if I get caught by Customs, I am going to be in BIG f**king trouble and I will also DIE because of not being able to go to Canada and get it. This is my last trip for a while as my husband will be picking up the March shipment as after three trips in a row they

MASS MURDERING DOCTORS: THE TRUTH ABOUT ONCOLOGISTS, CHEMOTHERAPY AND CANCER

looked hard at him and asked a lot of extra questions and spooked him a bit so I've made the last 2 trips by myself. I'm going to do this for them, but I shouldn't do it at all because it increases the risk and it's my 3rd trip in a row and I'm scared. I'm going to just have to pray and hope that my faith and that God will get me through it because it's for a good cause—to keep another terrified cancer patient from dying and to give someone hope who has none and save their life as part of it. Isn't that worth a chance? I'm so torn though—they tell me these people couldn't GET to Canada but I managed to get to Canada even though I had to go to Miami and get a same-day passport which was a massive up-charge for the same day service—a $120 passport ended up costing me just under $300 and then there's the $100+ for the rental car and another $75-100 for the hotel room for the night in Detroit plus I'm going to have to pay the duty on ALL the vials. I'm hoping they will change their minds and find another way because I'm too much of a terrified coward to pull this off and it could cost me my life if it causes me to be deprived of the GcMAF/Goleic while I am in PRISON for international smuggling. I was scared before just bringing back mine, but now there will be other people depending on me to get their GcMAF/Goleic back. I hope that they don't want me to smuggle a ton of it in because I can't explain why I would need THAT much insulin and it's imperative that I continue my treatment.

I receive an email and they want to ship an extra 10 bottles for me to get to someone else in the USA who cannot get to Canada to pick up their own. I am willing to do it, I would do ANYTHING for these people, I owe them my life and I will also be helping to save the life of another cancer victim. This is really the only thing that matters but if I get caught, I will be in BIG trouble, although I am confident in my cover story as it is rock solid thanks to my doctor being on board and helping me. John said he was going to make the March trip, but I still have to get this shipment across. I'm terrified, but I have to do it—there's no way I can say no to them—I owe them my LIFE as I should have died in November 2016 so I'm living on time THEY gave me. I told them that I will be dedicating the rest of my life to getting GcMAF/Goleic to be the only needed front-line cancer treatment and I'm going to enjoy the hell out of strolling into the medical board hearing on the complaint I made about Karuna Murray—who I am sure expects me to die before her medical board hearing. She's going to crap when I come stroking into the hearing and I want the b*tch's medical license for

MASS MURDERING DOCTORS: THE TRUTH ABOUT ONCOLOGISTS, CHEMOTHERAPY AND CANCER

trying to poison me when she KNEW—HAD TO KNOW—that her poison would do nothing but make me suffer and her a cool half million dollars, and if she DIDN'T know, she's got NO business being an oncologist so she's screwed no matter what.

John wanted to do the February smuggling run, but he doesn't know about the extra bottles and I am not going to tell him. It's between me and First Immune this time. I've been getting in touch with other anti-chemotherapy activists and the extra bottles are going to save the life of an infant who was chemo-ed NINE TIMES and was on death's door until he was given GcMAF/Goleic for two weeks, he's now tumor free in his belly and is being given GcMAF/Goleic via nebulizer to kill the cancer in his lungs and it's working. He looked like an Auschwitz baby 3 weeks ago, now he's all pink and plumping out—like a beautiful baby SHOULD look. To save the life of a baby, I WILL take the risk. They are sending 20 vials instead of 10 since I told them I could never explain more than 25 bottles because no one would carry that much insulin. I'll tell John when it's over and the delivery has been made because he will not be happy about my taking a bigger risk than necessary—not that it matters because if I get searched, I won't be in any more trouble than I already am for smuggling my OWN GcMAF/Goleic so it doesn't matter. It just makes my cover story a little less plausible, but I can also say that we just filled his prescription for the month and that he goes through 20 vials a month, after all there's only 2.2 mL of liquid in a vial—less than a ½ of a teaspoon. I will have to stick to my story like glue and have a refilled bottle with actual insulin if they decide to test it, but with the doctor's letter, the other diabetic medications that John actually DOES take, and the refilled bottle my cover should hold even with fairly close scrutiny. The only issue I will have is if they crack the seal on an unopened bottle because that would obviously NOT be insulin. This isn't even a DRUG—it's a Vitamin-D binding protein. I have GOT to get a meeting with President Trump and get this stuff available to cancer patients so that people can at least have a CHOICE other than the quackery that is chemotherapy. In the interim, I HAVE to get over on these guys again—my life depends on it. I just channel my inner CIA agent again and make up my mind to get over on them and laugh about it later. My LIFE hangs in the balance, so that's a LOT of pressure and they look for nervous people and ask nonsensical questions to see if you will lie. I play the role of earnest middle-aged citizen-shopper to perfection. I do stuff they don't expect. I

MASS MURDERING DOCTORS: THE TRUTH ABOUT ONCOLOGISTS, CHEMOTHERAPY AND CANCER

bought apples on the last trip and pretended to have a little freak out and turn myself in since the sign says "no fruits or vegetables" so I handed him the bag of 3 little apples and said "I'm really sorry—I—I didn't know they were forbidden and look scared. Honest people are ALWAYS afraid—scumbags have attitude. I learned that from my cop husband and he was right. When they asked me how much cash I had, instead of guessing, I whipped out my wallet and started counting it in front of him and he stopped me when I started counting the change in the ashtray. Honest people don't want to make mistakes either. What they don't know and hopefully will never find out is that I have CIA-level training and have a backup cover story that dovetails with idiot tourist woman persona and it's pretty ironclad and would be very difficult to disprove without a lot of research and they won't (hopefully) have the resources to check out. I'm a sly wench but I've never gotten so much as a parking ticket in my whole life, but I'm also now an international smuggler as well. Hard to reconcile and if my life didn't hang in the balance, I wouldn't do it, obviously. The good news is that they are not looking for affluent, middle-aged women shoppers and you'd never know I have cancer to look at me—because I refused chemo. I'm not the droids they are looking for and hopefully my Jedi mind tricks will get me back over the border for another month of the fight against the cancer trying to kill me—as desperately as I am trying to kill it. One of us is going to die before this is over, and it could EASILY be me. Interestingly, I came across the FDA regulations about bringing in GcMAF/Goleic. It is not illegal to bring in an unapproved drug (although GcMAF/Goleic isn't a drug, it's a vitamin D binding protein) under the following circumstances:

Is it legal for me to personally import drugs?

In most circumstances, it is illegal for individuals to import drugs into the United States for personal use. This is because drugs from other countries that are available for purchase by individuals often have not been approved by FDA for use and sale in the United States. For example, if a drug is approved by Health Canada (FDA's counterpart in Canada) but has not been approved by FDA, it is an unapproved drug in the United States and, therefore, illegal to import. FDA cannot ensure the safety and effectiveness of drugs that it has not approved. FDA, however, has a policy explaining that it typically does not object to personal imports of drugs that FDA has not approved under certain circumstances, including the following situations:

The drug is for use for a serious condition for which effective treatment is not available in the United States;

There is no commercialization or promotion of the drug to U.S. residents;

The drug is considered not to represent an unreasonable risk;

The individual importing the drug verifies in writing that it is for his or her own use, and provides contact information for the doctor providing treatment or shows the product is for the continuation of treatment begun in a foreign country; and

Generally, not more than a 3-month supply of the drug is imported.

Courtesy of the FDA website:
http://www.fda.gov/AboutFDA/Transparency/Basics/ucm194904.htm

Apparently it's not as illegal as I thought as long as I bring it in personally and if you have cancer, you should be able to hit on every single one of these qualifications to bring your GcMAF in from Canada to the USA. This takes the pressure down a few notches on the border crossing because apparently if the Customs officials find my GcMAF, I should be able to bring it into the USA without an issue. I need another letter from Dr. Janet, but I shouldn't have any issue getting it, and this information might make it easier for me to get this medicine into the USA.

The trip to Canada was harrowing to say the least! Security was tighter than I have EVER seen it at any entry port in any country. There were ICE agents walking through the cars waiting in line and going through them. They searched my car while I was in line and then when I pulled up to the booth, there was another search—and it was thorough. I was terrified beyond words, but I channeled my inner CIA-agent resolve not to die from the cancer and to make sure I got over on this guy. I had to get it through since I had my immuno-juice and brought over some extra for First Immune's other patients and shipped it to them on Monday. I didn't tell John I was doing this and it was even more pressure as there were other desperate and frightened cancer patients that need the GcMAF/Goleic just as badly as I do so I

MASS MURDERING DOCTORS: THE TRUTH ABOUT ONCOLOGISTS, CHEMOTHERAPY AND CANCER

couldn't say no to First Immune—I owe them my life! Normally I put the meds in my cooler as soon as I pick up, but a little voice in my head told me to get it out of there —and I was driving to the border and so I pulled over, got it out of the cooler and put it in John's backpack with his other diabetes meds. The voice in my head was correct as usual—I heard the ICE agent digging through the ice in the cooler and thumping the side panels looking for hidden compartments. I was scared to death but focusing on remaining cool while the agent searched the car for contraband for the second time. He opened the back passenger door and took out the backpack and asked me "What's in the backpack?" and I gave it a dismissive wave of my hand and said "It's my husband's junk, his computer and other stuff" and the ICE guy asked why I carried it around and I said "Because he won't leave it in the hotel room" and I guess this seemed reasonable. He put the pack back behind the seat, closed the door and walked around to the driver's side window. He asked me a couple more innocuous questions, then gave me back my passport, receipt for my Wal-mart purchases, car keys and told me I could go. I got about 100 yards away before I started shaking like a leaf, but I was safely through and another month closer to being cured. John is insisting that he should be the one to go next month, but I can't let him. He was beyond brave to take the risk of going over the border and getting it the first THREE times, but I CANNOT let him take the risk again. If I get arrested, it's not going to be that big of a deal since I will not go to prison and being self-employed I won't lose my job either. However, if JOHN were to get caught, he would lose his Top Secret security clearance, and with that would go his job and pension after 25 years in federal service. Our health insurance would be gone as well, so while it would be a headache for me to get caught, it would be a DISASTER if he did—and I can't let him take the chance.

I headed back to the hotel almost crying in relief for this trip being over and having successfully brought back my immuno-juice and enough extra to help 3 other people who were in desperate need of the vitamin D binding protein that is a PROVEN cancer cure. I ordered up some food and went to bed after I ate. I didn't sleep well, but got up at 5 am and headed out to get back to Illinois, which was an uneventful trip. I have an appointment with Dr. Janet on Tuesday and then I want to go back to Louisiana where I can freak out and stress out to my heart's content without John having to see it and be upset by it. He's housebreaking a pair of Siamese kittens we got for Christmas and Creole and Bayou take up a lot of his time.

CHAPTER 38: A YEAR INTO THE FIGHT, THE END IN SIGHT...?

After the Canadian adventure, I had an appointment with Dr. Janet that went very well. Even though I am getting very thin, it's not from the cancer, it's from the extremely low-carb diet I must remain on as sugar feeds cancer as we all know. I'm down to wearing size 6 jeans but I should be OK if I get the cancer cured. It's been a year since I started down this road with the "preventative" surgery that wasn't preventing ANYTHING.

Saw Dr. Janet today and spent about an hour with her. I was thoroughly poked, felt, prodded, manipulated, palpated and other assorted medical indignities for the better part of that time. She had the most interesting look of amazed wonder on her face when she finished and she said she is starting to believe that I might just pull this off. I continue to be totally symptom-free and so far, so good! She's ordering another MRI so we will know more in about 3 weeks when I get the results. I continue to feel fine with no pain, bloating or any kind of cancer symptom. I'm WAY over an IV injection every day, but it's what I have to do to survive, so that's what I'm doing. My loathing for salmon has not decreased one iota, but I'm still choking it down 5 times (or more) a week and following the protocol as closely as possible. No matter how much my back hurts, no matter how much I hate salmon, no matter how tired I am of being stuck with a needle in my vein on a daily basis—this STILL cannot possibly be as bad as the nightmare horrors of chemotherapy. Nothing is as bad as chemo, plus this actually works and cures cancer and a lot of other things in addition to cancer. It's nothing less than a medical revolution that leads to actual CURES for so many profitable chronic illnesses that it's no wonder BigPharma is in a panic over the thought that they could lose a penny from poisoning people for profit and the cozy chemo lobbying that keeps murdering cancer victims. It's worked on a lot of people and I hope and pray to GOD that it works on this cancer and cures it too.

The worst thing about cancer is the terrible fear that comes with it and the panic that comes with the fear. Every little twinge or pain brings on the terror that the cancer is bigger or your treatment isn't working. A strange pain brings on paralyzing panic attacks and it's exponentially worse when you are living on "borrowed time". I was supposed to die in November/December 2016. Since today is February 18, 2017 and I have zero symptoms, I am on borrowed time. I can't think about anything but how I have to keep fighting and that today is one year to the day that I found out I had cancer. Every day I feel my body for anything out of the ordinary. Is there bloating? A lump? Swollen lymph nodes in my groin, under my arms or in my neck? A gas pain causes me to start hyperventilating and my heart starts to pound and I know it's an anxiety attack I have to get under control before it gets out of control. I can't take any medication for it as it would affect the GcMAF/Goleic and could deactivate it so I force myself to chill and not give in to the panic. The sheer stress of battling a terminal cancer is almost overwhelming, without the terrible constant fear. It would be wonderful if I could just fill a prescription for GcMAF/Goleic at the local Walgreen's and know it will be there and I'll be able to have my lifesaving medication. It's horrifically stressful to have to go to Canada, a 1000 mile round trip, pick up the medication and smuggle it back into the USA because I cannot take the risk of losing it because my life depends upon it. DEPENDS ON IT. If they tell me I can't bring it into the USA, I will have to turn around and find a place to live in Canada until I am cancer free. It's terrifying and the stress is horrible and it's unbelievable that the government makes me go through this JUST TO STAY ALIVE. It's something I am going to do my best to put a stop to when I am cured as breaking the chemo lobby's stranglehold on the FDA and corrupt government is going to become my life's work when I am cancer-free. I will be dedicating the REST of my life to spreading the word that there IS A CURE and NO ONE needs to die from cancer ever again. I have to go to Canada again next week to bring home the juice and I am going to be carrying 10 extra bottles for people who can't go on their own because they are too sick. It adds to the pressure and the stress because I can't tell my husband I'm doing it and can't refuse because if I were depending on someone else to bring me lifesaving medication I'd hope that there would be someone like me that would bring it in for me so that I wouldn't DIE. It's adding to the pressure, but there's nothing I can do, I am on the side of the angels and hope that God takes that into consideration.

CHAPTER 39: DETROIT AGAIN, ANOTHER MRI AND A VISIT WITH ANDREA

MASS MURDERING DOCTORS: THE TRUTH ABOUT ONCOLOGISTS, CHEMOTHERAPY AND CANCER

So, getting ready for another MRI and another trip to the frozen tundra of Canada to smuggle back the only thing that has a chance to save my life from this pesky cancer that is so determined to kill me. My nerves are completely shattered as if this MRI is good, then my chances of surviving this cancer SKYROCKET and I will be able to actually BREATHE again. One improving MRI does not a cure make and I am so worried that the immuno-juice will stop working. I know I sound irrational, I have NO reason to think it's not working but the stress and fear screws with my head. I'm on borrowed time after all. I can only wait and see what happens. However, Big Pharma has intervened and shut down First Immune so I will have to stretch out my dosage. The government big pharma-owned scum shut down the place that makes my immunotherapy med and I am not going to be able to get it for the foreseeable future. I am fairly certain this means I will die from the cancer if they don't start production again. I'm pretty freaked out right now. I haven't told my parents and I'm not going to. There's nothing they can do and there's no point in making them worry. It's pointless—I wish I hadn't told them about the cancer. I don't know what else there is to say or do. I can only wait and see what happens. If they don't get back in business, I don't know that I will see 2018—it seems unlikely at this point. I'm scared to death—after all I've been through in this fight it seems that BigPharma is going to be able to silence me and shut down the cure. BASTARDS. I reached out to First Immune and hopefully their nutritionist will be able to help me. She's got a stockpile in her freezer and if I can get 20 vials, with the six I have left, I will be able to stretch it into a cure or until they start production again. If I have a good MRI and the cancer is almost gone, with any luck, I can stretch out the medicine enough to kill off the rest of the cancer and have a single vial left to do twice a week shots for the 8 weeks I have to continue it after the clear MRI. The original patients were cured on a dose far less than what I have been taking for 8 months so hopefully it will work out because if it doesn't I will die. If that's the case then David Noakes gave me an extra year of life for which I am grateful. I am also terrified because I don't want to die and frustrated as I stand poised to become the first and only known survivor of this killer cancer and now I may die because of the scumbags in the government who are on the payroll of Big Pharma. If I can't get any more GcMAF/Goleic, my cancer is going to come roaring back and kill me. It's the most aggressive cancer there is and there are NO

MASS MURDERING DOCTORS: THE TRUTH ABOUT ONCOLOGISTS, CHEMOTHERAPY AND CANCER

known survivors. I am a bundle of nerves and I am having my MRI today—a year to the day since my "staging surgery" with Dr. Xynos. This MRI needs to show the cancer almost gone in order for me to have a chance to survive it. If the cancer is almost gone, I have a chance—if I can get 20 more vials—to survive it. It also might hold me for a few months until First Immune re-opens and starts making immuno-juice again. However, it looks like they are done for good and I am going to die because of it then I have GOT to figure a way to get these tumors out of me. I got my MRI report today and I am not shrinking the tumors—they could be dying though. Maybe they are dead because they aren't growing and they aren't seeding the peritoneum. I have NO new tumors which is huge but when I use the last of the immuno-juice I'll be toast. I am flipped out beyond words but there's literally nothing I can do.

I'm semi-considering that perhaps chemo to get rid of The big two tumors like I tried to get them to do with this first started because I'm treading water there's too much cancer to kill off, but it's not spreading, I'm status quo. If I can get these two tumors gone which is going to require allowing them to chemo me I might be able to use the last of the immuno juice so I would have that I could just put it in the freezer and six weeks from now to wipe out the rest of the cancer and hope my body can take the damage it does. Tomorrow Detroit I'm going to talk to Andrea about this she's the greatest living expert on the substance of how it works so I will talk to her. I will talk to John before I make a decision on what to do though. It might work if I can do the absolute minimum chemo or since they're only doing it for the money, I'll show up and sign for the treatments and let them bill Blue Cross but stop the treatment. They hook you up to an infuser and walk away, I'll do something to prevent the infusion— I'll stab the bag with a 60 cc syringe and a 16 gauge needle and pull the crap out, hide the full syringes or pull the IV and drain it into a cup and dump them when I leave. My husband can go will me and be a lookout—2 or 3 treatments they'll be all happy and I'll have the surgery without letting the poison in me. I'm going to have to cancel seeing my parents this month and I am going to die before 2018 if I can't get this tumor removed or if I can't get any more Goleic/GcMAF to keep knocking it down until it disappears. Oddly in the last MRI, the tumors are not seeding new tumors and they are changing shape which means they could be dead. My visit with Andrea was productive, but I am still terrified. We did a livestream video where I went public and gave my name and Andrea is afraid that Big Pharma will try and kill me. 60 doctors using Goleic/GcMAF are now dead in the last 2 years. None of the murders have been solved and most have been covered up. David Noakes is in hiding and I am doing anything I can do to help him—I owe my life to him and First Immune.

CHAPTER 40: DID I COME ALL THIS WAY TO DIE WHEN THE CURE IS NEAR?

I have to find a surgeon to take out these tumors. I am in a blind panic—I can't sleep and I can't eat and if they all insist on chemo first I am in big trouble. My March MRI was almost the same as my November MRI, but the scattered tumors are definitely gone and the two bigger tumors haven't grown but have changed shape. They might be dead for all I know since they are supposed to double in size every 6 weeks or so but have not grown at all in 6 months—but they haven't shrunk much either. I wouldn't be worried about it if First Immune wasn't being fucked over by BigPharma's minions and there's NO MORE GcMAF/Goleic for love or money, so the 15 vials I have are ALL I am going to have and if these tumors are NOT dead then they will come roaring back and kill me after a year of fighting this killer disease that I am SO CLOSE to beating once and for all. Did I come all this way—eating wretched salmon, shots every day, smuggling the medicine in from Canada and more to die in the end when the cancer was beaten? I haven't had chocolate in a f**king year. I've eaten foods I strongly dislike and followed a protocol with all these supplements (and I hate taking pills—ugh!) not to mention being in miserable pain for a year from the woefully inadequate pain medicine that is Buprenorphine? Was it ALL for NOTHING??? Did God show me the cure but change his mind? WTF is going ON here?? I'm going to tell them I'm allergic to chemo drugs. They HAVE to believe me, they can't give me something I tell them I'm allergic to because the test could kill me from anaphylactic shock which is a risk they can't take. You can't give a patient something they tell you they are allergic to because if they die from it, which is a VERY real possibility, not only would the doctor be on the hook for medical malpractice but they could also be charged with murder because they caused the death of a patient through an overt act that the patient TOLD THEM would be harmful or fatal—that's NOT a chance these pussy poison pushers are willing too take, obviously. Besides, isn't EVERYONE allergic

MASS MURDERING DOCTORS: THE TRUTH ABOUT ONCOLOGISTS, CHEMOTHERAPY AND CANCER

to chemo? It makes you vomit, your hair falls out, mouth sores, intestinal lining sores, brain damage, Kidney damage, neuropathy in your hands and feet, liver damage, heart damage, eye damage and more. If THAT doesn't qualify as an allergy, I don't know what would!!!! That's way worse than some itchy hives!! I see the surgeon tomorrow at 4:30 pm and I am hoping to get the two tumors out next week and then seal the deal with the immuno-juice and become the Lone Survivor or die trying.

The surgeon was not willing to do the surgery because he didn't feel he was the right person, so my last hope is to go back to Dr. Xynos and see if he will take them out. I am not hopeful that he will since he tried to push me into useless chemo right out of surgery and I have no hope that he will do surgery—although I have no qualms about promising to do chemo AFTER the surgery if it gets me into the OR to get the two walnut-size tumors and then ghosting. This surgeon also thinks I have colon cancer due to a thickening in the sigmoid colon that was present on the cancer-free MRI I had in April (that he did not read) that has NOT progressed in a year, so I'm pretty sure he's wrong unless the immuno-juice stopped its progression for a year. However, since this cancer almost never invades the bowel and he's not an oncologist, just a general surgeon I disagree with his assessment. He also thinks I have cancer in my lymph nodes but I disagree again because there's no evidence of it. I am worried and scared because without access to the immunotherapy med—which I can't get any more and will maybe never get again, there's no surviving this because I have too much cancer to kill it off with what GcMAF I have left. I am combining some protocols to maximize the potential, but as aggressive as this cancer is, it will probably not be enough. No matter how it shakes out, I am glad I didn't do chemo and I am adamant that there will be NO chemo under any circumstances. If Dr. Xynos refuses to take out the tumors unless I have chemo first, then it's game over. If First Immune goes back up, I have a chance—but I'd be starting back at square one because I'd have a lot of cancer by then—but it would work then as it worked before. However, I don't know if that will be an option and right now doesn't look good. Since I doubt I'll be able to get it done as these greedy doctors are determined to make money from chemo and since everyone dies from this cancer, they want their cut of the chemo money and I will NOT let them chemo me. EVER. I've lived longer with NO chemo than people who GET chemo. The mother of one of the people that works for John was diagnosed with the same cancer 3 days after I was. She had a ton of chemo and is about to die with a belly full of cancer; while I am still asymptomatic and look exactly the same as I did a year ago when this started. If nothing else, I've gotten an extra year (so far) of high-quality life and will probably get another year assuming that Xynos refuses to remove the tumor and I can't get any more GcMAF. Best case scenario would be I get the tumors nipped out and First Immune starts production again, but that doesn't seem likely at this point. We'll see what happens—I'm not dead yet—and as ornery as I am, it might take a while—and the protocols are quite effective, but the biggest issue is that I had to cut my dose of immuno-juice by 2/3rds to stretch out what I have as long as possible. The key is going to be getting these tumors out ASAP but that's not likely so we'll just have to wait and see. I don't have anything left to fight WITH is the problem. For the first time I am weighing the odds of actually DYING from this wretched genetic defect and facing that I am now quite unlikely to survive this. However, I had a year of high quality life and we all DO die. I am pissed because I just got a handle on all of it in THIS life and now I don't know what it's like where I'll be and will I still be ME? It messes with your head, plus I'm stoned AF on medical weed—which is flipping AWESOME by the way. I'm glad they didn't have weed this good when we were kids, I'd have never amounted to ANYTHING LOL I'd have been like Tommy Chong in real life.

CHAPTER 41: BACK TO SQUARE ONE: DR. XYNOS FOR POSSIBLE SURGERY

I'm going to have to call that craphead Dr. Xynos again and tell him I have a recurrence and go see him but I am NOT going to the SLU-care medical mill again. EVER. I will go see him at his St Luke's office—it's a lot farther but it doesn't have the horrifying noise level and the "Take a number and shut the f**k up." attitude of the patient-churning, insurance-raping medical mill that is St. Louis University. I'd almost rather die than go back to see this miserable prick who is batcrap crazy on a good day and talks over me due to a raging God complex. I didn't like him last time and I don't trust him any more now than I did before. He's a chemo-pushing medical mill machine whose sole function in life is to poison as many people as possible for profit. I doubt he's going to operate on these tumors because he is going to insist on chemo

MASS MURDERING DOCTORS: THE TRUTH ABOUT ONCOLOGISTS, CHEMOTHERAPY AND CANCER

first—like whores who have to get their money up front because the payer isn't going to get what they want or need. He's a Big Pharma whore just like that miserable bitch Karuna Murray—they want your chemo money up front because they know chemo won't help you but they want their 75-100K a pop money for it even though it does nothing for the patient. I don't care if I die from the cancer, I am NOT having chemo. If I die, then so be it. I'm not going to die knowing these crapheads bought a new car with the money they got from poisoning me. I have an appointment with the gyno/onco that did my original staging surgery and with any luck will want to do another one which means he would also nip out the tumors and then try again to force me into chemo that I refused last March. If he gets the tumors, I might— MIGHT have enough immuno-juice to seal the deal and wipe out the last of the cancer. This is pivotal, as the key to my survival is getting them out. I think Dr. Xynos will probably want to go in for a look around as he insisted on this last year 3 weeks after my original hysterectomy and he likes to cut. It would be a robot surgery and then when he tries to toss me into chemo, I disappear into the sunset. However, if he doesn't do the surgery and First Immune doesn't start production soon, then it's going to be game over. No matter how much bullcrap they give me about chemo, I have read over 100 research papers that make 2 things crystal clear. First is that chemo doesn't touch or help this cancer. Period. I'm not going to spend the rest of the time I have left being poisoned. It's not going to happen. Second, and just as bad, there are no known survivors of the cancer I have. I have a chance if I can get the tumors out and can wipe it out with what I have left OR if First Immune starts production again. I've had many people contact me and they ALL just want more GcMAF and are desperate to get it because it WORKS—I'm living proof—I should have died months ago. It's out of my hands right now and I won't know more until I see the doctor tomorrow. However, I have history with this guy. The last time I saw him was 3 weeks after my original surgery and he INSISTED on a look-around or "staging" surgery. He likes to cut and he's good at it. IF he wants the staging surgery, he will try to remove as much cancer as possible as he will PROBABLY assume that I will let him chemo me since last time I refused chemo I was cancer-free. He's an old guy and this is the standard of care and he will assume that I am now terrified of dying and will let him poison me with chemo. It's not going to happen, but if I have to let

MASS MURDERING DOCTORS: THE TRUTH ABOUT ONCOLOGISTS, CHEMOTHERAPY AND CANCER

him think that, then so be it. I want these tumors OUT and if I have to shine him on to get rid of it, oh well, too bad. He'll get about 10 grand for a 90 minute surgery and if he believes there's another cool half million in chemo waiting for him on the other side, it gets my tumors out and I have a chance to survive, albeit a very small chance but still nonetheless, more of one than I have without the surgery. Life's a crapshoot and I rolled the dice with the immunotherapy to begin with, and the stakes were life and death from the get-go. I chose the immunotherapy and if I had it to do over again, I'd still refuse the chemo and make the same choice. I chose it because I knew that chemo couldn't cure me and that any extra time I might get from it would be poor quality life. I am NOT going to spend the last of my life vomiting, bald and suffering in the hope of a few more months of living in misery. That's not me, it never has been and never will be. I choose to live as I always have, and if I survive it then great, but if I succumb to the cancer, then so be it. I've had an amazing life and I've lived it on my terms and will continue to do so. I'm not interested in time for time's sake or a miserable, sick existence for a few extra months because I see no point to it. If I can't live as I always have—at 100 mph with my hair on fire—then there's no reason to grasp at straws and be sick and miserable with the end result being the same. Hopefully the onco/gyno Dr. Xynos will want another staging surgery before chemo, but if he insists on chemo first then that's the end of it. I'm not going to keep wasting my time and money seeing doctors who can't help me but want to profit from killing me with their ridiculously overpriced poison. I know this is hard to read, and believe me it was just as hard to write, but in the choice between ugly truth and sugar-coated bullcrap, I prefer the ugliest truth to the most gorgeous lie. Drug companies pay oncologists to promote (expensive) ineffective and toxic cancer drugs. Most oncologists don't make their money by treating patients, but by selling cancer drugs. In fact, according to the Journal of the American Medical Association, as much as 75% of the average oncologist's earnings come from selling chemotherapy drugs in his or her office, and at a substantially marked-up price.

Pharmaceutical companies not only hire charismatic people to charm doctors, exaggerate drug benefits and underplay side effects, but they also pay oncologists kickbacks to push their drugs. For example, *Astra Zeneca, Inc. had to pay $280 million in civil penalties and $63 million in criminal penalties to the federal government

MASS MURDERING DOCTORS: THE TRUTH ABOUT ONCOLOGISTS, CHEMOTHERAPY AND CANCER

after it paid kickbacks to doctors for promoting its prostate cancer drug. Many oncologists are criminals and bullies, not doctors (I can attest to this!!) Oncologists not only bully patients into taking the destructive route of chemotherapy, toxic drugs and surgery, but they also don't tell their patients the whole truth about the danger of these treatments, other available options, cancer survival statistics, and much more. An innumerable number of cancer patients have suffered needlessly at the hands of these so-called doctors, who are often really corrupt and immoral human beings that couldn't care less about the healing process of their patients. Many of these shameless oncologists deserve to be arrested and prosecuted immediately for the crimes they commit, yet they keep on sending patients down the same treacherous and painful road that has resulted in too many deaths to keep track of.

More and more patients are waking up to the truth about cancer treatment and educating themselves on the power of whole food nutrition and supplements—they are choosing doctors that educate and heal them rather than bully them into surgery and chemotherapy. The staggering documentary Cancer is Curable mentioned earlier interviews doctors who tell you how patients are often pressured by conventional oncologists; sometimes they're even hustled onto the operating table the day after their diagnosis without having any of their other choices explained to them. What's worse is that no matter how effective a treatment could be, conventional patients are still being killed by the food they are fed in hospitals. All the doctors in Cancer is Curable unanimously explain that sugar is the No. 1 killer for every cancer patient and although every medical doctor should know that fact, they still continue to give their patients tootsie rolls and candies in the chemotherapy room. Read more here: http://www.cureyourowncancer.org/exposing-the-fraud-and-mythology-of-conventional-cancer-treatments.html#sthash.wHlp5dX9.dpuf

There are a ridiculous number of false positives in cancer screenings. Among 1,087 individuals participating in a cancer screening trial who received a battery of tests for prostate, ovarian, colorectal and lung cancer, 43% had at least one false positive test result, according to a study published in an issue of Cancer Epidemiology, Biomarkers & Prevention. That's almost half of the patients who were tested! One of the obvious downfalls of this is the needlessly expensive medical care costs associated with false

MASS MURDERING DOCTORS: THE TRUTH ABOUT ONCOLOGISTS, CHEMOTHERAPY AND CANCER

positive cancer screenings. Considering the high cost of testing and treatments, the economic consequences of false-positive screening results are significant. Let's not neglect to mention the pointless emotional and physical suffering inflicted upon thousands of patients who are led to believe they have cancer. In the study mentioned above, men that specifically were given a false positive result for either prostate, lung or colo-rectal cancer averaged almost $2,000 in additional medical care expenditures compared to men with all negative screens. More than half (51%) of the men in the study had at least one false positive test. The lesson to take home from all this. These cancer cover-ups and myths are just a few basic examples of how corrupt and dishonest the cancer industry really is. This especially pertains to the oncologists, who are treating patients regardless of knowing the disturbing truth about the procedures, testing and treatment processes they so frequently push upon their patients.

While not all oncologists (only 99.9% to be STATISTICALLY fair) should be placed into the same category, a large majority of these criminal "doctors" should be held accountable and properly punished for the needless struggle they are inflicting upon thousands of cancer sufferers. If you know anyone who is being pushed into chemotherapy and other deadly and unnecessary "treatments," share the truth with them today and you could save a life. Fortunately, more and more people are waking up to these cancer lies and are looking into safer and more effective alternative treatment protocols and therapies. Ever since chemotherapy was introduced into the practice of western medicine, doctors and oncologists have been trying to answer this nagging question: Why does chemotherapy seem to work at first, but then cancer tumors cells grow back even more aggressively while the body becomes resistant to chemotherapy? It turns out that chemotherapy damages healthy cells, causing them to secrete a protein that accelerates the growth of cancer tumors. This protein, dubbed "WNT16B," is taken up by nearby cancer cells, causing them to "grow, invade, and importantly, resist subsequent therapy," said Peter Nelson of the Fred Hutchinson Cancer Research Center in Seattle. He's the co-author of the study that documented this phenomenon, published in Nature Medicine. This protein, it turns out, explains why cancer tumors grow more aggressively following chemotherapy treatments. In

MASS MURDERING DOCTORS: THE TRUTH ABOUT ONCOLOGISTS, CHEMOTHERAPY AND CANCER

essence, chemotherapy turns healthy cells into WNT16B factories which churn out this "activator" chemical that accelerates cancer tumor growth.

The findings of the study were confirmed with prostate cancer, breast cancer and ovarian cancer tumors. This discovery that chemotherapy backfires by accelerating cancer tumor growth is being characterized as "completely unexpected" by scientists. The chemotherapy fraud exposed and as Natural News has explained over the last decade, chemotherapy is medical fraud. Rather than boosting the immune response of patients, it harms the immune system, causing tumors to grow back. This latest researching further confirms what we've known for years in the holistic health community: That chemotherapy is, flatly stated, poison. It's not "treatment," it's not medicine, and it's not prevention or a cure. It's poison with virtually no medicinal value except in perhaps one to two percent of cancer cases. The No. 1 side effect of chemotherapy is, by the way, cancer. If you HAPPEN to survive the original cancer, you get a metachronous cancer about 5 years down the road from the chemotherapy and guess what they do for it? That's right: More Chemo! Talk about income security: oncologists give you chemo that causes cancer so they can rob you AGAIN down the road—although the vast majority of people who have been through cancer state they'd rather die than go through being voluntarily poisoned a SECOND or THIRD time! Cancer centers should technically be renamed "poison centers" because they are in the business of poisoning patients with a toxic cocktail of chemicals that modern science reveals to be a cancer tumor growth accelerant!
*http://www.cureyourowncancer.org/chemotherapy-backfires-causes-healthy-cells-to-feed-growth-of-cancer-tumors.html#sthash.PUCQaauB.dpuf

Don't take my word for it—go to the source. Here's some of the URLs of PubMed Cancer studies—and there are well over 100 that I have found with NO effort:

https://www.ncbi.nlm.nih.gov/pubmed/26198168

Conclusion: NAC 9 (*chemo first)* followed by IDS (*Interal debulking surgery=AFTER CHEMO)* provides equal survival compared with PDS (*surgery first)*. **Debulking to small residual tumors with a maximum diameter of less than 1 cm provides a smaller but still significant benefit for patients with PDS** (emphasis added) to improve the survival of patients with advanced ovarian cancer, the definition of "optimal" in IDS following NAC should be defined as no residual tumor.

There are dozens of research papers that all say the same thing. You can operate and poison with chemo but there are STILL NO KNOWN SURVIVORS with chemo and with no treatment everyone EXCEPT me has died. Every. Single. One. So, why am I still alive if GcMAF doesn't work—which is the claim Big Pharma and MHRA, et.al. Makes when they shut down biotechs who manufacture it. If it didn't work, I would be as dead as fried chicken—and here I am—calling them liars and murderers. Truth hurts, and it is especially painful to those who depend on mendacity.

I don't know ONE single cancer survivor who had chemo and they died FASTER with the chemo and they wanted to die because of the misery of chemotherapy. I've lived LONGER with NO chemo than my poor baby sister did with all the poison they could pump into her while lying to her and telling her that "the next chemo should be the cure" while they billed her for three quarters of a MILLION dollars to pump the poison that killed her into her. She was doomed from the get-go once the scumbags at Moffit Cancer Center in Tampa, FL started killing her slowly with their chemo poison.

CHAPTER 42: DR. XYNOS AND CHEMO/SURGERY; THE LADY OR THE TIGER?

The visit with Dr. Xynos did not go well. First he forced me to sign a second consent where I was forced to sign on to personal financial responsibility after I had declined it in the original signing—which my insurance company later took them to task for since they are UNDER CONTRACT to accept what the HMO pays. They are NOT allowed by law to bill you for one extra penny UNLESS YOU SIGN ON AND AGREE TO IT—hence the reason they forced me to sign it, it's all on tape where the nurse, Xynos and the office girl coerced me. He then proceeded to verbally abuse me for refusing chemo a year ago when he tried to force me to do it. I have the entire visit on tape, as I record ALL of my doctor visits in Missouri which is a one-party wiretap consent state. I called my insurance company to make a complaint about being coerced and have ALL of it on the recording after they came into the exam room and forced me to sign a new agreement accepting financial responsibility that I am not required to do. I am on an HMO and am not required to accept liability for anything past my contracted co-pays and monthly premiums. He told me how he'd cured cancer in "many many

MASS MURDERING DOCTORS: THE TRUTH ABOUT ONCOLOGISTS, CHEMOTHERAPY AND CANCER

people" with his poison. Dr. Xynos stood there and lied to me through his teeth telling me he had cured hundreds of cases of cancer. I've got to throw the bullcrap flag on that one—there's NO way, my cancer is incurable with chemo—everyone who has had this cancer is now DEAD. I am the LONE SURVIVOR with no chemo. Xynos stood there trying to bully me into chemo and lying to me about all the cancer he's cured with his million-dollar poison. I just got up and left. I am NOT doing chemo. I also called Blue Cross and told them about being forced to sign on to personal responsibility and they were extremely upset and said they would send their rep to talk to them. That doesn't address my current problem of getting this cancer cured though. I'm having to go back to the drawing board and hope for the best. The medical tourism hospitals are telling me I have to have surgery followed by chemo over there. WTF?? I could do that for FREE in America—I don't have to travel to a third world toilet and pay 20 grand in cash for "two weeks in the hospital." Two weeks? TWO WEEKS??? These people are out of their minds—I want a laparoscopic-assisted surgery to nip out the two big tumors and then I will find a way to seal the deal. I've found a product called Salicinium which is sold under the brand name Orasal and it's supposed to work differently than GcMAf/Goleic but with the same principle which is stopping the cancer from producing nagalase which allows the macrophages to kill the cancer. I've still got some GcMAF/Goleic left, I'd like to let them work together and I think it will work. It's expensive, but I've worked my whole life and if I die I can't take it with me, so I might as well see if my life savings will save my life. GcMAF wasn't cheap either—a lot more than the Salicinium and my husband has worked and saved the max in retirement funds and I'm his FIRST wife and he has NO children so he has plenty of money so if I spend every dime I have I'll still be well taken care of in my golden years. He's frantically trying everything he can think of to save my life, but I don't see the point in his bankrupting himself if I don't have a chance. We will see. I'm going to get some Orasal/Salicinium and use it with the GcMAF I have left and stretch out the doses so that I can get the maximum benefit of the salicinium. There was a clinic in AZ using this WITH the GcMAF and had a big success rate that they charged 50K to do. However they stopped using GcMAF when they stopped shipping it to the USA and now their patients are dying instead of getting better so I think it works only with it—however I have some. If I can stretch out the GcMAF with the Orasal it just might wipe it all out. I sure hope so as it's $250 for a Quart-size bottle and you need 2 bottles a month with some other products so it's not going to be cheap—but I have no other options and I'm scared to death. So, without further ado, let's look at how this works, courtesy of Perfect Balance, Inc. who is the patent holder on Salicinium marketed under the brand name of Orasal.

CHAPTER 43: THE SCIENCE OF HOW SALICINIUM WORKS

Here's the skinny on how salicinium is supposed to work. Every normal cell in our body takes in oxygen from our blood to perform its function; this is called respiration or an aerobic process and this process takes place in the mitochondria. Cells take in oxygen and perform their functions by producing a chemical called Adenosine tri-phosphate or ATP for short, which is the vital energy that runs our entire body.

Nobel Laureate Dr. Otto Warburg published in 1926 that by placing normal cells in a vacuum chamber and lowering oxygen content by 35%, normal cells had the ability to continue living without respiration: it is a survival process that every single cell in our body has the ability to do. This is called an anaerobic process meaning without oxygen or respiration. Every cell in our body has a completely different set of enzymes and a completely different way of living than by respiration which is quiescent until needed. We experience this every time we work or exercise too hard and our oxygen starved muscles become sore. The soreness is caused by the formation of Lactic Acid as some of our cells live anaerobically while returning to respiration.

Dr. Warburg realized that after a short time, measured in hours, one could add oxygen back and those cells would return to aerobic activity. However, if held in a reduced oxygen state long enough they become committed to being anaerobic cells. If oxygen is depleted long enough, cells lose their RNA and DNA identity and are permanently obligated anaerobic cells reproducing only other anaerobic cells. This new way of living for the formerly normal aerobic cell is called anaerobiasis and is accomplished by a process of fermentation. These cells now produce only five percent as much ATP or energy as formerly. They now ferment simple sugars—any sugar; it makes no difference to a fermenting cell what type of sugar. It is believed they have the ability to develop 19 times the number of sugar receptors on their surface as normal cells.

MASS MURDERING DOCTORS: THE TRUTH ABOUT ONCOLOGISTS, CHEMOTHERAPY AND CANCER

If it weren't for this low-energy phenomenon cancer would grow at the same rate as our normal cells and we would die very quickly. All dedicated or obligated fermenting cells have a universal co-enzyme called NAD+ and its function is very simple. Anaerobic or fermenting cells which include malignant cells all have a very acidic outside environment and an alkaline inside environment. The NAD+ co-enzyme travels the inside of the cell attaching itself to a hydrogen atom becoming NADH- and then transferring the hydrogen through the Trans Golgi Network to the outside by way of lactate and into the bloodstream. Taking the hydrogen from inside the cell to the outside, repeating this simple cycle of dismutation over and over again. A lack of hydrogen is alkaline and an abundance is acid. Medical science says there are 210 different types of cells. This means there are 210 different places or different cells in the human body for anaerobic (malignant or cancerous) cells to grow but the one function of the NAD+ co-enzyme is universal to all of those 210 different fermenting cells. Glycome means sugar. Salicinium is a Glycome; a complex molecule, the active ingredient being attached to a glycome. The sugar hungry malignant cell sees the glycome passing by in the blood, takes it in and very quickly another enzyme universal only to fermenting cells, beta-Glucosidase splits the sugar from the combined molecule. The NON-glycome material in Salicinium upon being released, attaches to the NAD+ coenzyme and disrupts the fermentation process by stopping dismutation. This is now the crux or turning point in the life of a fermenting cell. When a person first learns they have cancer their first question usually is: "How did I get it, where did it come from?" One forms cancer for the reason stated above and only this reason: A lack of oxygen to some certain set of the 210 different cells. This is called Hypoxia. Once the malignant process of cells changing from aerobic to anaerobic function is established those cells can then travel to other parts of the body causing the subject to have two or more forms of malignant cells. This is called metastasis. Up to this point we have discussed two types of universal enzymes specific to fermenting cells: Cancer specific NAD+ coenzyme and beta-Glucosidase. The third: alpha-N-acetylgalactosaminidase or for short – Nagalase. (Ah—nagalase—my old friend—Here you are again—which makes me think these people are on to something.)

As soon as a cell is forced into hypoxia and in order to survive by fermentation, the cell instantly begins to produce the Nagalase enzyme. Remember, this was a normal cell living by respiration and when it could no longer breathe properly it changed over to the fermentation of simple sugars in the liquid part of the cell or cytoplasm. Simple analogy: it is much like keeping a night light on: there is enough light to see how to get around but not enough to live and work by, but it will do until more light (oxygen) returns. At exactly the same time as fermentation begins, the now sickened, dysfunctional cell must also start protecting itself from the host immune system. It does so by producing Nagalase. The Nagalase enzyme travels through the Trans Golgi Network along with Lactate at approximately 7 pH. Nagalase completely shuts down the localized immune macrophages whose job is to destroy any harmed or not "self" dysfunctional cells. This is an easily understood function as, after all, when oxygen is returned to the cell and respiration begins again—whether in a few hours or a few days—the cell would return to its normal function. However, if the cell fails to return to normal and becomes a fully functioning anaerobe, the enzyme Nagalase continues to be produced and the anaerobic cancer process begins to expand. Anaerobic cells can only reproduce anaerobic cells thus the spread of cancer.

Salicinium, once binding the NAD+ co-enzyme, causes the cell to cease production of Nagalase. With Nagalase missing the innate immune macrophages return to their original function in the localized immune system. They recognize the sick, unprotected and dysfunctional cell and dispose of it as any other cell at the end of its life cycle. Salicinium has simply removed the protective barrier or "cloak" of the malignant cell thus modifying our own natural immune response enabling it to work as it should. Salicinium does not "kill" fermenting cells, the immune system does because now it can. By stopping Nagalase production Salicinium returns the immune system to a functional state. Since it is a complex sugar and normal aerobic cells have no bGlucosidase enzyme to split sugar for assimilation, healthy cells cannot assimilate it and do not absorb Salicinium. It is harmless to any normal cell in the human body. The Salicinium molecule is a very tiny molecule, able to go to any place in the body that blood or body fluids go including through barriers placed by the body for protection. This nutritive molecule is so small that with each gram reaching the bloodstream there are 2,120 quintillion individual opportunities for any fermenting cell to absorb it. The true number written out would be 2 sextillion, 120,000,000,000,000 quintillion per gram; the daily dosage is 3 grams. It is for this reason that control can be gained in as little as the three weeks of I.V. treatment. Salicinium is a prospective adjunct to Orthodox chemotherapy as neither interferes with the function of the other however by using Salicinium, chemotherapy may be reduced to a fractionated (10%/15%) amount. Salicinium is a "targeted" molecule for use in any fermenting process which eventuates in Nagalase and lactic acid. Salicinium has a half-life of approximately 24 hours. It has never had a known side-effect other than those functions allowed or caused by the Immune System.

Well, this is interesting. I think that if this works as advertised with the boost from the GcMAF/Goleic I have left, I might just survive this after all, assuming it works as described. If I don't do something and First Immune doesn't go back into production, I will be dead before 2018. I'm scared, but this science has brought me this far and I need to get this protocol started. I'm taking my GcMAF shot tomorrow so I want to do a shot of this Salicinium tonight and every 12 hours or so with the every three day injection of GcMAF. I'll know if it's working by the next MRI which I can have in early June, which if it shows a belly full of cancer—and it probably will, I'm going to have to call Hospice and make arrangements to go to Florida to die. My whole family is there and John can come down for the last couple of weeks or however long he wants. I'm not having a funeral—they are barbaric, and I don't feel like putting the family through it again. I want to be cremated and my ashes scattered wherever John and I decide is a special place for both of us. I ordered it and it is on the way, so I hope to be using it soon so hopefully I will have enough GcMAF left for my immune system to crush the cancer, but I am scared to death because I was doing so well on it until BigPharma decided that they had to stop David Noakes from saving people's lives with his amazing vitamin D binding protein and closed down his facility and put his people in jail on trumped up charges. It's outrageous and I have filmed a video deposition to support David Noakes since I literally owe him my life. No matter how this shakes out, I've had an extra year of high quality life I owe to him—no vomiting or bald head or ugly side-effects and if it turns out to be my time, then nothing will save me anyway, so I still have NOTHING to lose and everything to gain. I realize the odds are heavily against me surviving this cancer, but had I gone the chemotherapy route, I'd have died already. Living on borrowed time isn't optimum for someone like me. I'm a dedicated planner and I do my best to always have a contingency plan in place so "winging it" is never the way I like to do things!

CHAPTER 44: SALICINIUM, GcMAF & GOD, DO I LIVE OR DO I DIE?

No one is going to take these two tumors out without chemo first. They are bound and determined to get that chemo money no matter what. I find it SO refreshing that they are so willing to poison me for money after I hand them a stack of research papers from JAMA and NEJM clearly stating that chemo is totally ineffective against this cancer.

I've made some shifts in my treatment. I've cut my immunojuice dose from 1 mL/day x 5 week to .05 mL q 72 and I've added salicinium ($250 a quart!!!) to the regimen. Of all the research I have done, it's the only thing I've found that I thought was scientifically sound and mentions GcMAF as part of how it works. If it does what it says, then with a little luck and following the protocol I might be able to seal the deal with the GcMAF I have left. I'm also using high-dose CBD/THC cannabis oil to help it out since it seems to have so many anti-cancer benefits. I'm also still choking down wretched nasty salmon 5-10 times a week, no sugar, no carbs and it still sucks.

If all this works, I should be OK, but if not—and if First Immune either doesn't reopen or reopens after I pass the point of no return, then it was all for nothing and I will die before 2018. The next MRI is in June, if this doesn't work I'll be presenting the classic OVCA symptoms by then and will have about 4-6 months after that. I'm pretty scared but I'm certain that if I had let them force me to do chemo, I would be dead by now. I may die anyway, but I'm not going to die sick, bald and miserable and HAPPY to die to end it. I'm not about to make my last time on earth a bunch of unending medical appointments and bankrupt my husband to pay for this. If it comes down to it, I'm going to die drinking a Scotch and eating cake and so be it.

What bothers me the most is that I may not have the proof that the immuno-juice works—and I didn't do this just for me. I did it for the kids too—so that they would know that chemo wasn't the answer and that they didn't have to do it. I wanted this cure to be available to THEM too so that no one else would die from this and now I'm

MASS MURDERING DOCTORS: THE TRUTH ABOUT ONCOLOGISTS, CHEMOTHERAPY AND CANCER

distraught to think that after all I've done to try and prove this cure, I may lose because Big Pharma wants to protect their blood money.

I don't know what else to do. It's something I wanted and needed to try and do for the kids. I love them so much and if I can beat this, they can too—the same way. It was MORE than worth it to try and find the cure so that they can benefit from it as well and to show them that I lived longer with NO chemo than poor Lori after all she went through being poisoned for profit by greedy bastards. At any rate, time will tell me soon enough what I need to do, if I do beat this, it HAS TO BE NOW because if First Immune doesn't reopen and this cancer isn't gone by the next MRI, I won't have anything left to fight it with other than the salicinium and medical cannabis. Life's a crapshoot, and I'm still rolling the dice, we'll see what happens. It's been 14 months with no end in sight and I'm tired—but I can't quit now, I've come this far—but still so very far to go—and I am scared for all I put up a brave front. First Immune is done for the moment as they defend themselves against trumped-up charges from Big Pharma's minions in the MHRA and I could pay for this with my LIFE. Big Pharma is determined to prevent their chemo profits from disappearing with the cure that is GcMAF/Goleic and will do anything they can to force a cure from the market. They don't want to CURE cancer—they want to TREAT it with their million-dollar poisons that my DOCTORS tried to force me to take. I've lived longer with NO chemo than my poor doomed sister did with every bit of poison they could pump into her. With the owners and employees of First Immune under arrest on trumped up charges and the production of the GcMAF/Goleic shut down until all of this is resolved. The MHRA who are the English/UK version of the totally corrupt FDA accused First Immune of money laundering no less. How the f**k can they be laundering money when the only way to pay them was by bank wire transfer? The entire thing is absolute bullcrap and when they get their day in court, I can't wait to bring my medical records and testify for them and slam Big Pharma and the MHRA. I've had to change my cancer protocols to get GcMAF from other sources, and so far so good. Here's my complete protocol that I developed. In my cancer treatment, I look for 3 things: GcMAF (which is a natural substance) and things that boost production of T-cells, macrophages, dendritic cells, NK (natural killer) cells and macrophages along with things that prevent the cancer cells from making nagalase which is what shuts down the immune system. To

MASS MURDERING DOCTORS: THE TRUTH ABOUT ONCOLOGISTS, CHEMOTHERAPY AND CANCER

that end I have come up with a protocol to try and replace the GcMAF injections until First Immune comes back into production after the totally fabricated charges are resolved in David Noakes' favor. I am less concerned with eradication of the tumors at the moment because even if I'm only "treading water" it will keep me alive until I can start the injections again down the road. I'm NOT an oncologist or an MD but I have a hard science education and I'm using it along with every one of my IQ points to continue to try to stay alive and hopefully become cancer free at some point. First Immune was shut down before I could complete my cure, but my cancer—that kills with explosive exponential growth (rather than invading my other organs) that crushes out my visceral organ functions and that doubles in size every 6 weeks has NOT progressed at all in 9 months and the scattered miliary tumors that make this the only "weed and seed" cancer have disappeared. ANY advice that I give you is strictly based on my personal experience and shouldn't be considered medical advice because I am not allowed to give you medical advice, only a doctor is permitted and licensed to do that.

SIDEBAR: ALTERNATE CANCER TREATMENT UNTIL FIRST IMMUNE IS BACK

AHCC 750 mg caps: 2 caps 3 x a day to boost production of T-cells, macrophages, dendritic cells, NK (natural killer) cells and macrophages.

Salicinium: (Orasal) 1 ounce 2 x a day which contains a sugar molecule that anaerobic cancer cells grab since they "breathe" by fermentation rather than O2 as normal cells do. This shuts down their nagalase production which prevents the cancer cells from hiding from my immune system. There's no way to get it for less than retail as the company that makes it is the ONLY one and it's $250 a quart and you will need 2 quarts a month for active cancer. You won't need it if you are only wanting to rebuild your immune system.

Colostrum: 6 of the 500 mg caps 3x a day A natural source of GcMAF when used in in making yogurt (this is homemade Bravo GcMAF probiotic yogurt that is insanely overpriced by the health food shops that sell it) and I also make the yogurt which is stupid simple to make. I bought the 1 month Bravo yogurt kit from a supplier for 250 DOLLARS and all it contained was 4 small packets of colostrum and 4 small packets of yogurt starter!! I sent it back and bought the colostrum from a veterinary supply (my

MASS MURDERING DOCTORS: THE TRUTH ABOUT ONCOLOGISTS, CHEMOTHERAPY AND CANCER

cousin, a veterinarian told me it was exactly the same—which it is) for $75 for 2 POUNDS of colostrum—enough to make a TON of yogurt! You also don't need yogurt starter, all you need is about a Tablespoon of plain unflavored yogurt added to the milk and some time and you can use the last TBS of your GcMAF yogurt to ferment the next batch and if you forget, you can get a small cup at the store to start it for less than 75 cents. Here's the recipe: 2 cups milk, 1 heaping TBS plain yogurt, ½ cup of Bovine colostrum from a vet supply and 1 teaspoon of probiotic powder available on Amazon. Scald milk. Place in GLASS BOWL (not metal!!) Cool to room temp and whisk in the colostrum (it floats so I whisk it into a small amount of the milk and then add it back to the batch. Cover and place in your oven with the light turned on (just the right amount of heat) for 12-24 hours. Mine thickened in 7 hours, the longer you let it ferment the more tart it will be. I use whole milk to make my yogurt.

Vitamin D3: 10,000 IU EVERY DAY without fail—GcMAF will not work without it and you can take up to 20,000 IU daily if your levels are really low.

Vitamin K2: 500 mcg a day which helps the GCMAF work as well.

Metformin (Glucophage) 500 mg extended release pills, one per day. There's a ton of evidence that this old, cheap diabetes drug is effective against cancer since it helps starve cancer cells of sugar by making your body's natural insulin work better at keeping your sugar down. I am not a diabetic, but my doctor wrote the Rx for it instantly. I can't say enough good things about her, I would not have had even a chance to beat this terrible cancer without her. I may still die (and probably will) without the GcMAF/Goleic that BigPharma has successfully shut down with trumped up fake charges to prevent cancer victims from a REAL cure.

Forbidden: Sugar, carbs of any sort, alcohol, and opioid pain killers. You can use Buprenorphine which doesn't interfere and medical cannabis for pain. Try not to take ANY meds if you don't have to. If you are using Salicinium NO Vitamin C supplements as it negates the Salicinium. Don't gorge on high Vitamin C foods either. You should eat as much as you can of Salmon, nuts butter, cream, chicken livers and canned pigs brains for the lipids. I can't find the pig brains and doubt I could eat them if I did! No artificial sweeteners other than Stevia or Saccharine (pink packets i.e. Sweet-n-Low) and NO sodas with equal or splenda. I drink iced tea and unsweetened Kool-aid with a mix of stevia ($$) and cheap saccharine which is an OLD Atkins dieter's trick but it WORKS and it tastes very much like sugar.

HOW DO WE CHANGE THIS?

We need a large group and we need to go to DC and walk in to each and every one of our individual Congressional representatives. If we have 50 people, the entire group needs to descend upon the offices of 50 Congress(wo)men unless 2 happen to be from the same state/district. We need to bring petitions with lots of signatures. There are only 2 things they care about: campaign donations and getting re-elected. A social media campaign showering horrifying publicity on them is a plus. However, this won't happen. People are totally brainwashed that chemo is the only way and will NOT seek an alternative for a lot of reasons, but the biggest is the egregious behavior of oncologists desperate to protect their chemo blood money. The oncologists my insurance company has forced me to see have done everything but hold a gun to my head to try and force me into chemo. They've lied to me, threatened me, told me I'd die vomiting feces, told me "better call hospice since you'll die soon" and so on—and I am a medical professional. Think how this works on people who don't KNOW better, and doctors are TRUSTED for the most part by their patients, so they do as they're ordered to do like good little sheep. Second, I've desperately tried to save the lives of my friends and family who have cancer by telling them NO CHEMO and telling them about GcMAF. Right now I am a walking billboard for it, but you can't force them to seek an alternative. A guy that works for my husband for 10 years had his mother diagnosed with the exact same cancer I have THREE DAYS after I was diagnosed. I begged him to tell her about GcMAF and he did—repeatedly. I offered to talk to her, she wouldn't talk to me about it and she went the chemo route starting March 2016. Since then, he has watched ME be perfectly normal with no side effects, look great and feel great, while he watched in horror as chemo ravaged his poor mother. I set bucket after bucket of cool, tasty, life-saving water in front of them but they would not drink it. She continued on the chemo telling him that her doctor assured her the next chemo would "do the trick" just like they told my sister—who ALSO wouldn't listen to me. I told him she was being lied to because there are NO KNOWN SURVIVORS of the cancer she and I have and that chemo would not work. Again,

MASS MURDERING DOCTORS: THE TRUTH ABOUT ONCOLOGISTS, CHEMOTHERAPY AND CANCER

NOTHING. She died a couple of weeks ago, while I look the same as I always have with NO cancer treatments and feel fine, etc. I BEGGED my sister—on my KNEES—and crying—to listen to me and stop the chemo and she wouldn't do it. She died of a ruptured esophagus from chemo-induced vomiting, but of course her death certificate claims that her cause of death was "ovarian cancer".

The point is that the scumbags at the American Cancer Society, media, Big Pharma and the doctors spend all their time pushing chemo as a valid, effective treatment while trashing REAL cures like GcMAF and shutting down places like First Immune to protect their profits. They are not about to let another h.pylori scandal do to their oncologists what the h.pylori did to the gastroenterologists. Until the public perception of chemo as THE only treatment that has any chance of saving your life stops, we are screwed. That's why First Immune is trying desperately to keep me alive. I am their PRIZE lab rat because I have a "no known survivors" cancer AND I have NEVER had chemo or radiation. EVERY other cure they have came to them after being chemo-ed and radiated to death and sent home to die. Then when they were cured, big pharma spun it that it was the CHEMO that eventually saved them NOT the GcMAF which is total bullcrap but that's their narrative and they stick to it. However, if I survive the no survivors cancer with 100% irrefutable documentation that I've never had chemo or radiation then I bring the big pharma narrative crashing down. I fully expect them to try and kill me if I survive the cancer—my life—your life, anyone's life, means NOTHING to them when our survival takes 200 BILLION in ANNUAL profits out of their respective pockets. They are utter scum but they have convinced the population that CHEMO is an effective treatment and that there are no alternatives. Don't think they want to cure cancer—they do NOT. THEY WANT TO TREAT CANCER —FOR HUGE PROFITS. Also, chemo gives you MORE cancer down the road—so they get to ass-rape you again with MORE expensive chemo poison down the road caused by the "cure" of your original cancer. Second-time cancer patients are so damaged from the first time, a bigger percentage DIE from the second cancer chemo! That's why they shut down First Immune—because it WORKS and if I survive this crap I absolutely expect them to try and KILL me. Do you know that 61 doctors using GcMAF on their patients and curing them HAVE BEEN MURDERED in the last 2 years—ALL of them unsolved by the way. Our government and every facet of life from top to

MASS MURDERING DOCTORS: THE TRUTH ABOUT ONCOLOGISTS, CHEMOTHERAPY AND CANCER

bottom is rotted with abject and total corruption—and the sheeple keep signing up to be voluntarily poisoned. The oncologist I had to see 2 weeks ago told me he'd cured lots of people with my cancer—and I stood up and called him a lying cocksucker to his face. At this moment in time, 7/04/2017 I am the only known 18-month survivor with or without chemo. The ONLY ONE!!

The reason why you won't hear the truth from your mainstream doctor is because the government is overrun with corruption. President Roosevelt created the Food and Drug Administration (FDA) to protect the people of this country. Lincoln created the United States Department of Agriculture (USDA) and Nixon created the EPA for the same reason. Our government has become so corrupt that these same agencies that were created to protect you are now protecting industry instead. There is a cancer cabal in this country that prevents cancer patients from learning about treatments that can save their lives. This end-to-end corruption is going to be the death of America, but it will be the death of me first. I don't expect to survive this cancer without First Immune's GcMAF, so I am hoping and praying to be wrong. I knew chemo was bullcrap and I was desperate for a real cure. I want to survive this, but I also did it for those 3 known and potentially 6 BRCA1+ kids I love so much. I wanted to find a cure for Lori but when she wouldn't listen to me, and then I had to fight this as well, I wanted to do my best to find a cure so that this horrid cancer NEVER kills another member of my family.

If it turns out to be the cure and it goes mainstream as the front-line cancer treatment then they are safe. If it cures AD and my beloved John happens to get AD, I can keep what is happening to John's mom, my mother-in-law from happening to my beloved husband. I just had to have the guts to refuse the chemo and take the risk—and be willing to pay for it with my life if I was wrong—which I am willing to do since anything is better than chemo—even the certain DEATH my idiot oncologists keep telling me is coming if I don't have chemo. If it leads to a CURE for others—especially for the kids, then ANYTHING I have to do or go through is MORE than worth it. Whatever it takes to do this, I am willing to do—and then some. It was NEVER about just me and my life. It was always about protecting the next two generations of my family and their children who are potentially all BRCA1+ and while my brother wasn't

MASS MURDERING DOCTORS: THE TRUTH ABOUT ONCOLOGISTS, CHEMOTHERAPY AND CANCER

"gifted" the BRCA1+ defect, my sister passed it to all three of her children, two of which had children of their own before they realized they had it. If I survive the "always fatal" cancer with NO chemo and NO radiation—with nothing but the miracle of GcMAF/Goleic, I blaze the trail for their cure as well. It was NEVER just about me—it was for everyone I love and every cancer victim in the world.

The cytoxic effects of chemotherapy and radiation treatments for cancer are well-established, and increasingly more people are waking up to the fact that this conventional treatment model is a sure death sentence for most critically ill cancer patients. But a whole new level of evil is creeping its way into the conversation, with cancer doctors now administering these deadly treatments to healthy people who don't even have a legitimate cancer diagnosis.

One of these agents of death is Dr. Farid Fata of Michigan, who recently confessed to intentionally misdiagnosing healthy people with cancer in order to get them on chemotherapy treatments. By doing this, Dr. Fata, who demonically told a court that engaging in this type of depraved behavior "is my choice," was bilking the system for tens of millions of dollars in kickbacks. According to a recent USA Today report, Dr. Fata openly admitted that he administered chemo to patients for which it was "medically unnecessary." The married father of three, who was actively murdering patients for cash at Michigan Hematology Oncology Centers from 2009 to the present, had been treating roughly 1,200 patients for which he received more than $62 million from Medicare. Such evils are worthy of life in prison, according to U.S. attorney Barbara McQuade, who is quoted as saying that Dr. Fata's case is "the most egregious" case of medical fraud that her office has ever seen. Besides actively defrauding the government (taxpayers) of tens of millions of dollars, Dr. Fata was lying to patients who trusted him, and slaughtering them in the process.

"In this case, we had Dr. Fata administering chemotherapy to people who didn't need it, essentially putting poison into their bodies and telling them that they had cancer when they didn't have cancer," McQuade stated to the Free Press. "The idea that a doctor would lie to a patient just to make money is shocking......Dr. Fata was unique in that he saw patients not as people to heal, but as commodities to exploit. "Cancer doctors have a financial incentive to give you toxic chemotherapy treatments, even if

MASS MURDERING DOCTORS: THE TRUTH ABOUT ONCOLOGISTS, CHEMOTHERAPY AND CANCER

you don't have cancer! Dr. Fata is hardly alone in his wicked exploits. A 2012 survey of oncology doctors found that many of them recognize that they can make far more money by administering chemotherapy to their patients. The financial incentive to deceive patients for profit is high, in other words, and it is highly likely that there are many other doctors out there like Dr. Fata who are killing patients to feed their lust for money. "Many of these unscrupulous physicians are like businessmen without a conscience," said Dr. Sayed Mohammed, a retired oncologist who says he's been observing such evils taking place for more than a decade. "The only difference is they have your health and trust in their hands—a very dangerous combination when money is involved."

Sadly, chemotherapy is fraudulent regardless of whether or not a patient truly has cancer. Though you won't hear it from the mainstream media, the true statistical failure rate for this common treatment is an astounding 97 percent for long-term metastatic cancers, which means that a vast number of people who undergo chemotherapy won't be cured of their cancers, and will more than likely die early as a result of the treatment. "If [the mass media] did publish the long-term statistics for all cancers administered cytotoxic chemotherapy, that is 10+ years and produced the objective data on rigorous evaluations including the cost-effectiveness, impact on the immune system, quality of life, morbidity and mortality, it would be very clear to the world that chemotherapy makes little to no contribution to cancer survival at all," explains PreventDisease.com. This photo says it the best: I just love seeing my tax dollars at work, don't you?

Congressional Boot-Lickers Meeting With Big Pharma Lobbyists.

MASS MURDERING DOCTORS: THE TRUTH ABOUT ONCOLOGISTS, CHEMOTHERAPY AND CANCER

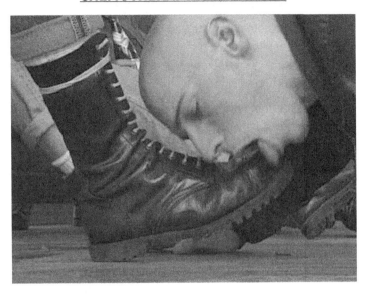

Here's another article just out today in the Telegraph (UK):

Chemotherapy may spread cancer and trigger more aggressive tumours, warn scientists. 5 JULY 2017 • 7:00PM http://stm.sciencemag.org/content/9/397/eaan0026

Chemotherapy could allow cancer to spread, and trigger more aggressive tumors, a new study suggests. Researchers in the US studied the impact of drugs on patients with breast cancer and found medication increases the chance of cancer cells migrating to other parts of the body, where they are almost always lethal. Around 55,000 women are diagnosed with breast cancer in Britain every year and 11,000 will die from their illness. Many are given chemotherapy before surgery, but the new research suggests that, although it shrinks tumors in the short term, it could trigger the spread of cancer cells around the body. It is thought the toxic medication switches on a repair mechanism in the body which ultimately allows tumors to grow back stronger. It also increases the number of 'doorways' on blood vessels which allow cancer to spread throughout the body.

Dr George Karagiannis, of the Albert Einstein College of Medicine of Yeshiva University, New York, found the number of doorways was increased in 20 patients receiving two common chemotherapy drugs. He also discovered that in mice with breast cancer chemotherapy increased the number of cancer cells circulating the body and in the lungs. Dr Karagiannis said women could be monitored during chemotherapy to check if cancer was starting to circulate and doorways were emerging.

"One approach would be to obtain a small amount of tumor tissue after a few doses of preoperative chemotherapy," he said.

"If we observe that the markers scores are increased we would recommend discontinuing chemo and having surgery first, followed by post-operative chemo. We are currently planning more extensive trials to address the issue."In this study we only investigated chemotherapy-induced cancer cell dissemination in breast cancer. We are currently working on other types of cancer to see if similar effects are elicited." The study was published in the journal Science Translational Medicine.

Had I acquiesced to the oncologists who were so desperate to chemo me for profit, I would be DEAD today! There needs to be a law against campaign bribes (donations) because it puts the average voter at the mercy of the very well funded lobbyists.

CHAPTER 44: LANETTE AND MAFACTIVE CREAM

Because I have not been silent about my treatment and the miracle of GcMAF as the ONLY cancer cure, many people have reached out to me in desperate attempts to find more GcMAF/Goleic even though there is none to be had for love or money until First Immune is cleared of these bogus charges and starts production again. However, there IS another source. There's a cream called MAF-active which contains a lot of GcMAF and was working wonders for many people, including autistic children and cancer patients. There's a lot of anecdotal evidence that the cream is just as effective as the injections and considerably less expensive. Lanette reached out to me and since she lives in Florida, we had lunch and compared notes. She's amazing and very talented in her own right as a medical tattoo artist who creates 3-D nipples on mastectomy patients after reconstruction and also covers scars to match your skin tones so that the scar just magically disappears. She's a true artist and an amazing person as well. She told me where to get the GcMAF cream and I have ordered some and am waiting to see how it works and I will cover this in another chapter later in the book. Suffice to say that if it works, it keeps me alive and kills this wretched cancer. I will be testing it on myself and hopefully it will keep me alive until First Immune can bring their production facilities back and supply the demand. More and more holistic practitioners are being murdered to facilitate Big Pharma's stranglehold on their chemo cancer blood money profits while they murder sick, innocent cancer victim. I truly do not think I could hold anyone in lower regard than I do the big drug companies for their organized and systemic murder of cancer victims that has been going on since the 1970s with their deadly overpriced poison. How they have managed to make this essentially useless poison with it's pathetic 2.1% cure rate the front-line treatment for all tumor cancers is a mystery until the lobbying of their paid scumbags to buy off OUR ELECTED REPRESENTATIVES becomes apparent. They are all bought and paid for and we are expendable tax slaves. However, with the internet (that they are trying to restrict more every day) a bright light of truth is being focused on the systemic corruption of the swamp that is our nation's capitol.

CHAPTER 45: GcMAF CREAM THAT JUST MIGHT SAVE MY LIFE

After much research looking for another source of GcMAF, God has led me to Lanette who is another First Immune patient. So many of the patients of First Immune have reached out to me desperate for GcMAF for their loved ones that if breaks my heart. I may not survive this terrible cancer but whether I do or not, I am doing my best to help the rest of the people left without their lifesaving medication by the fascist MHRA which is England's FDA/Big Pharma and they are scumbags indeed. They have faked ridiculous charges against David Noakes—the owner of First Immune—the man I owe my life to and I am going to England next year to testify in his trial unless I'm dead.B The charges are a lie—how can someone be money-laundering when the only way tore transfer? It's outrageous and shows that the greedy Big Pharma BASTARDS will stop at NOTHING to keep slaughtering and torturing innocent cancer victims for the OBSCENELY HUGE profits of the poison chemotherapy. I began using the cream sold under a different name and without any mention of the GcMAF that it contains to fight cancer. Two days after I began using it, my cancer symptoms that I was beginning to present disappeared and I began to feel better again other than the miserable side effects of the metformin pills (Metforming has a lot of anti-cancer properties and

MASS MURDERING DOCTORS: THE TRUTH ABOUT ONCOLOGISTS, CHEMOTHERAPY AND CANCER

"starves" the cancer cells). No avenue and no stone will I leave un-turned to fight the killer cancer that is trying to take my life. I view cancer as a problem and when I found the string that was GcMAF, I just kept pulling and pulling until I unraveled the entire thing and found what I needed. This isn't just about me—it was NEVER about just me. It's about my sister's kids—all three of them—every single one of them BRCA1+ who will likely have to fight cancer at some point in their lives. It's for all the frightened and desperate people who have reached out to me—and I want to help them. I never want to see "my" kids (they're orphans—lost BOTH parents to cancer before the youngest was 18) go through the horrors of chemo—and if I survive the cancer that killed their mother with chemo, they will KNOW they never have to be chemo-ed for cancer and will survive. For all the people who will survive because of this—and will spread the word—I will have some small part in taking down Big Pharma for their lies and mass murder of frightened desperate people who were sold poison and false hope and suffered horribly because of the chemo lies and poison. THAT'S what this is about for me. God brought me to this cure because He knows I have a big mouth and brass balls and don't back down. I'm scared but I'm mad and I have focused every bit of my German-English-Irish redheaded DNA on killing this miserable, wretched cancer that I hate—almost as much as the doctors who tried to murder me. I know what it feels like to be frightened and desperate for a cure that isn't going to kill me and most of the people who have reached out to me are the 98% of cancer patients that chemo didn't help and have been told that there's nothing more that can be done for them and they are going to die—after being screwed over for $750,000 is worthless chemo of which 700 THOUSAND went into their scumbag oncologist's pocket as they were sold false hope to keep them showing up to be voluntarily poisoned by chemo that is so ineffective that it would be removed from the market for lack of efficacy if it wasn't so incredibly profitable for the death merchants of Big Pharma and their boot licking oncologist murderers.

CHAPTER 46: ANOTHER 90 DAYS=ANOTHER MRI

I'm having my 90 day MRI at the most incompetent hospital on the planet. Possibly the worst hospital ever. In 6 months they STILL cannot figure out how to send a bill to my correct insurance company. This has caused me to have to forfeit HSA/FSA

MASS MURDERING DOCTORS: THE TRUTH ABOUT ONCOLOGISTS, CHEMOTHERAPY AND CANCER

reimbursements for MRI co-pays. They consistently continue to bill the WRONG insurance company. Dozens of phone calls and explaining to them EVERY SINGLE TIME I have to have an MRI that they keep billing the wrong insurance company. They are either ridiculously incompetent or flat out stupid. They send the wrong codes, bill the wrong company, and no matter how many times I try to correct this, IT KEEPS HAPPENING. I have never in my life seen such horrifying incompetence in what is supposed to be a PROFESSIONAL medical organization! Even my wonderful VETERINARIAN manages to get the billing correct and I have MORE confidence in the care my house pets receive than what I get at this place. Either their entire computerized system was installed by someone incorrectly or they are hiring illiterates for their billing. I am appalled at the STAGGERING incompetence but there's nothing I can do about it. It's driving my poor husband crazy.

OK, the MRI is done and the report shows that one of my tumors is slightly larger, my lymph nodes are slightly smaller and I am essentially treading water. It's not as good as I had hoped, but not NEARLY as bad as I had feared. Considering the gap in medication along with the 75% reduction in dosage to stretch out what I had left, it could have been FAR worse. Hopefully I will get what I need on my trip as I am leaving Saturday. It progressed a little bit, but this cancer doubles in size every 6 weeks, and in 12 weeks it should be a lot larger, but is not, so cutting down the dosage and stretching it out appears to have been effective enough to prevent the explosive growth it is so famous for doing as it's method of killing victims. The problem is not whether or not it will work—I KNOW it works or I would have died last December like they told me I would without chemo. The problem is getting it back here in a large enough quantity to seal the deal and save my life. Also, I started putting the cream on my goddaughter-niece, Tiffany who has a ZZ genetic defect that presented right after she became pregnant for the first time—which means her body produced—wait for it—NAGALASE for the first time when she became pregnant with her son. Nagalase keeps your immune system from killing the fetus because it's only HALF yours—the other half comes from the father so if it weren't for the nagalase shutting down your immune system, it would attack the fetus and kill it. Her symptoms started almost immediately after she became pregnant and subsequently miscarried and became pregnant AGAIN within 3 months of the miscarriage and her immune system started attacking her liver since what she has MUST BE an auto-immune disorder since she has colitis—also an auto-immune disorder to go with it. She's going to die from this genetic disorder caused by her body attacking her liver which was (I believe) triggered by the nagalase from the pregnancy. If the GcMAF resets her immune system the way I believe it will, she will be all right and her cirrhotic liver will cure itself when her body stops attacking it—plus she has other issues and she's got zero immune system so the idiot doctors fed her Cipro NON-STOP for the past few years to try to keep her from getting opportunistic infections because she has no immune system left. What does GcMAF do? It resets and rebuilds her immune system so that her body can heal itself and then she doesn't need a transplanted new liver—she will be OK from what is considered a terminal condition. If I am right, she lives out her normal life span, if I am wrong, she had nothing to lose and everything to gain. I am hoping and praying this will work for her and that it will be the magic bullet we so desperately need to save both of our lives, providing Big Pharma doesn't crash my plane to England later today. I hate flying more than anything else as the TSA are world class assholes who abuse ordinary travelers and give special preference and treatment to anyone in a burqa while strip searching the elderly and infirm along with small children. I wish I could drive to England, it would be a much more pleasant journey! I'm on Thomas Cook Airlines and it is much nicer than I thought it would be. After 2 meals and 3 movies, I arrive at Gatwick Airport in London where I meet the man to whom I owe my life, the CEO of First Immune, the maker of the GcMAF and my personal hero. I am here to testify in his upcoming trial which was delayed for a month so I am furious that I will not get to testify in his behalf. I am going to do a video deposition and let the chips fall where they may. Update: Tiffie is doing much better! She's apparently on the road to recovery and I will update as I write—I wasn't 100% sure the GcMAF would help her, but I knew it wouldn't hurt her. Her blood counts have doubled in less than three weeks!!

CHAPTER 47: OFF TO ENGLAND TO TESTIFY FOR FIRST IMMUNE AND MORE

Here I am in merry old England with David Noakes, the owner of First Immune biotech and his family. While I am here, he is busy injecting me with a double dose of GcMAF daily and I will be taking some back to the USA and hopefully completing the

MASS MURDERING DOCTORS: THE TRUTH ABOUT ONCOLOGISTS, CHEMOTHERAPY AND CANCER

cure when I return. It's a lovely home in Dover, Kent with the white cliffs and the North Sea and English channel making for a stunning view. The home/clinic is on some amazing property and the former English Lord that lived here must have been ridiculously rich. The main house is the size of Buckingham Palace and the caretaker's "cottage" is a huge 8 bedroom home that is on some interesting geographical energy lines that run through a thousand year old church. It was a super visit but I still have to smuggle the GcMAF back to America, and I have chosen to leave through a gateway city that has huge amounts of international tourists daily so that I can get lost in the massive numbers of tourist. The flight home is comfortable and my seatmate is a pleasant young man in the restaurant business, so we have a nice conversation. I am again impressed with the cleanliness of the plane and the food was also good. The scone and clotted cream snack an hour before landing was very tasty and the flight was smooth and the pane was clean. Getting off the plane and heading for Customs and the FDA, I have my paperwork to import the GcMAF but I am not going to show it unless they open my bags. I have hidden the vials in my laundry bag and put my dirty panties on top to discourage rooting through it—and I know—it's gross, but it's my LIFE hanging in the balance so I'll just have to be yucky and disgusting. Going through Customs I am nervous but being casual and the Customs agent stamps my passport and they wave me through. My beloved sister Sarah snatches me up from the curb about 5 minutes after I get there and I am home free with 2 months worth of GcMAF but I am going to have to go back to get the rest. After that, I am going to retire from my "career" as an international smuggler, which is definitely nerve-wracking and not something I ever wanted to do. It's amazing to me that I have been able to find the nerve and resolve to boldly break all kinds of laws in order to save my life. As a lifetime law-abiding citizen, I have always looked down on criminals and I am sad that I have had to become one to save my own life. The Chemo lobby is the most powerful one in the world and they do not want to lose their stranglehold on the 200 billion dollars of revenue that the chemotherapy LIES generate every year while trashing real cures. I can't decide whom is the most monstrous—the FDA, Big Phama or the scumbags calling themselves "doctors" who prey on the sickest and most desperately frightened members of society. Only cancer patients will submit to being voluntarily poisoned by these criminal charlatans

MASS MURDERING DOCTORS: THE TRUTH ABOUT ONCOLOGISTS, CHEMOTHERAPY AND CANCER

masquerading as "healers" who bully, lie and threaten terrified patients in order to enrich themselves selling their chemo poison. It's unconscionable that they are allowed to continue this and the associated charities promote the mass murder of cancer patients with chemotherapy without mentioning how totally ineffective and pathetic the cure rate is. If the FDA followed their own rules which means removing any drug or treatment that has a less than 5% efficacy rate, chemo would be outlawed and removed as a legitimate treatment. However, when the profits for the scumbag oncologists and Big Pharma are so massive, they leave it on the market because they are bribed to do it.

CHAPTER 48: LIVING, LAUGHING AND CURSING THE ONCOLOGISTS

I am doing great since my return from England. I successfully smuggled in the medication I needed that was a gift from David Noakes. I have been using it in conjunction with the cream and I continue to be symptom free. I have turned my attention and time to helping other cancer patients who have refused the lie of poison chemotherapy and have sought alternatives to being poisoned for profit by greedy oncologists (who hate my guts for not dying from my 100% fatal cancer). I was told I would die in six months without the chemo they were desperate to force me to undergo and here I am 18 months later and now the longest-known survivor of ovarian high-grade serous carcinoma of the ovary/uterus recurring as peritoneal carcinomatosis—and in NO danger of dying anytime soon. I am certain that my next MRI in October will show a marked improvement in my tumors—that have either been resolved (the scattered miliary tumors) or halted from metastasizing throughout my pelvis and crushing the visceral organ function through explosive growth. I find it amazing and miraculous that tumors that are supposed to double in size every 6 weeks have NOT progressed in 18 months—they are still the same size as they were in July of 2016. This is irritating to the oncologists who were so desperate to try and kill me with chemo—like they killed my sister. She'd be alive today if she had listened to me instead of her idiot ex-husband and scumbags calling themselves "doctors" who chemo-ed her for profit until they killed her with it. I am confident that my decision to refuse chemo is the reason I am alive today and in exceptionally good health for someone who was repeatedly told that death would occur in 6 months if I refused the

MASS MURDERING DOCTORS: THE TRUTH ABOUT ONCOLOGISTS, CHEMOTHERAPY AND CANCER

chemo poison they were so desperate to administer to me. Here's some hard truth, courtesy of CancerTutor.com:

Since the 1920s medical progress in curing cancer has come to a virtual dead end. The reason: surgery, chemotherapy and radiation treatments are so, so profitable for pharmaceutical companies, chemical companies, petroleum companies, doctors, hospitals, medical equipment makers, charities, media companies, and many other industries. The most important concept in chemotherapy is the concept of "remission." However, remission, response, tumor markers, etc. are terms that are meaningless. They are supposed to equate to "length of life since diagnosis," but in fact there is no correlation between being in remission and "length of life since diagnosis."

"Cure rates" are another deception tactic of orthodox medicine. Rather than use the logical concept of "length of life since diagnosis," orthodox medicine uses a meaningless statistic based on the percentage of people who live for 5 years between diagnosis and death. This statistic is easily manipulated to make orthodox treatments look more and more effective. But the only thing that really improves is their ability to deceive. Chemotherapy drugs are evaluated by the FDA based on tumor size reduction and other irrelevant measurements, not on the basis of extending the life of the patient compared to a person not taking orthodox treatments. When they talk about extending a person's life, it is based on comparing one or more toxic poisons to another group of toxic poisons.

In most cases a person would live longer, and have a far higher quality of life, if they took no orthodox treatments for cancer. Chemotherapy generally does far more harm to a patient than good. It destroys the immune system, making it more difficult for some alternative treatments to work, loses valuable time for the patient to take more effective treatments, causes people to die of complications directly and indirectly from chemotherapy, causes enormous pain and sickness, etc. Chemotherapy is virtually worthless, but it is very profitable.

The uselessness of surgery, chemotherapy and radiation is hidden behind a maze of very sophisticated false and misleading statistics, misleading definitions, meaningless concepts and many other techniques. Above all, there is a complete failure to compare chemotherapy to the statistics of people who refuse orthodox treatments and there is

MASS MURDERING DOCTORS: THE TRUTH ABOUT ONCOLOGISTS, CHEMOTHERAPY AND CANCER

an intentional failure to meaningfully compare the Big 3 to alternative treatments. Cancer research today is largely a fraud. If only a small percentage of research money were spent on studying alternative treatments, known to work, cancer would be a sad footnote in history books within 10 years. (Note: It is absolutely critical that alternative health zealots control research and money or it will be just another scam.)

In comparing Vitamin C, and perhaps by taking a few other vitamins and minerals with Vitamin C, patients who avoid orthodox treatments would live several times longer than similar patients who took orthodox treatments. They would have a far better immune system, have far less pain (zero pain from the treatment), feel better and have a much higher quality of life. In other words, Vitamin C therapy is far superior to the Big 3—and so the FDA outlawed IV Vitamin C in mid 2017—God forbid it should cure one patient and make some scumbag oncologist forgo a million bucks for chemo!

Yet Vitamin C therapy, even with the Hoffer nutrients added, is not EVEN one of the "top 100" alternative treatments for cancer. It's cure rate is far too low to make that list. Bogus scientific studies have been commissioned by the NIH specifically to discredit valid studies and the testimonies of tens of thousands of patients cured of cancer with alternative treatments. The media are nothing but worthless whores. They sell-out to the highest bidder, which is always the corrupt pharmaceutical industry. Everything they say is aimed to please those that pay the most. The media has many different techniques they routinely use to brainwash the general public. They can all be summarized in two words: "whited sepulcher." They lie, withhold information, deceive you, tell half-truths, and so on. The job of the FDA, NIH and NCI is to suppress the truth about alternative treatments for cancer. Their number one job is to insure there is "no scientific evidence" for alternative treatments so that alternative treatments can be legally suppressed. They are corrupt to the core and are directly responsible for the deaths of hundreds of thousands of Americans every year. The reason for the FDA, etc. suppressing the truth of alternative medicine is so they can continue to suppress the availability of alternative medicine substances and so the AMA can suppress the availability of patients to get alternative treatments from medical doctors. They also just outlawed IV Vitamin C which was curing many cancer patients.

MASS MURDERING DOCTORS: THE TRUTH ABOUT ONCOLOGISTS, CHEMOTHERAPY AND CANCER

Congress, whose job is to protect Americans and eliminate the corruption in Government, are largely inept and could easily be accused of intentionally "looking the other way" at what the FDA is doing, just as they have been "looking the other way" at what the tobacco industry has been doing for over 70 years. Not only does the media provide a lot of misinformation, but the internet also has an enormous amount of misinformation about alternative treatments. Universities frequently pass on this bogus information. The scientific evidence for alternative treatments for cancer is overwhelmingly superior to the scientific treatments for orthodox medicine. For those who understand statistics, the difference is greater than 1,000 standard deviations in some comparisons. Alternative treatments are so good, many thousands of people cure their own cancer without any medical help. The primary way the medical establishment tries to suppress the tens of thousands of testimonials of people cured of their cancer by alternative medicine (most of them were sent home to die by orthodox medicine before they started alternative treatments) is to talk about "spontaneous remission." The joint concepts of "spontaneous remission" and "psychological remission" are statistical nonsense and are nothing more than overt lies to protect the obscene chemo profits.

I fully expect the thug minions of Big Pharma to try and murder me as they murdered so many other alternative medicine practitioners, 62 since 2015 with the most notable being Dr. Jeffrey Bradstreet who managed to "commit suicide" by shooting himself in the chest and then throwing himself into a river where his body was found. Take note: I will not die via suicide. I am not suicidal, nor am I depressed. I am getting better and my mission in life is the bring the true cure for disease, immunotherapy via GcMAF, to cancer patients who need it. Every cancer patient that I help to cure, nicks about a million dollars from the TWO HUNDRED BILLION in profits they take in from cancer treatments EVERY YEAR. Every oncologist in America derives 80% of their annual income from failed chemotherapies. EIGHTY PERCENT of their income from killing their patients with the lie that is chemotherapy. Google h.pylori scandal and see how the Big Pharma scumbags tried to suppress that a week's worth of antibiotics cured ulcers—they suppressed it because the gastroenterologists were having people come to their office every month for prescription antacids (at the time Tagamet was the best selling drug in the world—for YEARS) AND THEY NEVER GOT ANY BETTER—

MASS MURDERING DOCTORS: THE TRUTH ABOUT ONCOLOGISTS, CHEMOTHERAPY AND CANCER

but Tagamet was STILL the number one most profitable drug in the world. Then the word got out and the jig was up. It cost every gastroenterologist in America about 28% of their net income when their ulcer patients were cured—there's NO money to be made from healthy people. Chemo is the most profitable treatment that exists, bar none, and oncologists are MASS MURDERERS. There's no other way to put it—and that's the ugly truth. Here's a list of the most common cancers:

Here's a look at the 10 cancers that killed the most people in the United States between 2003 and 2007, the most recent data available, according to the National Cancer Institute (NCI).

1. Lung and bronchial cancer: 792,495 lives

Lung and bronchial cancer is the top killer cancer in the United States. Smoking and use of tobacco products are the major causes of it, and it strikes most often between the ages of 55 and 65, according to the NCI. There are two major types: non-small cell lung cancer, which is the most common, and small cell lung cancer, which spreads more quickly. More than 157,000 people are expected to die of lung and bronchial cancer in 2010.

2. Colon and rectal cancer:268,783 lives

Colon cancer grows in the tissues of the colon, whereas rectal cancer grows in the last few inches of the large intestine near the anus, according to the National Cancer Institute. Most cases begin as clumps of small, benign cells called polyps that over time become cancerous. Screening is recommended to find the polyps before they become cancerous, according to the Mayo Clinic. Colorectal cancer is expected to kill more than 51,000 people in 2010.

3. Breast cancer: 206,983 lives

Breast cancer is the second most common cancer in women in the United States, after skin cancer, according to the Mayo Clinic. It can also occur in men – there were nearly 2,000 male cases between 2003 and 2008. The cancer usually forms in the ducts that carry milk to the nipple or the glands that produce the milk in women. Nearly 40,000 people are expected to die from breast cancer in 2010, according to the NCI.

MASS MURDERING DOCTORS: THE TRUTH ABOUT ONCOLOGISTS, CHEMOTHERAPY AND CANCER

4. Pancreatic cancer: 162,878 lives

Pancreatic cancer begins in the tissues of the pancreas, which aids digestion and metabolism regulation. Detection and early intervention are difficult because it often progressives stealthily and rapidly, according to the Mayo Clinic. Pancreatic cancer is expected to claim nearly 37,000 lives in 2010, according to the NCI.

5. Prostate cancer: 144,926 lives

This cancer is the second-leading cause of cancer deaths in men, after lung and bronchial cancer, according to the NCI. Prostate cancer usually starts to grow slowly in the prostate gland, which produces the seminal fluid to transport sperm. Some types remain confined to the gland, and are easier to treat, but others are more aggressive and spread quickly, according to the Mayo Clinic. Prostate cancer is expected to kill about 32,000 men in 2010, according to the NCI.

6. Leukemia: 108,740 lives

There are many types of leukemia, but all affect the blood-forming tissues of the body, such as the bone marrow and the lymphatic system, and result in an overproduction of abnormal white blood cells, according to the NCI. Leukemia types are classified by how fast they progress and which cells they affect; a type called acute myelogenous leukemia killed the most people – 41,714 – between 2003 and 2007. Nearly 22,000 people are expected to die from leukemia in 2010.

7. Non-Hodgkin lymphoma: 104,407 lives

This cancer affects the lymphocytes, a type of white blood cell, and is characterized by larger lymph nodes, fever and weight loss. There are several types of non-Hodgkin lymphoma, and they are categorized by whether the cancer is fast or slow-growing and which type of lymphocytes are affected, according to the NCI. Non-Hodgkin lymphoma is deadlier than Hodgkin lymphoma, and is expected to kill more than 20,000 people in 2010.

8. Liver and intrahepatic bile duct cancer: 79,773 lives

Liver cancer is one of the most common forms of cancer around the world, but is uncommon in the United States, according to the Mayo Clinic. However, its rates in

America are rising. Most liver cancer that occurs in the U.S. begins elsewhere and then spreads to the liver. A closely related cancer is intrahepatic bile duct cancer, which occurs in the duct that carries bile from the liver to the small intestine. Nearly 19,000 Americans are expected to die from liver and intrahepatic bile duct cancer in 2010, according to the NCI.

9. Ovarian cancer: 73,638 lives

Ovarian cancer was the No. 4 cause of cancer death in women between 2003 and 2007, according to the NCI. The median age of women diagnosed with it is 63. The cancer is easier to treat but harder to detect in its early stages, but recent research has brought light to early symptoms that may aid in diagnosis, according to the Mayo Clinic. Those symptoms include abdominal discomfort, urgency to urinate and pelvic pain. Nearly 14,000 women are expected to die of ovarian cancer in 2010, according to the NCI.

10. Esophageal cancer: 66,659 lives

This cancer starts in the cells that line the esophagus (the tube that carries food from the throat to the stomach) and usually occurs in the lower part of the esophagus, according to the Mayo Clinic. More men than women died from esophageal cancer between 2003 and 2007, according to the NCI. It is expected to kill 14,500 people in 2010.

All of these are treated exactly the same way: The 39-year old platinum-based chemotherapy protocol with it's totally ridiculous 2.1% survival rate—which if you remove the Hodgkin's people, is actually 1%. However, at 75-100 thousand dollars per chemo with most of that going in the oncologist's pocket, there's not going to be any changes. They do not want to **CURE** cancer—they want to **TREAT** cancer. Your very best hope for survival is the refuse the chemo and go with a holistic naturopath and to get yourself some GcMAF—otherwise, put your affairs in order and get ready for a lot of visits from people who care about you who will be watching you die one day at a time: bald, vomiting, skinny and brain-damaged and ultimately GLAD to die.

CHAPTER 49: IN CONCLUSION

MASS MURDERING DOCTORS: THE TRUTH ABOUT ONCOLOGISTS, CHEMOTHERAPY AND CANCER

This book was a labor of love and pain. It started as a loving tribute to my baby sister who died from chemo poisoning fighting for her life and to raise awareness of the incredible danger of being BRCA1+ which is well-known to Angelina Jolie and Christina Applegate who managed to survive chemo and Angelina who is what is called a "previvor" by having her entire reproductive system ripped out along with a double mastectomy but still can develop primary peritoneal carcinoma which means she can STILL get ovarian cancer—even though she had no ovaries. If nothing else, I hope and pray that this book will help people realize that chemo is a bullcrap lie and that their best hope is not having it—even in terminal cases. My mother said my sister only got really sick AFTER she started the chemo—she would have had the same lifespan, less suffering and a LOT more money if she hadn't wasted SEVEN HUNDRED AND FIFTY THOUSAND DOLLARS on the chemo that killed her while the lying oncologists sold her poison and false hope. It doesn't have to be that way—and you know that now. Use it to your advantage—and remember—if you have cancer you are far better off NOT to do chemo. You will live longer, have better quality of life and the possibility of a cure—NONE of which will happen if you agree to be voluntarily poisoned by greedy "doctors" who make a living poisoning desperately ill and very frightened people. There's a special place in HELL for them—and they richly deserve it for lying and MURDERING their patients. May they burn in hell for it!

CHAPTER 50: NEED HELP? HERE'S WHERE TO GET IT

You are welcome to reach out to me for help. My email address is: TeriDavisNewman@aol.com and has been for over a decade. Thousands of people email me for help every month and I promised God I'd help anyone who needed it if He would show me the way to the cure. While I am not cured yet, I am in no danger of dying anytime soon and my life's work is to help every cancer patient I can—with no chemo! If I put oncologists out of business, so be it. Big Pharma will try to kill me and again, so be it. I'm on the side of the angels and always have been. Thank you!

{part two}

MASS MURDERING DOCTORS: THE TRUTH ABOUT ONCOLOGISTS, CHEMOTHERAPY AND CANCER

CHAPTER 51: KILLING THE TUMORS!

I am just trying to kill off these tumors once and for all. I have the tumors under control and I stopped the spread and all the NEW tumors that were starting up are all gone and have been since last November but to two golf ball size ones aren't shrinking—but when you consider that they should be basketball size, (and I should be dead) I cannot complain. I have a 6 pack of apple juice, a pint of pharmaceutical grade DMSO and pound of pure Vitamin C. I'm going to use the Apple juice as a Trojan horse to make the cancer cells grab it for the sugar, C is just like sugar to cancer cells and the DMSO to drive it in to the tumors. If this doesn't start shrinking the tumors I will try something else. This has a lot of scientific stuff behind it though. Mix 1 TBS C, 4 oz apple juice and teaspoon of DMSO and down the proverbial hatch! I just mixed up a yummy Trojan horse cocktail for them. 10 oz apple juice divided, 5 grams pure Vitamin C (7500% of MDR) and a teaspoon of pharmaceutical grade DMSO. Vitamin C and DMSO kill cancer cells. The sugar in the apple juice will make the cancer cells grab it the DMSO will drive the C into the cancer cells and since C is chemically very close to sugar they will think it's Sunday dinner for the cancer family Robinson and KABOOM. Or so it is supposed to work. Tasted horrible though. I mixed 4 ounces of juice with the C and DMSO and then drank the other 6 ounces to kill the taste. Pretty yukky but it's my life at stake so if I have to drink this crap so be it—NOTHING can be as bad as chemo. NOTHING! I'm due for an MRI in about 2 weeks so hopefully it will show some progress shrinking the tumor if I do this for 2 weeks and if not and they stay the same, I'll just keep treading water until I get a surgeon to take them out. Tomorrow I'm mixing it in 2 oz of apple juice so there's less of it to choke down. It's even nastier than salmon if that's possible, I may have to stop bitching about the wretched fish and kvetch about the rotten Apple cancer cocktail. My aversion to chemo continues unabated as I approach the 90-day MRI point where I will find out if the changes to my immunotherapy protocol are working. I've tweaked it by adding Metformin—an old and cheap diabetes drug that has a great deal of anti-cancer efficacy as it seems to "starve" the cancer cells of the sugar that they are desperate to have and I've added Cucurmin, magnesium, DMSO and vitamin C to the GcMAF because I'm tired of treading water. I've done the impossible according to my doctors by holding this cancer at bay and preventing not only the

MASS MURDERING DOCTORS: THE TRUTH ABOUT ONCOLOGISTS, CHEMOTHERAPY AND CANCER

growth of the two larger tumors, but also managing to eradicate the tumors that were beginning and prevented any new ones from starting. I am hoping that the additions to the protocol will actually start shrinking and resolving the two golf-ball size tumors in my pelvis and that I can shut this cancer down and get back to work and normal life—which for me means NEVER eating another bite of salmon as long as I live. I've decided that apple juice has too much sugar and I'm not really sure if it binds to the vitamin C and DMSO (another miracle drug suppressed by the FDA—originally to protect the profits of aspirin makers in the 1930's which is how LONG out government has been corrupt) and I'd rather not feed the bastards so I just mix it will water— about two Tablespoons so that I can hork it down. I thought salmon tasted terrible until now—which just goes to show you things can always be worse! The other thing I did was read my sister's journal at CaringBridge.org which just ripped my heart to pieces. Reading in her words how she was so certain she was going to survive, how miserable the chemo treatments were—and worst of ALL how those lying oncologist scumbags at the Moffit cancer center kept feeding her false hope when they KNEW she had no chance to survive. They kept telling her all these lies to keep her showing up to be poisoned on a regular basis. I am crying so hard I can barely see to type this and it's a good thing I don't know who her oncologists were because I want to tear them to pieces with my bare hands for lying to her while they slowly murdered her. She was beautiful and kind and everyone loved her and she trusted and believed them when all they cared about was that 75 grand they were banging her insurance to pay every week—they are the utter scum of the earth. Every word she wrote rang with hope and courage and the utter trust she had in these bastards while they were murdering her for money. I know it's wrong to wish them ill but I can't help myself. They KNEW all along she never had a chance and they viewed her as a revenue source and lied to her for a year, sold her false hope along with their overpriced poison and to read her words—and how much she trusted and believed them is beyond wrenching. There's cold anger and hot rage—and right now all I feel is rage. It's wrong to hate and be this angry and I know that but I can't help myself. I never even looked at her caring bridge journal until today which is almost two years since they murdered her and orphaned her children. I can't even look at Total Image when I drive by either—as long as I don't go in the building I can wallow in the denial that

MASS MURDERING DOCTORS: THE TRUTH ABOUT ONCOLOGISTS, CHEMOTHERAPY AND CANCER

she's still inside.   I can see her at her station with her hands in someone's hair and that's what sustains me—I know deep down she's gone but I am allowing myself the luxury of denial-that she's still there doing hair and I will stop and see her tomorrow. As we all know, tomorrow never comes. It helps me cope with losing her, but it does nothing for the fury over her being murdered for profit by mercenary scum that she TRUSTED to be curing her and I couldn't convince her that they were going to kill her until it was too late and they succeeded. I hope God will forgive me for my blind rage and hatred of them. It's wrong, it's un-Christian and I DON'T CARE. They earned it and on judgment day I'll pay for it but they murdered her; I'm just mad about it. Big difference—huge actually. I find it ironic that in her entire journal she never mentions me at all when I managed to write an entire book about her. It underscores the fact that we had almost no contact and no real relationship to speak of other than she was my hairdresser. I also find it ironic that the entire time I was trying to convince her to save her own life, the same cancer was trying to kill me and I had NO idea. If she hadn't been tested for BRCA1 and told me to get tested, I would not have found out about my cancer in time to intervene. It has been heartbreaking to read her journal at the caring bridge website. To read how happy she was to hear her lying sacks of shit oncologists tell her she was going to be fine when they HAD to know she had no chance to survive her cancer just enrages me all over again. They sold her a ton of false hop along with more than 25 rounds of chemo—they gave her MORE chemo after she was in HOSPICE for God's sake! Apparently the greed of these scumbags has no limits and God will punish them for murdering her and so many others.

CHAPTER 52: JUST WHEN YOU THOUGHT IT COULDN'T GET ANY WORSE...

Just tripped over a brand new study published in July 2017. It says what I've been saing all along: Chemo makes cancer immortal. From the web; NaturalSociety.com: http://naturalsociety.com/chemotherapy-makes-cancer-far-worse/

A team of researchers looking into why cancer cells are so resilient accidentally stumbled upon a far more important discovery. **While conducting their research, the team discovered that chemotherapy actually heavily damages healthy cells and subsequently triggers them to release a protein that sustains and fuels tumor growth. Beyond that, it even makes the tumor highly resistant**

MASS MURDERING DOCTORS: THE TRUTH ABOUT ONCOLOGISTS, CHEMOTHERAPY AND CANCER

to future treatment. Reporting their findings in the journal Nature Medicine, the scientists report that the findings were 'completely unexpected'. Finding evidence of significant DNA damage when examining the effects of chemotherapy on tissue derived from men with prostate cancer, the writings are a big slap in the face to mainstream medical organizations who have been pushing chemotherapy as the only option to cancer patients for years.

The news comes after it was previously ousted by similarly-breaking research that expensive cancer drugs not only fail to treat tumors, but actually make them far worse. The cancer drugs were found to make tumors 'metasize' and grow massively in size after consumption. As a result, the drugs killed the patients more quickly.

Known as WNT16B, scientists who performed the research say that this protein created from chemo treatment boosts cancer cell survival and is the reason that chemotherapy actually ends lives more quickly. Co-author Peter Nelson of the Fred Hutchinson Cancer Research Center in Seattle explains:

"WNT16B, when secreted, would interact with nearby tumor cells and cause them to grow, invade, and importantly, resist subsequent therapy." The team then complimented the statement with a word of their own: "Our results indicate that damage responses in benign cells... may directly contribute to enhanced tumor growth kinetics." Meanwhile, dirt cheap substances like turmeric and ginger have consistently been found to effectively shrink tumors and combat the spread of cancer. In a review of 11 studies, it was found that turmeric use reduced brain tumor size by a shocking 81%. Further research has also shown that turmeric is capable of halting cancer cell growth altogether. One woman recently hit the mainstream headlines by revealing her victory against cancer with the principal spice used being turmeric.

This accidental finding reached by scientists further shows the lack of real science behind many 'old paradigm' treatments, despite what many health officials would like you to believe. The truth of the matter is that natural alternatives do not even receive nearly as much funding as pharmaceutical drugs and medical interventions because there's simply no room for profit. If everyone was using turmeric and vitamin D for cancer (better yet cancer prevention), major drug companies would lose out.

MASS MURDERING DOCTORS: THE TRUTH ABOUT ONCOLOGISTS, CHEMOTHERAPY AND CANCER

Additional sources: Pubmed/21775121 Pubmed/19138983

CHAPTER 52: TIME TO SLIDE INTO THE MRI TUBE AGAIN!

Once again it is time to see Dee for my 90-day MRI. I change into the baggy hospital gown and pants ensemble that was obviously tailored for someone about 200 pounds heavier than I am. There's the blood draw to make sure my kidneys are OK to use the contrast dye and Dee makes sure I'm comfy and I roll in for a 90 minute experience that always reminds me of being in a metal garbage can while someone beats the outside of it with a club. Ear plugs and music through the headphones make it tolerable and Dee is so kind to me—she's done the vast majority of my MRIs and she's so nice and very good with the IV stick and draw. I'm a little claustrophobic but with the blindfold, I get through it nicely. I focus on remaining as motionless as possible and try and doze off but I can't sleep. I didn't take my usual painkillers prior to the MRI and I cut my patch dosage to 40 mcg per hour from 60 with the last change. I've lost 40 pounds with the low carb, so I want to see how my back is doing and to my surprise I am comfortable on a 35% medication reduction which tells me I'm probably not looking at major (if any) progression of the tumors—and that my back problems are affected by my weight loss which gives me hope of a normal life without painkillers down the road when this is over. Meanwhile, back in the tube, the banging stops, Dee rolls me out and I'm done for another 90 days. Never get a CT scan, the radiation is much to high—MRIs may be more expensive but there's no radiation to exacerbate your cancer (or give you cancer) and I will also never have another mammogram for the same reason. Had my 90-day MRI today. Waiting to get the results. I'd sure like to see some shrinkage on the two tumors. I remain totally asymptomatic so I'm not in a blind panic like I usually am, but I always hate getting an MRI on Friday—but they called me last night to schedule it and had an 8 am this morning so I snagged it—but I usually can get the results the next day. Now I have to wait until Monday to see what's going on. The waiting is unsettling. I don't know the radiologists, they work for the hospital you never see them or talk to them. They send the results to my doctor right away but the hospital is like 2 minutes drive so I just run over and pick them up, the girl in the scheduling is friendly with me and she calls me when she gets the report and I go pick it up and in about a week my doctor's office mails me a copy, if it were bad they'd call me. The MRI tech said they looked about the same, so we'll see. I'd like to see my lymph nodes shrink because that would be a sign the tumors are dying because they are seeding the peritoneum but the GcMAF is keeping it from sticking and forming new tumors and converting the omentum to omental cake which is what it's called when the fat is turned into cancerous tumor. However, if they get overwhelmed, then I'll be in trouble because they could start to stick but it's out of my hands really. I can only do what I'm doing-- but I look at it this way: If it goes south, I'll have about a year and I'm already 9 months past my "expected terminating event" I'm not suffering, bald or sick. If I had gone the chemo route, I would already be dead—a long time ago too—and would have suffered horribly. So, every day is a gift. I'm taking life a little slower and appreciating how blessed I am and hoping for the best and I have prepared for the worst. We all bebop along every day never giving a thought about a lot of things because we all think we have all the time in the world and la-dee-dah I'll get to it when I have time in a day/week/whenever. Then the phone rings and a voice on the other end says "Hey—guess what? YOUR time may be just about up". It's life-changing, there's no other way to say it.

After a weekend of stressing over the possible results of the MRI, again my tumors appear to be stable. The doctors are also assuming that I have cancer in my lymphatic system as well, but they are wrong. I have two swollen lymph nodes in my pelvis which are carrying away the cancer cells, but they are the ONLY two and they are just doing their job of disposing of the cells that the two tumors are seeding my peritoneum with but they aren't implanting and forming new tumors because the GcMAF is preventing that, but the other tumors aren't being resolved so I have to break the fibrins and the digestive enzymes aren't doing the job so I am going to unleash the fire and fury (thanks President Trump!) of Vitamin C and DMSO on them. I started with the DMSO about 3 days before the current MRI and one of my tumors really lit up with the contrast medium so that tells me that they may be starting to break down from the DMSO/vitamin C assault. One of them apparently grabbed a LOT of the contrast medium--enough that the radiologist commented on it--which has never happened. When they start to break down do they grab more of the dye? I have no idea--but I am dissolving 10 grams of Vitamin C in a little Kool-aid and a

MASS MURDERING DOCTORS: THE TRUTH ABOUT ONCOLOGISTS, CHEMOTHERAPY AND CANCER

teaspoon of DMSO 2x a day and drinking it down. I think that it may have broken the fibrins because DMSO targets cancer cells and drags the C right in with it--which theoretically the cancer should grab because sugar and Vitamin C are so chemically similar. Vitamin C is a powerful anti-oxidant than given intravenously has been shown to cure cancer, so the FDA outlawed IV administration of Vitamin C and of course DMSO has been shelved since the 1930s to protect the profits of aspirin makers. It's somewhat discouraging to discover that the government has been corrupt for nearly 100 years, but apparently it has. DMSO is harmless and targets cancer cells and drags other substances like the vitamin C into the cancer cells and kills them. It was also used in potentiated chemotherapy with very low doses which bypassed healthy cells and targeted cancer cells. Of course this cured cancer on with very tiny doses of the poison, so naturally the treatment was outlawed. One treatment of a tiny amount of poison isn't nearly as profitable as 25 or more at 75-100 THOUSAND per treatment and since it will CURE the patient, it simply cannot be allowed. God forbid they actually cure some poor bastard in one treatment and cut their chemotherapy profits by 99% as that just doesn't fit their business model! Anyway. I'm going to tweak my protocol again. I bought the strongest cream they make today—15K milligrams which is like nuclear strength--it was $800 but it's so much stronger that it's actually the best deal by far. I just send my whole paycheck to Visa these days. I'm on the "buy what you need send them every penny you make" payment plan. Here's my current protocol: (I'm making this up as I go. I'm in totally uncharted waters here—NO one has ever survived this long with this cancer without chemo—and I'm going to be the longest survivor of anyone with or without if I make another year.) My protocol may not be right for you, but I view it with the AA's creed: Take what you need and leave the rest. This is what I do on a daily basis:

15,000 IUs Vitamin D3,

200 mcg Vitamin K2,

400 ng GcMAF (via cream)

500 mg Metformin ER,

400 mg Magnesium,

MASS MURDERING DOCTORS: THE TRUTH ABOUT ONCOLOGISTS, CHEMOTHERAPY AND CANCER

1 good quality multi-vitamin,

1 B-12 supplement,

4 curcumin capsules,

2 AHCC (750 mg) capsules,

2 500 mg caps of colostrum,

Medical cannabis oil (orally for pain and sleep)

High CBD cannabis oil suppositories (add oil to melted cocoa butter and put in a mold)

Medical cannabis (vaped for appetite stimulation) as low carb kills your appetite;

1 88 mg thyroid pill*,

37.5 mg Triamterine* (diuretic—keeps ascites down by keeping fluids down);

10 grams pure vitamin C (pharmaceutical grade); (Up from 5 grams once a day) mixed with 1 tsp pharmaceutical grade DMSO mixed with the C and 2 TBS of Kool-aid twice a day—and it tastes godawful!! I thought salmon was horrid till I tasted this! Drink it fast and chase it with something that tastes good! Plus I continue on the ketogenic diet—no sugar, no carbs, no liquor, no diet soda, no sweeteners other than Stevia and I also dip my fingers in DMSO and rub it over the cream to drive it into the bloodstream! I am also buying the 15,000 MILLIGRAM cream—massively stronger than the 8,000 nanogram cream I have been using. We will see what happens!

*Pre-cancer medications—that I was taking before my cancer diagnosis.

I got caught totally flat-footed when First Immune was shut down and had NO idea where to find anything to replace it with and was freaked out beyond words. I found 20 vials and paid ten grand for them—money I had to come up with in 24 hours. I stretched them out and tried to figure out some way to make GcMAF at home and did some other things and then I found Lanette who told me about the cream and that led me to you but I go through 4 jars a month but I realized that I really should switch to the 15000 milligram cream as it's so much stronger that a jar would last me 3-4 months easily which would cut my cost from $600 month to $200 a month with MORE medication, so that's what I am going to do with the next order. I keep a dozen jars in

MASS MURDERING DOCTORS: THE TRUTH ABOUT ONCOLOGISTS, CHEMOTHERAPY AND CANCER

case of emergency, civil war, riots, hurricanes and snowstorms so that no matter what, I have it. It's called paranoia and fearing for your life, but I've been freaked out and scared to death and holding my breath and living 90 days at a time—that's how often I have an MRI. When I get it and I don't have a belly full of cancer and the tumors are stable, I can breathe for a few days—but then it starts all over again. I've been battling this bastard for 19 months—and I'm tired. I'm scared. I don't know how this ends. My poor husband is scared too—I'm his first wife, we will have our 10th anniversary next month—in about 3 weeks. Last year he was so scared I wouldn't make the 10th, he went nuts making #9 special because that's just how he is. He thinks I don't know he's scared, but I do. He lost his dad to lung cancer 11-11-11 so I hate to put him through this nightmare again—and possibly with the same ending. I've moved up the food chain to the 15,000 MILLIGRAM strength cream which is 1,000,000 times stronger than the 15,000 nanogram cream so I will actually save money even though it's $800 a jar as opposed to the $150 a jar and I use 4 jars per month so that's $600 but the $800 jar will last for 3-4 months so hopefully between that, the DMSO and Vitamin C and the metformin along with the zero-carb diet I can get these tumors to start resolving because even though they are stable instead of doubling in size every 6 weeks with a bunch of new ones starting up (which is normal for this very very aggressive cancer) it will eventually overwhelm my lymphatic system and I will succumb to this cancer. I'm fighting tooth and nail, but it may not be enough. However, I have lived longer at this point than any other chemo-naive victim of this most aggressive of all cancers, so there's that, plus my quality of life has been exactly the same as if I didn't have cancer at all. Even if I do end up dying from this cancer, I do not regret not having chemo and if I had it to do over again, I'd still refuse the chemo poison.

I freaked out over my last MRI because I'm still just treading water and eventually the cells the tumors are spraying will overwhelm my system (I already have 2 big lymph nodes that the oncologist thinks are cancerous but I disagree—they're just getting clogged with cancer cells which are huge spheroids compared to regular cells) because if my lymphatic system was malignant, I'd have swollen nodes everywhere and I don't. However, I can no longer risk waiting because they will eventually become malignant if I don't knock this cancer out. I've held it at bay for 20 months,

MASS MURDERING DOCTORS: THE TRUTH ABOUT ONCOLOGISTS, CHEMOTHERAPY AND CANCER

but I haven't been able to kill it off, so even though I should be dead already it's not good enough and eventually it will beat me. The good news is that I started drinking a Trojan horse cocktail of 10 grams of pure Vitamin C in a TBS of juice and a tsp of DMSO 4 days before the MRI on the 15th of September. For the first time, one of the tumors LIT UP like a light bulb to the point where the radiologist remarked on it in the report. A pathologist friend of mine told me that necrotic tissue will grab dye like that, so I hope and pray it means that it's FINALLY starting to break down—and] the DMSO binds chemically with the C and drags it into the cells and because Vitamin C is so chemically similar to SUGAR that the cancer cells EAT it UP and it kills them. There's no other plausible explanation for what was on the CD—NONE. So, extrapolating everything I figured that I'd need the super-strong GcMAF to demolish the tumors that the C/DMSO is breaking apart because NOTHING I have previously done would break the fibrins protecting them. I'm making this up as I go—I research this constantly but I think I'm right. I will never kvetch about having to eat the wretched salmon again. I hate salmon because it's icky and fishy-tasting and I don't like that. However, DMSO and C are vile-tasting beyond words—but to kill this cancer I would drink NUCLEAR WASTE! We'll see what happens. My husband has a fit every time he sees me drinking DMSO because he thinks it's poison but it's not toxic (which he won't believe) or I'd be dead. You should look into DMSO—an amazing substance that also got screwed by the FDA back in the 1930's to protect the aspirin company's profits. It's disheartening to realize that the government corruption goes back a hundred years!! I've been unable to break the fibrins but I think the DMSO is doing that. If I'm right—and I have to be if I am going to survive this—the December MRI will show progress on resolving the tumors. I also went to the nuclear strength GcMAF cream—my dose has been 1000 nanograms a day with the 8000 nG cream but I went to the 15,000 mg cream which is exponentially stronger. I use a lot less of it obviously, but my neck was sore—and I thought it was from a crick or something stupid like that until I realized that it was the lymph nodes that were painful—a sure sign they were becoming malignant. Good news: the nuclear strength cream resolved the pain and the nodes in a few days and if the DMSO is breaking the protective fibrins on the tumors then I have a chance to win this—but I'm literally in uncharted territory. NO one has ever survived this cancer to this point and I am literally making this up as I go. I research through PubMed constantly—all day every day to try to find the answer I KNOW must be here somewhere but this is the best I can do. My fear

MASS MURDERING DOCTORS: THE TRUTH ABOUT ONCOLOGISTS, CHEMOTHERAPY AND CANCER

is that it may not be enough—this cancer is so aggressive and no one survives it. I have to make medical history (and I already have) every day just to keep breathing—that's some stress for real. I am certain of one thing—I would be dead if I had gone the chemo route.

I am waiting for my December MRI to decide on more tweaks to my protocols. On the outside chance that my pain medication (I've been in multiple car crashes resulting in 5 back surgeries and two fusions) I've decided to kick my narcotic painkillers after 21 YEARS which I am sure will be a lovely withdrawal experience that I am not looking forward to experiencing but I have to give the GcMAF cream every chance to cure me. If it doesn't work, then at some point I will be on a narcotic drip as I die from the cancer that can very easily still kill me; the fact that my tumors are stable and not increasing doesn't change the fact that I can still die from this. The tumors are spraying my peritoneal cavity with cancer cells that are starting to clog my lymphatic system and can very well metastasize there and then I've got an aggressive as hell ovarian cancer in my lymphatic system which will be a BITCH to eradicate but I can't stop now. Every doctor I see tells me I should be dead as a door nail and that what I have done is nothing short of miraculous, but I'm not yet cancer-free but I am working on it! I wrote this book because I want to help others who might need the information I spent over a year researching and writing down. My oncologists LIED to me, bullied me and coerced me to try and FORCE me to have chemo. I can't be the ONLY one they did this too. I'm looking to share the TRUTH that I spent over a year—when I didn't know if it would be my LAST YEAR so that others could benefit. People supported me when I was weak and I made a promise to GOD that I would try and help everyone I possibly could if he would show me the way to a cure. I'm NOT cured but I am alive and my tumors—that kill with explosive growth and double in size every six weeks while forming new tumors to crush out visceral organ function—have NOT progressed in 19 months. My non-oncologist doctors and my doctor friends tell me I'm a walking miracle and I want to share that to HELP EVERYONE I POSSIBLY CAN. I've been lied to and threatened by my DOCTORS and I had to learn on my own how to keep alive. Sharing that is my sole motivation. If you bought a copy of the book, I'd make 41 cents—but I will sent it to ANYONE who asks for it because the information is solid TRUTH that people NEED TO KNOW! I paid for this information with tears and fear—not knowing if the next MRI would tell me I had 90 days to live. If it helps ONE person survive then it was worth the effort of hundreds of hours of research and typing over 300 pages to share with other cancer victims. For the Trojan Horse

MASS MURDERING DOCTORS: THE TRUTH ABOUT ONCOLOGISTS, CHEMOTHERAPY AND CANCER

cocktail, you need Pharmaceutical grade DMSO. DO NOT USE PLASTIC TO MIX IT OR LATEX OR NITRILE GLOVES as it will drag the toxic chemicals in the gloves/plastic right into your bloodstream. Also, do not use within 2 hours of taking prescription medications of any kind as it will drag those into your bloodstream as well with potentially fatal results from overdosage. Don't be alarmed if the skin "peels" in a few days, it's harmless; no worse than the peeling you get from a sunburn—because DMSO draws the moisture from the skin cells so they dry out and slough off. Do this EVERY day for two weeks and depending on the amount of improvement you can adjust the dosage frequency it needed. To break the tumor fibrins down to let the GcMAF work, this is what I did:

Oral Dosage: Mix 1.5 TBS (20 mL) distilled water, 1 tsp (5mL) DMSO and 10 grams of powdered pure vitamin C. Put the 10 grams of vitamin C in the water (2 level teaspoons is usually 10 grams but check the label on the package, add the DMSO (in a glass container and measure with METAL or GLASS spoons—NO PLASTIC!! You will have to stir it for a couple of minutes to make it totally dissolve because it's such a supersaturated solution but it's the worst-tasting stuff you'll ever drink so I make a minimal amount to get it DOWN in one swallow. I have new wrinkles from the face it causes me make, but I am ALIVE to make that face so I drink it down and chase it with something nice-tasting and have it close enough to grab quickly.

I bet my life on this protocol and I was supposed to die year ago, but I feel GREAT, and the cancer that's supposed to double in size every 6 weeks has not progressed in 20 months. I am hoping and praying you have the same success and I think you will. The DMSO/C drink kills the cancer you can't see. The fluorouracil/DMSO will kill the cancer on the skin you CAN see. The GcMAF should rebuild the bone marrow and immunity issues that allowed metachronous cancer to recur so that this time it is a CURE—not a treatment. I also received a great phone call from a cardiologist friend of mine that went over my MRI images with his brother, a colo-rectal surgeon and they are BOTH of the opinion that the DMSO/Vitamin C Trojan Horse Cocktail I dreamed up is ripping the tumors apart—so color me HAPPY!! Of course I am getting brand new wrinkles from the face I make from the taste of it, but wrinkles are the road map of a life well-lived! At this point I wouldn't have surgery anyway as I am

MASS MURDERING DOCTORS: THE TRUTH ABOUT ONCOLOGISTS, CHEMOTHERAPY AND CANCER

pretty sure that I am on track to demolish the tumors. I look at it this way. There are no known chemo naive 20 month survivors of this and if it goes south it would still be another couple of years before it actually kills me--which it might. However, they killed my sister in 11 months—diagnosis to grave. They told me I'd live 6 months without chemo. I've had almost 2 years of very high quality life (despite having to eat all that wretched salmon) and I will have a minimum of another year and maybe two if it goes bad, and it was on my terms. I didn't spend what was left of my time getting chemo and suffering for a cancer that no one survives once it recurs as peritoneal carcinomatosis. John and I celebrated our 10th wedding anniversary Friday October 13th 2017 that he and I didn't expect to happen. My beloved goddaughter is getting married in March and I will most likely get to attend, and my elderly parents may predecease me so that I don't have to put them through the agony of losing a second child. Also, my Alzheimer's stricken mother in law may predecease me as well—but in all likelihood won't be put into a home prematurely because hubby can't care for her. I got to re-establish a relationship with some estranged family members and in general everyone I love knows that I do. I'm so very blessed to have been able to do that and to have had the health to enjoy it—that if I do end up dying from this it's just simply my time. There will be another edition of this book or a sequel to this one. I wanted to put this one out so that I would be able to help others and by not waiting two more years, I might be able help people that wouldn't have had 2 years without the information in the book. I remain willing to help anyone who reaches out to me.

EPILOGUE

My beloved sister—I miss you so much. I'm fighting your battle too—but I have a chance because you told me you were BRCA1+ and that I needed to be tested and you were right. I'm also BRCA1+ and the "preventative" surgery revealed that we have the same cancer—and I can't even tell you about it because you aren't here to tell. 90 days to the day after you died and I had to tell Mom and Dad I've got the same cancer that took you. I hate my oncologists, they are assholes who are lying to me about being cured when I know there are NO survivors. I will pick up the torch babe—I got this—and you inspire me every day. I will not let this cancer win and I will NOT do chemotherapy. They murdered you with their million-dollar poison while they

MASS MURDERING DOCTORS: THE TRUTH ABOUT ONCOLOGISTS, CHEMOTHERAPY AND CANCER

lied to you and sold you false hope of a cure and they deserve to burn in hell for their lies which kept you from listening to me and finding a REAL cure. I wrote a book about you and us and this wretched cancer, I didn't know I would be part of it, it was supposed to be a loving tribute to you and to raise awareness of the danger of being BRCA1+ but I had to become part of the story that was supposed to be about you. I know you're watching—and I will not let you down. I'm now the longest-known non-chemo-ed survivor of our cancer, High-grade serous adenocarcinoma, and you saved my life by telling me to get tested baby sis. You paid for my chance to survive with your life. The book I wrote about us came out today and your picture is on the front cover because it was supposed to be about you, not me or us. I know you are watching from above and I am still fighting for my life—but I wouldn't have made it this far without you telling me to get tested for BRCA1 and if I win my fight it will be only because of your intervention that gave me the chance to fight back—a chance you never had. Here's our story, hope Amazon delivers to heaven! Love you and miss you baby sis—more than anyone but the two of us know.

Made in the USA
Monee, IL
20 October 2020